Neurosurgery Research Progress

nova
Medicine & Health

Neurosurgery Research Progress

Advances in Neurosurgery Research
Amit Agrawal, MD, Pradeep Chouksey, MD, Adesh Shrivastava, MD, Sumit Raj, MD, Rakesh Mishra, MD
2022. ISBN: 978-1-68507-859-1 (Hardcover)
2022. ISBN: 979-8-88697-061-6 (eBook)

The Handbook of Neuromodulation (2 Volume Set)
Albert J. Fenoy, MD, Georgios Matis, MD, PhD, Pritam Majumdar, PhD, Sait Ozturk, MD (Editors)
2022. ISBN: 978-1-68507-617-7 (Hardcover)
2022. ISBN: 978-1-68507-789-1 (eBook)

Neuroendoscopic Procedures and Challenges
Soner Duru, MD (Editor)
2021. ISBN: 978-1-68507-092-2 (Softcover)
2021. ISBN: 978-1-68507-155-4 (eBook)

Craniospinal Vascular Diseases and Endovascular Neurosurgery
Xianli Lv MD (Editor)
Guihuai Wang MD (Editor)
James Wang MD (Editor)
2021. ISBN: 978-1-53619-342-8 (Hardcover)
2021. ISBN: 978-1-53619-357-2 (eBook)

More information about this series can be found at
https://novapublishers.com/product-category/series/neurosurgery-research-progress/

Amit Agrawal, Pradeep Chouksey, Adesh Shrivastava, Sumit Raj and Rakesh Mishra
Editors

Neurosurgery Research: An Update

nova
Medicine & Health

DOI: https://doi.org/10.52305/QKZG9560

Library of Congress Cataloging-in-Publication Data

ISBN: 978-1-68507-837-9

Published by Nova Science Publishers, Inc. † New York

Contents

Preface

There has been an exponential rise in neurosurgical literature in the last decade. Such enormous scientific text makes it impossible to keep abreast with the recent developments in the dynamic field of neurosurgery. Almost all the subspecialties in neurosurgery have changes in guidelines, recommendations and standard of care. We pre-presented the updates on general neurosurgery, neurosurgical oncology, and functional neurosurgery in our previous book, *Advances in Neurosurgery Research*. In this book, chapters covering the broad areas in spinal neurosurgery, pediatric neurosurgery, and peripheral nerve surgery are included. Not all the chapters in which evidence are well established are included. We have presented the chapters which have been of active interest in academia for the last couple of decades. We hope to avoid duplication from other neurosurgical texts and enhance the present text's utility and readability. We hope that with the sincere efforts of the authors of each chapter, we will be able to make this text comprehensive and a source of archival value. These chapters will provide a framework of current understanding and available evidence, which will help interested readers understand the area in more depth. These advances in neurosurgery should be available for access at the same time worldwide, enabling all neurosurgeons to be on the same page.

Chapter 1

Recent Advancements in the Management of Primary Spinal Tumors

Orlin Pavlov[1], MD

[1]Department of Neurosurgery, Helios Klinikum Krefeld, Germany

"If I could give a pill to a patient with malignant spinal tumor and he is going to be okay, I would gladly give my job away"
Jeremy Reynolds, Consultant Spinal Surgeon, Oxford University

Abstract

The advances in the treatment of primary spinal tumors encompass the advances in the pharmacological and in surgical treatment. There is limited data regarding the targeted therapy for primary spinal tumors. With the progress of the targeted therapy in patients with spinal metastasis, a partial success in the treatment of primary spinal tumor has been achieved. Denosumab has already been approved for the treatment of giant-cell tumors of the spine. Everolimus, which is an mTOR inhibitor, shows promising results in the treatment for recurrent ependymoma in children. The advances in the surgical treatment are based on the development of strict protocols for patient selection and surgical decision-making. The evaluation of patients with primary spinal tumours consists of four parts: 1. Clinical assessment, 2. Biopsy, 3. Local staging and 4. Systematic staging. The clinical assessment begins with careful history and neurologic status. The biopsy itself could be percutaneous, open or excisional. The basic rules for biopsy are applied here as well, including: obtaining a representative material, avoiding contamination and tumour spread. The local staging is one of the most important for the surgical planning. The tumour staging is the last part of the initial process of tumour evaluation. PET-CT (Positron emission tomography plus CT) is turning to be one of the most elaborate methods

In: Neurosurgery Research
Editors: Amit Agrawal, Pradeep Chouksey, Adesh Shrivastava et al.
ISBN: 978-1-68507-837-9

to achieve a complete tumour staging. During this stage, the possible treatment with biological therapies (targeted therapies) must be also considered. Lastly, in this stage, the patient performance status has to be evaluated, in order to sort out the surgical candidates.

Recent Advancement in Primary Spinal Tumors

The precise incidence of primary spinal tumors remains unknown, with reporting incidence in literature from 4% to 13% of all CNS tumors (Char, Cross, and Persaud 1987, Wen-qing et al. 1982, Hirano et al. 2012). These tumors are divided in two groups, according to their histopathologic patterns:

Table 1. Benign and malignant primary spinal tumors

Benign primary spinal tumors	Malignant primary spinal tumors
Aneurysmal Bone Cyst (ABC)	Chordoma
Hemangiomas	Chondrosarcoma
Osteoid osteoma and Osteoblastoma	Osteosarcoma
Enchondroma	Ewing's Sarcoma
Osteochondroma	Plasmacytoma and Multiple Myeloma
Chondroblastoma	Malignant Astrocytomas
Giant Cell Tumor	Anaplastic Ependymoma
Meningiomas	Anaplastic Oligodendroglioma
Nerve Sheath Tumors (NSTs)	Anaplastic Ganglioglioma
Myxopapillary ependymomas	Malignant Peripheral Nerve Sheath Tumors
	Malignant Meningeoma
	Primary Spinal Melanoma

Recent Advances in Targeted Therapy for Primary Spinal Tumors

There is limited data, regarding the targeted therapy in primary spinal cord tumors. With the progress of the targeted therapy in spinal metastasis (See Chapter Spinal Metastasis), a partial success in the treatment of primary spinal tumors has been achieved.

Spinal Giant-Cell Tumor (GCT)

The spinal localization of this tumor is uncommon. This tumor is malignant in behavior. The majority of the experience with giant-cell tumors (GCT) is derived from the orthopedics, where these tumors are more common; axial skeleton remains one of the last locations. The local recurrence risk is associated with the extent of soft tissue infiltration (Klenke et al. 2011), observed in 20% to 25% of all GCT. Osteoclasts play a very important role in the pathogenesis of GCT, causing osteolysis. RANKL (receptor activator of nuclear factor kappa B ligand) is one of the factors for osteoclast differentiation and activation and thus target for the monoclonal antibodies, such as Denosumab (Morgan et al. 2005). This antibody was recently approved by the FDA (Food and Drug Administration) for the treatment of GCT. The therapy with Denosumab is currently used in tumors, which are unresectable or when surgical resection is deemed inappropriate due to high risk of surgery-associated mortality and morbidity. *Thomas et al.* published their results from the first open-labeled Phase II clinical trial with Denosumab, where 86% of the patients exhibited clinical benefit from it (Thomas et al. 2010). The results were confirmed by a second Phase II clinical trial, conducted by *Chawla et al.*(Chawla et al. 2013), where 96% of the patients had no disease progression over 13 months. The authors conclude that Denosumab is a new treatment option for the patients with GCT. Regarding the spinal GCT, there are multiple case reports, which are citing a progression free period between 8 and 14 months (Kelly et al. 2016).

Ependymoma

Recurrent ependymoma represent a significant surgical challenge due to adhesions and the risk for neuronal injury. As an alternative to surgery, a PDGF-receptor-targeted agent (Imatinib) could be used to achieve a partial remission (Fakhrai et al. 2004). Other pharmacological agents, used in the molecularly-guided therapies are: mammalian target of rapamycin (mTOR) inhibitors and bevacizumab. NF2 gene encodes merlin protein, thus forming the basis of mTOR inhibitors in the cases of NF2 mutated spinal ependymoma. A phase II clinical trial is carried out, assessing the treatment with Everolimus in the cases of recurrent ependymoma in children. Bevacizumab was recently used in patients with NF 2 and spinal ependymomas by *Morris et al.* (Morris 2017). The authors report an improvement in the clinical status of the patients in 7 from 32 cases. *Kalamarides et al.* conducted a multicenter retrospective review comparing the surgical management of NF2-associated spinal ependymomas with bevacizumab. Despite the numerous flows in the study design, the authors were still able to deduct useful data, including the fact that the patients, who are not surgical candidates would benefit from therapy with bevacizumab.

Astrocytoma

Astrocytoma represents the most common pediatric intramedullary spinal cord tumor (IMSCT), with slight male predominance (Luksik et al. 2017). Achieving a gross total resection is the treatment of choice. However, due to the infiltrative nature of this tumor and the absence of clear plane of dissection, a residual tumor is often observed. With the better understanding of the genomics of these tumors, the options for genotype-directed and targeted therapy need to be considered. The BRAF alterations, which are often found in WHO I and II tumors, suggests that a treatment with BRAF-MEK inhibitors is possible. *Kaley et al.* published the results in 2018 from the VE-BASKET study (Kaley et al. 2018). In some patients with BRAFV600-mutant gliomas, an antitumor activity of selective BRAFV600 inhibition was observed. However, the authors conclude that further studies are required, in order to confirm, which patients are going to clinically benefit from this therapy. Inhibition of histone deacetylase and histone demethylase in patients with diffuse intrinsic pontine glioma, which harbors the H3F3A K27 mutation, could also bring therapeutic benefit (Grasso et al. 2015). One of the novel treatments for spinal cord glioma is genetically modified *Salmonella typhimurium* A1-R tumour-targeting bacterium strain (Kimura et al. 2010). It was administered systemically or intrathecally in orthotopic mouse models. The authors found out that intrathecally treated animals had a significantly better survival than the systematically treated group and the control group (Kimura et al. 2010). Another novel approach to the treatment of spinal astrocytoma was introduced in 2016 by *Ropper et al.* (Ropper et al. 2016). The authors used a dual gene-engineered human neural stem cell regimen, 5-fluorocytosine and ganciclovir for five days in rats, previously injected with human glioblastoma cell lines. The rats under the dual gene-engineered human neural stem cell regimen had a prolonged survival and better motor and autonomic functions than the control groups (Ropper et al. 2016). Immunotherapy has offered several possible novel approaches to these tumors, including: immune checkpoint inhibitors, chimeric antigen receptor (CAR)-T therapy and vaccine therapy (Wang, Bandopadhayay, and Jenkins 2019). Targets of the checkpoint inhibitors are: PD-1, PD-L1, and CTLA-4. The expression of these molecules correlates positive with the tumour grade. The combination of anti-PD-1 and anti-CTLA-4 has shown to stop tumour growth in the preclinical setting (Reardon et al. 2016). However, due to the difficulties in recreating an actual tumour microenvironment, the clinical data is still limited. Nivolumab and pembrolizumab, both of which are monoclonal antibodies used to block PD-1, are under investigation in clinical trials. Nivolumab failed to demonstrate a prolonged survival and pembrolizumab showed a limited benefit to the overall survival (Cloughesy et al. 2019, Weller et al. 2013). Chimeric antigen receptor (CAR) T cell therapy is also a part of the immunotherapy, where T cells are able to recognize tumour-specific surface antigens without the need for major histocompatibility complex antigens. *Mount et al.* conducted a study in 2018, suggesting that H3K27M in high grade spinal gliomas could be a potential target for CAR-T cell therapy (Mount et al. 2018). The research in this area is still in preclinical setting. H3K27M in high-grade spinal gliomas is also the target in development of vaccines, with very promising preclinical results. *Ochs* et al. conducted a study, where they were able to prove that H3K27M can be targeted by mutant specific peptide vaccines and thus induce specific T cell responses. Their vaccine was able to reduce tumour growth in mouse models (Ochs et al. 2017). Their work laid the basis for the development of vaccines targeting H3K27M.

Hemangioblastoma

The association between hemangioblastoma and von Hippel-Landau (VHL) syndrome is well established. This represents the familial form of hemangioblastomas, accounting for 20% to 40% of all hemangioblastomas. Around 20% of these lesions are located in the spinal cord (Gläsker 2005, Ostrom et al. 2013). The surgical resection of hemangioblastoma and the following radiotherapy are currently golden treatment standard. However, genotype-directed therapy and targeted agents could be used in the cases of VHL syndrome and associated hemangioblastoma. Bevacizumab, a VEGF receptor blocker, has been used in numerous cases, where a surgical resection of the tumor is not feasible (Omar 2012). Thalidomide is another pharmacological agent, which has shown an anti-angiogenic effect and has been used in the treatment of multifocal and recurrent hemangioblastoma. A recently conducted Phase II trial with Pazopanib, which is a tyrosine kinase inhibitor that limits tumor growth by targeting angiogenesis through inhibition of enzymes such as VEGFR, platelet-derived growth factor receptor (PDGFR), c-KIT and FGFR, has shown a limited effectiveness on the CNS hemangioblastomas. Among 49 CNS hemangioblastomas, only two showed responsiveness to the treatment with Pazopanib. Another discouraging fact here is that one patient died because of CNS bleeding in this single-arm study (Jonasch et al. 2018).

Schwannoma

The standard treatment strategy for spinal schwannoma remains maximal safe surgical resection. In patients with NF2 with recurrent schwannoma, a gross total resection is not easily achievable (Safaee et al. 2015). In the cases, where safe resection is not possible, stereotactic radiosurgery remains a feasible option.

The molecular characterization of these tumors laid the groundwork for the possible genotype-directed therapy and targeted agents. One of the recent studies by *Agnihotri et al.* found out that the expression of the SH3PXD2A-HTRA1 fusion resulted in elevated phosphorylated ERK, increased proliferation, increased invasion and in vivo tumorigeneses (Agnihotri et al. 2016). The authors suggested that by targeting the MEK-ERK pathway with trametinib, which is a MEK-Inhibitor, could be an affective therapeutic strategy. However, the authors found out that only 10% of the cases were harbouring the SH3PXD2A-HTRA1 fusion.

Chordoma

Chordomas are locally invasive tumours with high rates of local recurrence. Chordomas are located in 32% of the cases in skull-base, mobile spine in 32, 8% and in sacrum in 29, 2% of the cases (McMaster et al. 2001). Therapy of choice remains en block resection of the tumour with wide margins. Achieving a wide margin of surgical resection assures a 5-year local control rate of 100% (Fuchs et al. 2005). However, in many cases en block resection is not possible due to the tumour's size and invasion of neuronal structures. *Walcott* et al. conducted a retrospective review of the cases, in which an en block resection was possible. A gross total resection was possible only in 50% of the cases of sacral chordoma and much less in the mobile spine (Walcott et al. 2012). High-dose photons or protons radiation used as an adjuvant therapy, brings a local control rate of 85, 4% over 5 years (Kabolizadeh et al. 2017). The conventional chemotherapy has little to no effect in the treatment of chordoma (Walcott et al. 2012). The outlined problems show the necessity to approach these tumours differently. So far, two promising targets for genotype-directed therapy and targeted agents have been identified: 1. Somatic mutations in PI3K signalling genes and 2. LYST mutations (Tarpey et al. 2017). Four pharmacological agents have been tested in patients with chordomas: 1. Imatinib, 2. Afatinib. 3. Lapatinib and 4. Sorafenib (Bompas et al. 2015, Stacchiotti et al. 2013). Imatinib, Lapatinib and Sorafenib are already through Phase 2 clinical trials, where Imatinib, which is a tyrosine-kinase inhibitor, showed 64% clinical benefit rate (Stacchiotti et al. 2012).

Ewing's Sarcoma

Ewing's sarcoma (ES) is one of the most aggressive forms of neoplasm, with high local recurrent rate and distant metastasis. Despite heroic efforts for maximal tumor resection and reconstruction of the segment, this entity remains the most malignant primary bone tumor. It is estimated that only 8% of ES arise primary from the spine (Zuberi et al. 2018). Only 69 case reports have been identified in the literature, describing neurologic deficits from tumor infiltration from ES (BOUSSIOS et al. 2018). That is why most of the novel therapies for spinal ES are derived from the orthopedic ES. The understanding of the genetics of the tumor and tumor growth pathways have led to the identification of EWS/FLI translocation as a sole genetic aberration that drives Ewing's sarcoma oncogenesis (Pishas and Lessnick 2016). *Toretsky* et al. identified a small molecule- YK-4-279, which was able to effectively dissociate EWS/FLI from RNA helicase A (RHA) (Erkizan et al. 2009) and thus reducing the EWS/FLI-driven transcriptional activation *in vitro* (Barber-Rotenberg et al. 2012). A problem in the preclinical trials was the low oral bioavailability and the short plasma half-life (Hong et al. 2014). To overcome part of the pharmacokinetic drawbacks of YK-4-279, TK216 (clinical derivative of YK-4-279) was created. It undergoes a phase I clinical trial (NCT02657005) with dose escalation in patients with relapsed or refractory Ewing sarcoma. Other possible ways for targeted therapy in ES are: 1. Reversing EWS/FLI gene signatures 2. Inhibitors of lysine-specific demethylase 1 and 3. Inhibitors of poly-ADP ribose polymerase. These strategies are currently in development and are still undergoing early preclinical trials.

Recent Advances in Surgical Strategies for Primary Spinal Tumours

Williams et al. developed a comprehensive algorithm for the treatment of primary spinal tumours. The algorithm is based on the basic principles of oncologic surgery (Williams, Foote, and Deverall 2012). The process begins with tumour evaluation, which consists of four parts: 1. Clinical assessment, 2. Biopsy, 3 Local staging and 4. Systematic staging. The clinical assessment begins with careful history and neurologic status. Pain is one of the major symptoms of primary spinal tumours. Anamnesis for "Red Flags" is important, when initiating a CT or MRI. Biopsy is the second step in the proposed algorithm. The biopsy itself could be percutaneous, open or excisional. The basic rules for biopsy are applied here as well, including: obtaining a representative material and avoiding tumor spread. The local staging plays important role in the process of surgical planning. The Weinstein-Boriani-Biagini (WBB) anatomical classification of tumor invasion gives the surgeon viable information about the surgical strategy and possible difficulties. The tumor staging is the last part of the initial process of tumor evaluation. PET-CT (Positron emission tomography plus CT) is turning to be one of the most elaborate methods to achieve a complete tumor staging. During this stage, the possible treatment with biological therapies (targeted therapies) must be also considered. Evaluation of the patient's performance status has to be carried out at this stage, in order to sort out the surgical candidates. Two scales are vastly used and validated by multiple studies- Eastern Cooperative Oncology Group (ECOG) score (Oken et al. 1982) and the percentage-based Karnofsky score (Karnofsky 1949).

In the second part of the algorithm, a treatment strategy has to be developed, including neoadjuvant, surgical and adjuvant therapy. Sometimes, the initial therapy would begin with neoadjuvant therapy, depending on the histology of the tumor. The rationale behind this strategy is shrinkage of the tumor and achieving a gross total resection. This strategy is commonly used in the cases of ES. After neoadjuvant chemotherapy, the bone mineral density could be further diminished, which could bring further biomechanical problems. Benign lesions are typically managed by an intralesional resection or marginal resection. The lesions, with a high rate of local recurrence, such as aggressive osteoblastoma and giant cell tumor are best to resected with a wide margin. The malignant lesions, which are considered resectable, need to undergo an *en block* resection with wide margin. After the surgical resection for malignant tumors, an adjuvant therapy is recommended- chemotherapy and/or radiation therapy.

Osteoid-Osteoma (OO)

Being a benign and relatively common tumour of the musculoskeletal system, the spine surgeons have a lot of experience, dealing with this pathology. In the spine, OO occurs almost exclusively in the posterior elements. OO is histologically similar to the osteoblastomas but the latest shows a higher local recurrence rate. The OO is best treated with intralesional excision, whereas osteoblastomas needs to undergo an *en block* resection. To achieve a full intralesional excision, it is recommended to use a portable gamma probe with intraoperative radioisotope localization (Osebold et al. 1993). At our institution, a spinal neuronavigation (CT or MRI) is used to achieve a complete resection of the nidus.

Hemangiomas

The hemangiomas are also a common incidental finding. The author sees them as a *locus minoris resistance* because of the thinned bone at the level. The bone hemangiomas could evolve in the so called "aggressive" hemangioma, where neural structures are being compressed. Moreover, a collapse of the vertebral body is sometimes observed, resulting in axial pain. A treatment of choice is stabilization of the segment and decompression. For less aggressive lesions, *Kawahara et al.* proposed a "closing-opening wedge" osteotomy technique (Kawahara et al. 2001).

Chordomas

The surgical resection of chordomas is treatment of choice in all surgical candidates. This strategy has been confirmed by *Jawad et al.* by analysing 962 patients from the SEER database of the National Cancer Institute (Jawad, Haleem, and Scully 2011). The authors found that- age < 59 years, Hispanic ethnicity, size < 8 cm and gross total surgical resection have a positive prognostic impact. *Boriani et al.* reported their results, after analysing the cases with chordoma over a 50-years period, treated at the same institution (Boriani et al. 2006). They report that disregarding radiation therapy after intralesional resection, all patients had a local recurrence in period of 2 years. Bergh et al. analyzed retrospectively 69 cases of chondrosarcoma, finding that the factors, like reoperations, positive margins and higher tumor volume have a negative prognostic impact.

Ewing's Sarcoma

Due to the limited data in the literature, regarding spine ES treatment, the data was insufficient till the publication of *Bacci et al.* (Bacci et al. 2009). They analysed 43 patients. 26 underwent radiotherapy alone and 17 underwent surgical treatment. The authors didn't find a statistically significant difference in the overall survival at 5- and 10-year mark, which was 42% and 32% respectively. Lesions in the non-mobile spine are carrying the worst prognosis of all. In one of the recent reviews of *Sciubba et al.*, there was strong evidence supporting that the ES should undergo neoadjuvant chemotherapy (Sciubba et al. 2009). As a standard therapy for ES, a gross total resection should be aimed, avoiding simple debulking. *Zhang* et al. have conducted a statistical analysis of 39 patients with spinal ES, concluding that R0 resection, followed by induction chemotherapy is strongly recommended when technically achievable (Zhang et al. 2018).

Conclusion

The future development of the treatment for primary spinal tumours is strictly connected to progress in tumour biology and cell-signalling. Denosumab has shown to be a viable treatment option in patients with GCT. On the other hand, the other targeted therapy agents need to undergo further investigation in preclinical trials, before jumping to clinical trials. In the cases of neurologic deficit and biomechanical instability, surgery remains a treatment of choice, followed by chemotherapy and/or radiation therapy.

References

2017. "The response of spinal cord ependymomas to bevacizumab in patients with neurofibromatosis Type 2." *J Neurosurg Spine* 26 (4):474-482. doi: 10.3171/2016.8. spine16589.

Agnihotri, S., S. Jalali, M. R. Wilson, A. Danesh, M. Li, G. Klironomos, J. R. Krieger, A. Mansouri, C. Khan, Y. Mamatjan, N. Landon-Brace, T. Tung, M. Dowar, T. Li, J. P. Bruce, K. E. Burrell, P. D. Tonge, A. Alamsahebpour, B. Krischek, P. K. Agarwalla, W. L. Bi, I. F. Dunn, R. Beroukhim, M. G. Fehlings, V. Bril, S. M. Pagnotta, A. Iavarone, T. J. Pugh, K. D. Aldape, and G. Zadeh. 2016. "The genomic landscape of schwannoma." *Nat Genet* 48 (11):1339-1348. doi: 10.1038/ng.3688.

Bacci, G., S. Boriani, A. Balladelli, E. Barbieri, A. Longhi, M. Alberghini, K. Scotlandi, C. Forni, P. Pollastri, D. Vanel, and M. Mercuri. 2009. "Treatment of nonmetastatic Ewing's sarcoma family tumors of the spine and sacrum: the experience from a single institution." *Eur Spine J* 18 (8):1091-5. doi: 10.1007/s00586-009-0921-0.

Barber-Rotenberg, J. S., S. P. Selvanathan, Y. Kong, H. V. Erkizan, T. M. Snyder, S. P. Hong, C. L. Kobs, N. L. South, S. Summer, P. J. Monroe, M. Chruszcz, V. Dobrev, P. N. Tosso, L. J. Scher, W. Minor, M. L. Brown, S. J. Metallo, A. Üren, and J. A. Toretsky. 2012. "Single enantiomer of YK-4-279 demonstrates specificity in targeting the oncogene EWS-FLI1." *Oncotarget* 3 (2):172-82. doi: 10.18632/ oncotarget.454.

Bompas, E., A. Le Cesne, E. Tresch-Bruneel, L. Lebellec, V. Laurence, O. Collard, E. Saada-Bouzid, N. Isambert, J. Y. Blay, E. Y. Amela, S. Salas, C. Chevreau, F. Bertucci, A. Italiano, S. Clisant, and N. Penel. 2015. "Sorafenib in patients with locally advanced and metastatic chordomas: a phase II trial of the French Sarcoma Group (GSF/GETO)." *Ann Oncol* 26 (10):2168-73. doi: 10.1093/annonc/mdv300.

Boriani, S., S. Bandiera, R. Biagini, P. Bacchini, L. Boriani, M. Cappuccio, F. Chevalley, A. Gasbarrini, P. Picci, and J. N. Weinstein. 2006. "Chordoma of the mobile spine: fifty years of experience." *Spine (Phila Pa 1976)* 31 (4):493-503. doi: 10.1097/01. brs.0000200038.30869.27.

Boussios, Stergios, Catherine Hayward, Deirdre Cooke, Nikolaos Zakynthinakis-Kyriakou, Alexandros K. Tsiouris, Aikaterini A. Chatziantoniou, Foivos S. Kanellos, And Afroditi Karathanasi. 2018. "Spinal Ewing Sarcoma Debuting with Cord Compression: Have We Discovered the Thread of Ariadne?" *Anticancer Research* 38 (10):5589-5597. doi: 10.21873/anticanres.12893.

Char, G., J. N. Cross, and V. Persaud. 1987. "Tumours of the central nervous system. Analysis of 476 cases observed at the University Hospital of the West Indies." *West Indian Med J* 36 (3):140-9.

Chawla, S., R. Henshaw, L. Seeger, E. Choy, J. Y. Blay, S. Ferrari, J. Kroep, R. Grimer, P. Reichardt, P. Rutkowski, S. Schuetze, K. Skubitz, A. Staddon, D. Thomas, Y. Qian, and I. Jacobs. 2013. "Safety and efficacy of denosumab for adults and skeletally mature adolescents with giant cell tumour of bone: interim analysis of an open-label, parallel-group, phase 2 study." *Lancet Oncol* 14 (9):901-8. doi: 10.1016/s1470-2045(13)70277-8.

Cloughesy, T. F., A. Y. Mochizuki, J. R. Orpilla, W. Hugo, A. H. Lee, T. B. Davidson, A. C. Wang, B. M. Ellingson, J. A. Rytlewski, C. M. Sanders, E. S. Kawaguchi, L. Du, G. Li, W. H. Yong, S. C. Gaffey, A. L. Cohen, I. K. Mellinghoff, E. Q. Lee, D. A. Reardon, B. J. O'Brien, N. A. Butowski, P. L. Nghiemphu, J. L. Clarke, I. C. Arrillaga-Romany, H. Colman, T. J. Kaley, J. F. de Groot, L. M. Liau, P. Y. Wen, and R. M. Prins. 2019. "Neoadjuvant anti-PD-1 immunotherapy promotes a survival benefit with intratumoral and systemic immune responses in recurrent glioblastoma." *Nat Med* 25 (3):477-486. doi: 10.1038/s41591-018-0337-7.

Erkizan, H. V., Y. Kong, M. Merchant, S. Schlottmann, J. S. Barber-Rotenberg, L. Yuan, O. D. Abaan, T. H. Chou, S. Dakshanamurthy, M. L. Brown, A. Uren, and J. A. Toretsky. 2009. "A small molecule blocking oncogenic protein EWS-FLI1 interaction with RNA helicase A inhibits growth of Ewing's sarcoma." *Nat Med* 15 (7):750-6. doi: 10.1038/nm.1983.

Fakhrai, N., P. Neophytou, K. Dieckmann, A. Nemeth, D. Prayer, J. Hainfellner, and C. Marosi. 2004. "Recurrent spinal ependymoma showing partial remission under Imatimib." *Acta Neurochir (Wien)* 146 (11):1255-8. doi: 10.1007/s00701-004-0374-5.

Fuchs, B., I. D. Dickey, M. J. Yaszemski, C. Y. Inwards, and F. H. Sim. 2005. "Operative management of sacral chordoma." *J Bone Joint Surg Am* 87 (10):2211-6. doi: 10.2106/jbjs.d.02693.

Gläsker, S. 2005. "Central nervous system manifestations in VHL: genetics, pathology and clinical phenotypic features." *Fam Cancer* 4 (1):37-42. doi: 10.1007/s10689-004-5347-6.

Grasso, C. S., Y. Tang, N. Truffaux, N. E. Berlow, L. Liu, M. A. Debily, M. J. Quist, L. E. Davis, E. C. Huang, P. J. Woo, A. Ponnuswami, S. Chen, T. B. Johung, W. Sun, M. Kogiso, Y. Du, L. Qi, Y. Huang, M. Hütt-Cabezas, K. E. Warren, L. Le Dret, P. S. Meltzer, H. Mao, M. Quezado, D. G. van Vuurden, J. Abraham, M. Fouladi, M. N. Svalina, N. Wang, C. Hawkins, J. Nazarian, M. M. Alonso, E. H. Raabe, E. Hulleman, P. T. Spellman, X. N. Li, C. Keller, R. Pal, J. Grill, and M. Monje. 2015. "Functionally defined therapeutic targets in diffuse intrinsic pontine glioma." *Nat Med* 21 (6):555-9. doi: 10.1038/nm.3855.

Hirano, Kenichi, Shiro Imagama, Koji Sato, Fumihiko Kato, Yasutsugu Yukawa, Hisatake Yoshihara, Mitshuhiro Kamiya, Masao Deguchi, Tokumi Kanemura, Yuji Matsubara, Hidefumi Inoh, Noriaki Kawakami, Tetsuro Takatsu, Zenya Ito, Norimitsu Wakao, Kei Ando, Ryoji Tauchi, Akio Muramoto, Yukihiro Matsuyama, and Naoki Ishiguro. 2012. "Primary spinal cord tumors: review of 678 surgically treated patients in Japan. A multicenter study." *European spine journal: official publication of the European Spine Society, the European Spinal Deformity Society, and the European Section of the Cervical Spine Research Society* 21 (10):2019-2026. doi: 10.1007/s00586-012-2345-5.

Hong, S. H., S. E. Youbi, S. P. Hong, B. Kallakury, P. Monroe, H. V. Erkizan, J. S. Barber-Rotenberg, P. Houghton, A. Üren, and J. A. Toretsky. 2014. "Pharmacokinetic modeling optimizes inhibition of the 'undruggable' EWS-FLI1 transcription factor in Ewing Sarcoma." *Oncotarget* 5 (2):338-50. doi: 10.18632/ oncotarget.1495.

Jawad, M. U., A. A. Haleem, and S. P. Scully. 2011. "Malignant sarcoma of the pelvic bones: treatment outcomes and prognostic factors vary by histopathology." *Cancer* 117 (7):1529-41. doi: 10.1002/cncr.25684.

Jonasch, E., I. E. McCutcheon, D. S. Gombos, K. Ahrar, N. D. Perrier, D. Liu, C. C. Robichaux, M. F. Villarreal, J. A. Weldon, A. H. Woodson, P. G. Pilie, G. N. Fuller, S. G. Waguespack, and S. F. Matin. 2018. "Pazopanib in patients with von Hippel-Lindau disease: a single-arm, single-centre, phase 2 trial." *Lancet Oncol* 19 (10):1351-1359. doi: 10.1016/s1470-2045(18)30487-x.

Kabolizadeh, P., Y. L. Chen, N. Liebsch, F. J. Hornicek, J. H. Schwab, E. Choy, D. I. Rosenthal, A. Niemierko, and T. F. DeLaney. 2017. "Updated Outcome and Analysis of Tumor Response in Mobile Spine and Sacral Chordoma Treated With Definitive High-Dose Photon/Proton Radiation Therapy." *Int J Radiat Oncol Biol Phys* 97 (2):254-262. doi: 10.1016/j.ijrobp.2016.10.006.

Kaley, T., M. Touat, V. Subbiah, A. Hollebecque, J. Rodon, A. C. Lockhart, V. Keedy, F. Bielle, R. D. Hofheinz, F. Joly, J. Y. Blay, I. Chau, I. Puzanov, N. S. Raje, J. Wolf, L. M. DeAngelis, M. Makrutzki, T. Riehl, B. Pitcher, J. Baselga, and D. M. Hyman. 2018. "BRAF Inhibition in BRAF(V600)-Mutant Gliomas: Results From the VE-BASKET Study." *J Clin Oncol* 36 (35):3477-3484. doi: 10.1200/jco.2018.78.9990.

Karnofsky, David A. 1949. "The clinical evaluation of chemotherapeutic agents in cancer." *Evaluation of chemotherapeutic agents*:191-205.

Kawahara, N., K. Tomita, H. Baba, T. Kobayashi, T. Fujita, and H. Murakami. 2001. "Closing-opening wedge osteotomy to correct angular kyphotic deformity by a single posterior approach." *Spine (Phila Pa 1976)* 26 (4):391-402. doi: 10.1097/00007632-200102150-00016.

Kelly, Deirdre, Sarah Mc Erlean, Danielle Byrne, Peter Mac Mahon, and John Mc Caffrey. 2016. "A case of thoracic giant cell tumor of bone and discussion of radiological features and current management practices." *Radiology case reports* 11 (3):222-226. doi: 10.1016/j.radcr.2016.04.009.

Kimura, H., L. Zhang, M. Zhao, K. Hayashi, H. Tsuchiya, K. Tomita, M. Bouvet, J. Wessels, and R. M. Hoffman. 2010. "Targeted therapy of spinal cord glioma with a genetically modified Salmonella typhimurium." *Cell Proliferation* 43 (1):41-48. doi: https://doi.org/10.1111/j.1365-2184.2009.00652.x.

Klenke, F. M., D. E. Wenger, C. Y. Inwards, P. S. Rose, and F. H. Sim. 2011. "Giant cell tumor of bone: risk factors for recurrence." *Clin Orthop Relat Res* 469 (2):591-9. doi: 10.1007/s11999-010-1501-7.

Luksik, A. S., T. Garzon-Muvdi, W. Yang, J. Huang, and G. I. Jallo. 2017. "Pediatric spinal cord astrocytomas: a retrospective study of 348 patients from the SEER database." *J Neurosurg Pediatr* 19 (6):711-719. doi: 10.3171/2017.1.peds16528.

McMaster, M. L., A. M. Goldstein, C. M. Bromley, N. Ishibe, and D. M. Parry. 2001. "Chordoma: incidence and survival patterns in the United States, 1973-1995." *Cancer Causes Control* 12 (1):1-11. doi: 10.1023/a:1008947301735.

Morgan, Teresa, Gerald J. Atkins, Melanie K. Trivett, Sandra A. Johnson, Maya Kansara, Stephen L. Schlicht, John L. Slavin, Paul Simmons, Ian Dickinson, Gerald Powell, Peter F. M. Choong, Andrew J. Holloway, and David M. Thomas. 2005. "Molecular profiling of giant cell tumor of bone and the osteoclastic localization of ligand for receptor activator of nuclear factor kappaB." *The American journal of pathology* 167 (1):117-128. doi: 10.1016/s0002-9440(10)62959-8.

Mount, C. W., R. G. Majzner, S. Sundaresh, E. P. Arnold, M. Kadapakkam, S. Haile, L. Labanieh, E. Hulleman, P. J. Woo, S. P. Rietberg, H. Vogel, M. Monje, and C. L. Mackall. 2018. "Potent antitumor efficacy of anti-GD2 CAR T cells in H3-K27M(+) diffuse midline gliomas." *Nat Med* 24 (5):572-579. doi: 10.1038/s41591-018-0006-x.

Ochs, K., M. Ott, T. Bunse, F. Sahm, L. Bunse, K. Deumelandt, J. K. Sonner, M. Keil, A. von Deimling, W. Wick, and M. Platten. 2017. "K27M-mutant histone-3 as a novel target for glioma immunotherapy." *Oncoimmunology* 6 (7):e1328340. doi: 10.1080/2162402x.2017.1328340.

Oken, M. M., R. H. Creech, D. C. Tormey, J. Horton, T. E. Davis, E. T. McFadden, and P. P. Carbone. 1982. "Toxicity and response criteria of the Eastern Cooperative Oncology Group." *Am J Clin Oncol* 5 (6):649-55.

Omar, A. I. 2012. "Bevacizumab for the treatment of surgically unresectable cervical cord hemangioblastoma: a case report." *J Med Case Rep* 6:238. doi: 10.1186/1752-1947-6-238.

Osebold, W. R., E. L. Lester, J. H. Hurley, and R. L. Vincent. 1993. "Intraoperative use of the mobile gamma camera in localizing and excising osteoid osteomas of the spine." *Spine (Phila Pa 1976)* 18 (13):1816-28. doi: 10.1097/00007632-199310000-00018.

Ostrom, Q. T., H. Gittleman, P. Farah, A. Ondracek, Y. Chen, Y. Wolinsky, N. E. Stroup, C. Kruchko, and J. S. Barnholtz-Sloan. 2013. "CBTRUS statistical report: Primary brain and central nervous system tumors diagnosed in the United States in 2006-2010." *Neuro Oncol* 15 Suppl 2 (Suppl 2):ii1-56. doi: 10.1093/neuonc/not151.

Pishas, Kathleen I., and Stephen L. Lessnick. 2016. "Recent advances in targeted therapy for Ewing sarcoma." *F1000Research* 5:F1000 Faculty Rev-2077. doi: 10.12688/f1000research.8631.1.

Reardon, D. A., P. C. Gokhale, S. R. Klein, K. L. Ligon, S. J. Rodig, S. H. Ramkissoon, K. L. Jones, A. S. Conway, X. Liao, J. Zhou, P. Y. Wen, A. D. Van Den Abbeele, F. S. Hodi, L. Qin, N. E. Kohl, A. H. Sharpe, G. Dranoff, and G. J. Freeman. 2016. "Glioblastoma Eradication Following Immune Checkpoint Blockade in an Orthotopic, Immunocompetent Model." *Cancer Immunol Res* 4 (2):124-35. doi: 10.1158/2326-6066.cir-15-0151.

Ropper, A. E., X. Zeng, H. Haragopal, J. E. Anderson, Z. Aljuboori, I. Han, M. Abd-El-Barr, H. J. Lee, R. L. Sidman, E. Y. Snyder, M. S. Viapiano, S. U. Kim, J. H. Chi, and Y. D. Teng. 2016. "Targeted Treatment of Experimental Spinal Cord Glioma With Dual Gene-Engineered Human Neural Stem Cells." *Neurosurgery* 79 (3):481-91. doi: 10.1227/neu.0000000000001174.

Safaee, M., A. T. Parsa, N. M. Barbaro, D. Chou, P. V. Mummaneni, P. R. Weinstein, T. Tihan, and C. P. Ames. 2015. "Association of tumor location, extent of resection, and neurofibromatosis status with clinical outcomes for 221 spinal nerve sheath tumors." *Neurosurg Focus* 39 (2):E5. doi: 10.3171/2015.5.focus15183.

Sciubba, D. M., S. H. Okuno, M. B. Dekutoski, and Z. L. Gokaslan. 2009. "Ewing and osteogenic sarcoma: evidence for multidisciplinary management." *Spine (Phila Pa 1976)* 34 (22 Suppl):S58-68. doi: 10.1097/BRS.0b013e3181ba6436.

Stacchiotti, S., A. Longhi, V. Ferraresi, G. Grignani, A. Comandone, R. Stupp, A. Bertuzzi, E. Tamborini, S. Pilotti, A. Messina, C. Spreafico, A. Gronchi, P. Amore, V. Vinaccia, and P. G. Casali. 2012. "Phase II study of imatinib in advanced chordoma." *J Clin Oncol* 30 (9):914-20. doi: 10.1200/jco.2011.35.3656.

Stacchiotti, S., E. Tamborini, S. Lo Vullo, F. Bozzi, A. Messina, C. Morosi, A. Casale, F. Crippa, E. Conca, T. Negri, E. Palassini, A. Marrari, E. Palmerini, L. Mariani, A. Gronchi, S. Pilotti, and P. G. Casali. 2013. "Phase II study on lapatinib in advanced EGFR-positive chordoma." *Ann Oncol* 24 (7):1931-1936. doi: 10.1093/annonc/mdt117.

Tarpey, P. S., S. Behjati, M. D. Young, I. Martincorena, L. B. Alexandrov, S. J. Farndon, C. Guzzo, C. Hardy, C. Latimer, A. P. Butler, J. W. Teague, A. Shlien, P. A. Futreal, S. Shah, A. Bashashati, F. Jamshidi, T. O. Nielsen, D. Huntsman, D. Baumhoer, S. Brandner, J. Wunder, B. Dickson, P. Cogswell, J. Sommer, J. J. Phillips, M. F. Amary, R. Tirabosco, N. Pillay, S. Yip, M. R. Stratton, A. M. Flanagan, and P. J. Campbell. 2017. "The driver landscape of sporadic chordoma." *Nat Commun* 8 (1):890. doi: 10.1038/s41467-017-01026-0.

Thomas, D., R. Henshaw, K. Skubitz, S. Chawla, A. Staddon, J. Y. Blay, M. Roudier, J. Smith, Z. Ye, W. Sohn, R. Dansey, and S. Jun. 2010. "Denosumab in patients with giant-cell tumour of bone: an open-label, phase 2 study." *Lancet Oncol* 11 (3):275-80. doi: 10.1016/s1470-2045(10)70010-3.

Walcott, B. P., B. V. Nahed, A. Mohyeldin, J. V. Coumans, K. T. Kahle, and M. J. Ferreira. 2012. "Chordoma: current concepts, management, and future directions." *Lancet Oncol* 13 (2):e69-76. doi: 10.1016/s1470-2045(11)70337-0.

Wang, S. S., P. Bandopadhayay, and M. R. Jenkins. 2019. "Towards Immunotherapy for Pediatric Brain Tumors." *Trends Immunol* 40 (8):748-761. doi: 10.1016/j.it.2019.05.009.

Weller, M., T. Cloughesy, J. R. Perry, and W. Wick. 2013. "Standards of care for treatment of recurrent glioblastoma--are we there yet?" *Neuro Oncol* 15 (1):4-27. doi: 10.1093/neuonc/nos273.

Wen-qing, H., Z. Shi-ju, T. Qing-sheng, H. Jian-qing, L. Yu-xia, X. Qing-zhong, L. Zi-jun, and Z. Wen-cui. 1982. "Statistical analysis of central nervous system tumors in China." *J Neurosurg* 56 (4):555-64. doi: 10.3171/jns.1982.56.4.0555.

Williams, Richard, Matthew Foote, and Hamish Deverall. 2012. "Strategy in the surgical treatment of primary spinal tumors." *Global spine journal* 2 (4):249-266. doi: 10.1055/s-0032-1329886.

Zhang, Jianjun, Yujing Huang, Jing Lu, Aina He, Yan Zhou, Haiyan Hu, Zan Shen, Yuanjue Sun, and Yang Yao. 2018. "Impact of first-line treatment on outcomes of Ewing sarcoma of the spine." *American journal of cancer research* 8 (7):1262-1272.

Zuberi, Jamshed, Mariam Selevany, Farooq Shahzad, Lena Qasem, Fatema Saloukha, and Manrique Guerrero. 2018. "A typical presentation of Ewing sarcoma in a pediatric patient: A case report." *Adv Surg Tech Proc* 1 (1):8-11.

Chapter 2

Advances in Spinal Metastasis

Orlin Pavlov[1], MD and Kalina Koleva[2], MD, PhD
[1]Department of Neurosurgery, Klinikum Fulda, University Medicine Marburg, Germany
[2]Department of Pharmacology and Toxicology Medical University of Sofia, Bulgaria

Abstract

One of the most problematic facts in spinal metastasis surgery is evaluating the patient's life expectancy and whether to operate or not. There are multiple classifications, developed trying to answer the question: 'How long is the patient going to live?' With the development of the new targeted therapies, this answer is becoming even harder to answer because many patients are going to benefit from this new approach. For instance, patients with non-small cell lung carcinoma could be treated with Pembrolizumab, which has been approved as a first line treatment, improving overall survival and progression-free survival (PFS) significantly. On the other hand, currently 3 new pharmacological agents (Palbociclib, Ribociclib, Abemaciclib) and 1 new group (CDK4/6 inhibitors) are being used in the cases of metastatic breast cancer, improving PFS. The advances in the targeted therapy lead to advances in the surgical strategies as well. That is why the paradigm is shifting to a more aggressive approach in the treatment of spinal metastasis. The NOMS (Neurologic, Oncologic, Mechanical, and Systemic) decision framework revises all the possible treatment modalities (separation surgery, stabilization, external beam radiation, and radiosurgery), taking in regard the tumour's and patient's specifications. The development of strict protocols in patient selection is of utter importance for the outcome after the surgical treatment. To overcome the limitations of the titanium screws, which are commonly used in stabilization procedures, the

In: Neurosurgery Research
Editors: Amit Agrawal, Pradeep Chouksey, Adesh Shrivastava et al.
ISBN: 978-1-68507-837-9

radiolucent carbon fiber-PEEK screws were introduced in the cases of radiotherapy. The traditional titanium or stainless-steel screws had two major disadvantages in radiotherapy – planning and delivery of the radiation. The new type of implants aims to improve the conditions for the following radiotherapy.

Introduction

The recent advances in the treatment of spinal metastasis could be divided into two groups: 1. Advances in the pharmacological treatment of the patients and improvement of life expectancy, quality of life, tumour-free period etc., and 2. Surgical advances in the treatment of spinal metastasis. Spine is the most common place for bone metastasis and ca. 10% of the patients with tumours develop symptomatic spinal metastasis (Sundaresan et al., 1991), where the thoracic region is the most commonly affected, followed by lumbar and cervical spine (Sundaresan et al., 1991, Algra et al., 1992, Togawa and Lewandrowsky 2006). More than 50% of the patients with spinal metastases have multiple levels involvement. The lung and breast cancers metastasize preferably in the thoracic region because of the venous drainage of the breast through the v. azygos (Togawa and Lewandrowsky 2006, Batson 1942, Maccauro et al., 2011). The metastases from prostate carcinoma give metastasis in the lumbar and sacral region via plexus of Batson. The most common primary tumours predominantly metastasizing to the spine in descending order are: breast (21%), lung (19%), prostate (7.5%), renal (5%), gastrointestinal (4.5%), and thyroid (2.5%) (Ziu, Viswanathan, and Mesfin 2021).

Advances in the Pharmacological Treatment of Tumours

One of the most problematic facts in spinal metastasis surgery is evaluating the patient's life expectancy. There are multiple classifications, developed to answer the question: 'How long is the patient going to live?' At the moment, there is no score able to assess the life-expectancy of the patient with metastatic spinal disease with 100% accuracy (Tokuhashi, Uei, and Oshima 2017, Karhade, Shin, and Schwab 2019), which roots in the inability to understand the tumourbiology to the fullest. In 2018, Uei et al., developed a new prognostic scale for the patients with lung cancer and spinal metastasis

(Uei and Tokuhashi 2018). This new classification is based on the revised Tokuhashi score. In this new score system, two very important factors are considered and precisely – the histology of the tumour (adeno vs non-adenocarcinoma) and the ability to use molecular target drug therapy. With 6 points, the patients have a life-expectancy over 1 year, between 3 and 5 points – less than a year and less than 2 points – less than 6 months. The authors recognise the importance of the molecular target drug therapy in the life expectancy of the patients.

The identification of specific receptor gene mutations (protein kinases or other membrane receptors) played a very important role in understanding the tumourbiology of non-small cell lung cancer (NSCLC). The second step was creating a specific targeted therapy, like tyrosine kinase inhibitors (TKIs) and monoclonal antibodies directed against specific receptors, in order to improve the overall survival rate. The mutation of epithelial growth factor receptor (EGFR) is a predictor for clinical benefit in patients with NSCLC (Goodwin et al., 2016). TKI in patients with EGFR mutations enhance apoptosis while conversely decreasing cell growth, metastases, and angiogenesis (Pirker and Filipits 2009). The TKI ensure a longer progress free survival (PFS) compared to the traditional chemotherapy. In the group without EGFR mutations, the PFS was longer with conventional chemotherapy (Savas, Hughes, and Solomon 2013). With EGFR inhibitors, the median overall survival was improved up to 36 months (Helissey, Champiat, and Soria 2015). Combating the drug-resistance in one of the key factors in achieving a 'stable disease' in patients with NCCLC. One of the mechanisms for drug-resistance is T790M. Osimertinib, which is a third-generation EGFR TKI, proved to be effective in T790M + advanced NSCLC (Mok et al., 2017). Angiogenesis, on the other hand, is one of the hallmarks of tumor expansion and progression. Bevacizumab is an inhibitor of the vascular endothelial growth factor A (VEGF-A). Bevacizumab improves significantly the PFS and OS in patients with NSCLC (Lauro et al., 2014). This VEGF-A inhibitor is also used in the cases of malignant brain tumors, achieving the so-called pharmacological debulking. Two monoclonal antibodies directed against the programmed death 1 receptor (anti-PD1), Pembrolizumab and Nivolumab, were approved for the treatment of NSCLC (Cofano et al., 2019). In patients with metastatic NSCLC overexpressing PD-ligand 1 (L1), Pembrolizumab has been approved as a first line treatment, improving OS and PFS significantly (Reck et al., 2016).

Breast cancer has a heterogeneous biology, which influences the therapeutic strategies. The most important classification of BC (Table 1) is based on the expression of hormone receptors (HRs) and on the amplification/expression of the HER2 gene/protein (Tong et al., 2018, Cofano et al., 2019):

Table 1. Types of breast cancer

Type:	Characteristics:
Luminal A	HR + /HER2−
Luminal B	HR + /HER2 +
HER2 type	Overexpression of HER2/ERBB2 oncogene
Triple negative	HR−/HER2−

The tumourbiology has a predictive value in the overall survival outcome. Luminal A type tumours behave less aggressively than the luminal type B. The triple negative type is the most aggressive type of tumour and remains difficult to treat because of early drug resistance. Overcoming the endocrine resistance in metastatic breast cancer is one of the key factors for a successful systematic therapy. Currently 3 new pharmacological agents (Palbociclib, Ribociclib, Abemaciclib) and 1 new group (CDK4/6 inhibitors) are being used in the cases of metastatic breast cancer, improving PFS (Shah and Cristofanilli 2017, Sledge et al., 2017). Targeting the mutated phosphatidylinositol 3-kinase-catalytic subunit p110 α with Buparlisib, Alpeisib and Talesisib has shown promising results and it is currently under investigation. For the patients with HER2 type breast cancer, the anti-HER 2 monoclonal antibodies represent the therapy of choice. Currently, two pharmacological agents are used-Trastuzumab and Pertuzumab, which are acting on different binding sides. To overcome the Trastuzumab-resistance, novel therapies are applied, including phosphoinositide 3-kinase (PI3K) inhibitors, such as Buparlisib and Pilaralisib. The targeted therapy in breast cancer was further expanded with the introduction of the inhibitors of HER-family receptors, including Neratinib, Patritumab and Margetuximab. Each of these pharmacological agents shows different predilection towards HER1, 2, 3 and 4 receptors. The immunotherapy has made success with the introduction of Nelipepimut-S, which is a peptide, derived from HER2, used as a vaccine in order to prevent recurrence of breast cancer. It is currently undergoing Phase IIb clinical trial (Fisk et al., 1995).

The prostate cancer is the second most common malignant tumour in men. These tumours are characterised by slow growth and *per se* the patients have a good OS. The blockade of androgen pathways is a treatment of choice in these patients, independent from the tumour status (advanced or metastatic). There are three ways to block the androgen pathway (Klotz et al., 2008): 1.

LHRH ligand, 2. Blockade of androgen synthesis, 3. Antiandrogens that antagonize the androgen receptor (Attard et al., 2009). In order to reach the androgen-resistant stage, the androgen synthesis pathway is further changed throughout the following mechanisms: 1. Mutation of androgen receptor, 2. Overexpression of the androgen receptor, 3. Upregulation of the androgen receptor coactivators (Bousset et al., 2018). Two pharmacological agents are used to stop the cascade from intratumoral overproduction of active androgens Cabazitaxel and Mitoxantrone, where the first showed a better OS (de Bono et al., 2010). For the patients with bone metastasis, Denosumab is used to inhibit osteoclast proliferation and survival and thus improving the function outcome of these patients (Smith et al., 2012). Immunotherapy is also used in the treatment of prostate cancer, where currently an FDA-approved vaccine, Sipuleucel-T, is being used to further improve the OS (from 4 to 13 months) (Redman, Gulley, and Madan 2017). Another achievement of the immunotherapy is the development of engineered immune cells, which are used currently in patients with myeloproliferative diseases. The trials with engineered immune cells for prostate cancer are completed in Phase I clinical trial (Junghans et al., 2016, Priceman et al., 2018) and Phase 2 is planned to commence.

The spinal metastases from renal cell carcinoma present a challenge to the spine surgeon due to the vascularity of the tumour. The prognosis of the patients was extremely poor till the introduction of the targeted therapy against VEGF. The tyrosine-kinase inhibitors, such as Sunitinib have become a standard treatment of those patients. Other agents from this group are: Pazopanib, Axitinib, or Sorafenibm (Escudier, Eisen, et al., 2007). Of course, Bevacizumab, as mentioned previously, is one of the monoclonal antibodies against VEGF, used in different malignancies is also used for the treatment of renal cell carcinoma (Escudier, Pluzanska, et al., 2007).

Advances in Surgical Treatment of Spinal Metastasis

In 2013, a new algorithm for the treatment of spinal metastasis was introduced by Bilsky et al., incorporating the milestones in decision-making process. The NOMS (Neurologic, Oncologic, Mechanical, and Systemic) decision framework revises all the possible treatment modalities (separation surgery, stabilization, external beam radiation, radiosurgery) in regard to tumour's and patient's specifications.

The neurological assessment consists of two phases – neurological examination (myelopathy, radiculopathy) and radiological assessment of the degree of epidural spinal cord compression (ESCC). The degree of ESCC plays a very important role in the decision-making process. Spine Oncology Study Group (SOSG) developed a six-point score system for the assessment of ESCC, using axial T2 weighted images (Table 2).

Table 2. ESCC scale by Bilsky et al.

Grade	Description in MRI:
0	Disease limited in the bone
1A	Epidural impingement, no deformation of thecal sac
1B	Deformation of thecal sac, no spinal cord abutment
1C	Deformation of thecal sac, with spinal cord abutment, no cord compression
2	Spinal cord compression, CSF still visible
3	Spinal cord compression, CSF is no longer visible

Grades 0, 1a, and 1b and generally considered for radiation, in the cases of absence mechanical instability. The higher Grades- 2 and 3 describe the surgical candidates, where decompression surgery is required prior to radiotherapy.

The oncological assessment is based on the ability to achieve a local tumour control with radiation. The limiting criterion in this case is spinal cord in the radiation field. To overcome this limitation, a novel image-guided radiation therapy was introduced, being able to deliver higher dosage of radiation in close proximity to the spinal cord, without damaging it. From oncological point of view, the tumours are divided in two groups: radiosensitive and radioresistant. Radiosensitive tumours are: lymphoma, seminoma, myeloma, breast, prostate, ovarian, and neuroendocrine carcinomas (Gerszten, Mendel, and Yamada 2009). In the group of radioresistant tumours are: renal carcinoma, hepatocellular, colon, NSCLC, sarcoma and melanoma. Depending on this grouping, the therapeutic strategies are further divided. The patients with lymphoma, seminoma and myeloma undergo cEBRT, regardless of ESCC. The solid radiosensitive tumours undergo cEBRT or SRS, where the radioresistant solid tumours must undergo an SRS to achieve a good local tumour control.

The assessment of the mechanical stability relies on the spinal instability neoplastic score (SINS). In this score both radiological and clinical criteria are considered in order to assess the mechanical stability of the affected segment (Fisher et al., 2010). Lesions with score between 0 and 6 are generally considered stable and don't require a surgical stabilization. On the other hand, lesions with score between 13 and 18 are unstable and require a stabilization procedure. Of course, there is a wide window from 6 and 13. The patients falling in this group are going to need further assessment to assure the mechanical stability. However, when considering this score, one must also take in account also the surgical decompression technique, meaning what kind of surgery-attributed instability will be added to the score, after a simple decompression. In a case of patient with a prostate carcinoma with two metastatic lesions in L2 and L4, wide epidural compression and SINS score of 7. In this case, because of relatively low SINS, one could decide to offer only decompressive surgery to the patient, however, when the surgeon revise his operative plan and see that extensive laminectomies are required to achieve a good decompression, the surgical strategy needs to be altered and stabilization is required.

The systemic assessment is based on assessment of tumour burden and comorbidities. Multiple scales for life-expectancy prognosis have been proposed, as stated above. The systematic assessment is to be performed by oncologist and internist, being able to surgically stratify the patients in regard of the tumour burden and comorbidities. As mentioned above, the novel techniques for systemic, which improve the life-expectancy, are rapidly evolving and thus the spine surgeons are not always up to date. A multidisciplinary team approach is required to assure that the best therapeutic strategy has been chosen.

After the introduction of separation surgery, the spine oncological surgery has further evolved. The concept of separation surgery lies in decompression of the spinal cord and creation of a safe target for SRS or SBRT by creating a corridor of at least 2-3 mm between the spinal cord and tumour mass. The extended approaches, such vertebrectomy and extended intralesional removal of the vertebral body have lost their values and should be performed only in selected cases (Barzilai et al., 2019). Such cases are the patients with a single metastasis from radiosensitive tumours or in the cases of metastasis of radioresistant tumours, where the full potential of the therapy with SRS or SBRT could not be achieved (Di Perna et al., 2020). As a first step of separation surgery a dorsal stabilization has to be performed, as suggested by Barzilai et al., (Barzilai et al., 2018), in order to achieve a relief of mechanical pain. A long segment fixation should be aimed, meaning a dorsal fixation two levels above and below the affected level, followed by a circumferential decompression of the spinal cord without the need for extensive intralesional removal of the vertebral body or vertebrectomy. Barzilai et al., reported that by following this protocol a local recurrence rate of 2.1% and 4.3% at 6 months and 12 months, respectively was achieved (Barzilai et al., 2017). The main concern, using separation surgery with SRS or SBRT is of course hardware failure due to: 1. Lack of ventral stabilization. 2. Inability to achieve fusion due to chemotherapy and shorter life expectancy in cancer patients 3. Radiation therapy. One of the largest retrospective studies, conducted by Amankulor et al., has evaluated the hardware patients in 318 patients over 7 years, registering only 2,8% of hardware failure incidence (Amankulor et al., 2014).

To overcome the limitations of the titanium screws, the radiolucent carbon fiber-PEEK screws were introduced. The traditional titanium or stainless-steel screws had two major disadvantages in radiotherapy- planning and delivery of radiation. The postoperative CT images contain artefacts because of the titanium/stainless steel screws, interfering with the software for dose calculation, which could lead to under dose/overdose of radiation in the region of interest. Secondly, the metal implants cause dispersion from therapeutic megavolt beams, where due to the attenuation effect and a dose reduction between 5% and 10% behind the screws is reported (Mesbahi and Nejad 2007, Mian et al., 1987, Nevelsky et al., 2017). Numerous authors have proven that the carbon fiber-PEEK screws have multiple advantages on the imaging modalities, including- Fleege et al., in 2020 (Fleege et al., 2020). There is no level 1 or 2 evidence supporting the superiority of the carbon fiber PEEK cages over the titan cages for radiotherapy. In terms of hardware failure, the carbon fiber PEEK screws demonstrated equal results compared to the titanium screws, confirmed in multiple biomechanical studies (Lindtner et al., 2018).

In our institution, we conducted a retrospective analysis of the patient with spinal metastasis, who underwent a circumferential reconstruction of the segment (ventral stabilization with expandable cage on one or more levels because of en block vertebrectomy and dorsal stabilization). From 2012 to 2020, only 9 patients underwent the most extensive surgical approach for resection of spinal metastasis. Sex, age operative time, SINS, Tokuhashi score, tumour histology was assessed. Tokuhashi Score Mean was 6,5, ± 3,3; Standard error-1,1 and SINS: Mean 11,7; ± 3,66, Standard error-1,22. The high SINS score indicated that the patients had a very high instability in the segment. For illustration purposes, the following case will be presented. A patient with breast tumour presents in the emergency room because of severe pain in the thoracic spine with myelopathy signs and paraparesis. The patient was in good general condition- ECOG score of 1 (Eastern Cooperative Oncology Group).

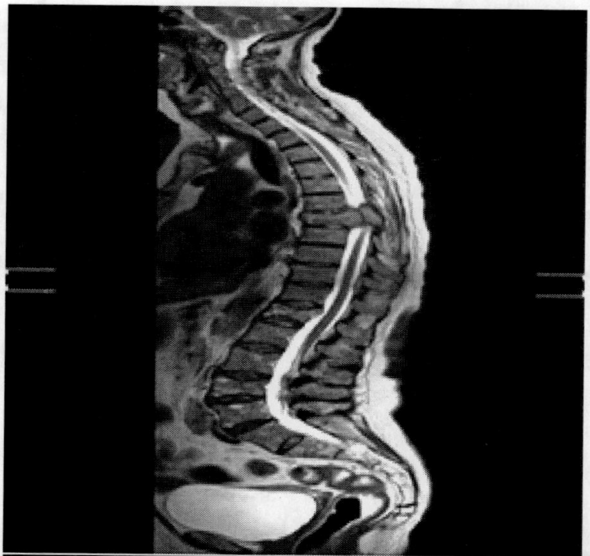

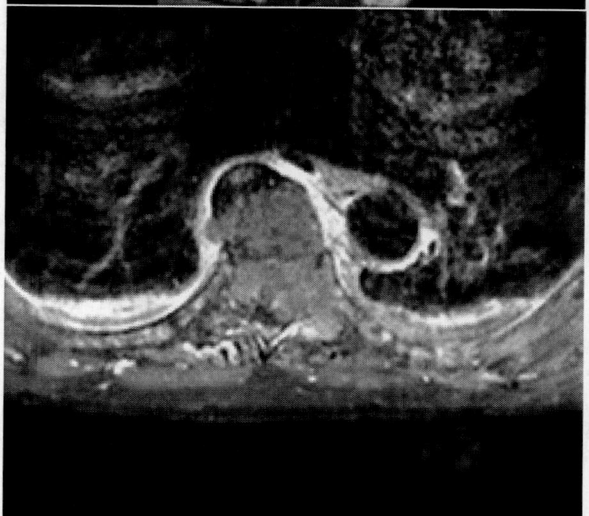

Figure 1. (Sagital) and **Figure 2.** (Axial) MRI of the spine, depicting a metastastis in 7th thoracic vertebrae. **Author's arcive, all rights reserved.

Due to the acute neurological deficit-myelopathy and paraparesis for two days, an emergency surgery was carried on the same day.

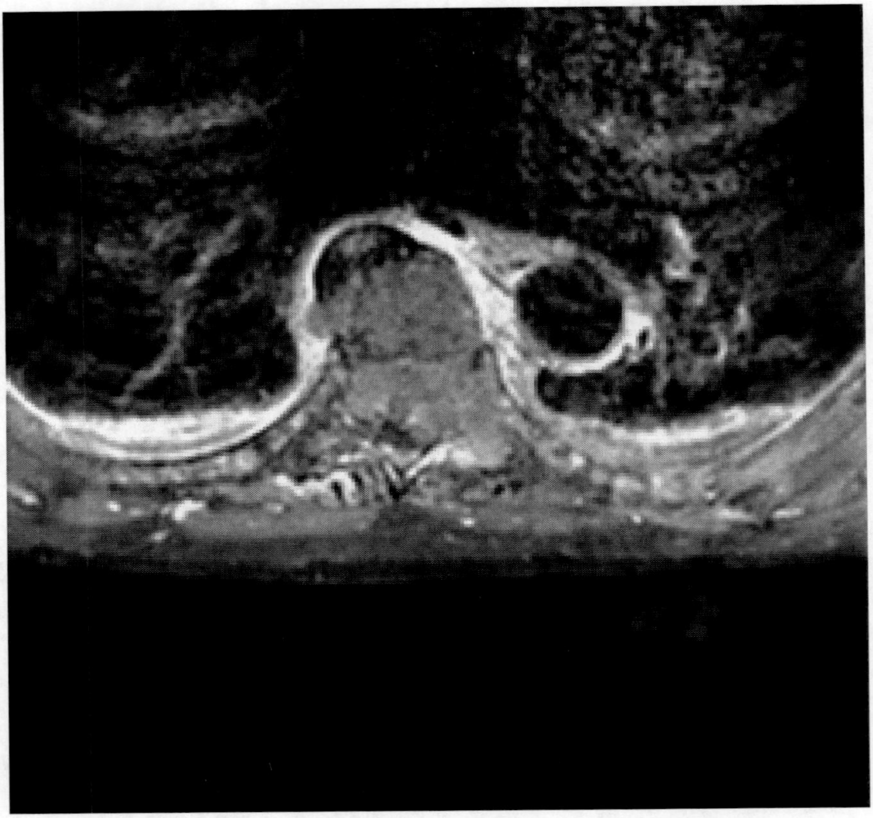

Figure 3. Sagial X-Ray depicting a dorsal stabilization with screws and ventral reconstruction with expandable cage after en block vertebrectomy. **Author's arcive, all rights reserved.

The operation was performed through a costotransversectomy approach with stabilization two levels above and below and implantation of expandable cage for ventral support. Based on author's research for his PhD Thesis, the author developed a protocol for circumferential reconstruction of the affected segment:

Through a careful patient selection and assessment of individual risk factors of the patients, the perioperative mortality and morbidity could be reduced to a minimum.

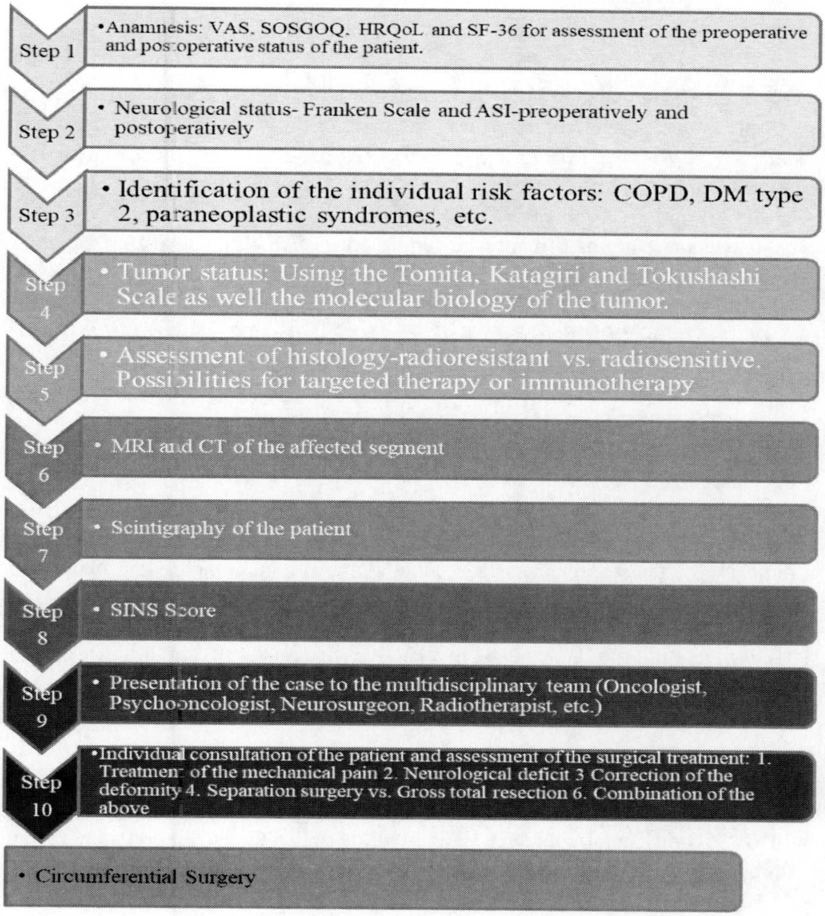

Figure 4. Protocol for circumferential reconstruction of the affected segment.

Conclusion

The approach to the patients with spinal metastasis is changing rapidly and surgery is often indicated, especially in the cases with favourable histology and tumourbiology. The limitation of the titan screws could be overcome by the new carbon-fiber PEEK screws, making the postoperative local control of the tumour longer, ensuring a longer life-expectancy with a good quality of life. In some carefully selected cases, however, the circumferential reconstruction of the segment is the best treatment choice.

References

Algra, P. R., J. J. Heimans, J. Valk, J. J. Nauta, M. Lachniet, and B. Van Kooten. 1992. "Do metastases in vertebrae begin in the body or the pedicles? Imaging study in 45 patients." *AJR Am. J. Roentgenol.* 158 (6):1275-9. doi: 10.2214/ajr.158.6.1590123.

Amankulor, Nduka M., Ran Xu, J. Bryan Iorgulescu, Talia Chapman, Anne S. Reiner, Elyn Riedel, Eric Lis, Yoshiya Yamada, Mark Bilsky, and Ilya Laufer. 2014. "The incidence and patterns of hardware failure after separation surgery in patients with spinal metastatic tumors." *The Spine Journal* 14 (9):1850-1859. doi: https://doi.org/10. 1016/j.spinee.2013.10.028.

Attard, G., A. H. Reid, R. A'Hern, C. Parker, N. B. Oommen, E. Folkerd, C. Messiou, L. R. Molife, G. Maier, E. Thompson, D. Olmos, R. Sinha, G. Lee, M. Dowsett, S. B. Kaye, D. Dearnaley, T. Kheoh, A. Molina, and J. S. de Bono. 2009. "Selective inhibition of CYP17 with abiraterone acetate is highly active in the treatment of castration-resistant prostate cancer." *J. Clin. Oncol.* 27 (23):3742-8. doi: 10.1200/jco.2008.20.0642.

Barzilai, Ori, Mary-Kate Amato, Lily McLaughlin, Anne S Reiner, Shahiba Q Ogilvie, Eric Lis, Yoshiya Yamada, Mark H Bilsky, and Ilya Laufer. 2017. "Hybrid surgery–radiosurgery therapy for metastatic epidural spinal cord compression: A prospective evaluation using patient-reported outcomes." *Neuro-Oncology Practice* 5 (2):104-113. doi: 10.1093/nop/npx017.

Barzilai, Ori, Stefano Boriani, Charles G. Fisher, Arjun Sahgal, Jorrit Jan Verlaan, Ziya L. Gokaslan, Aron Lazary, Chetan Bettegowda, Laurence D. Rhines, and Ilya Laufer. 2019. "Essential Concepts for the Management of Metastatic Spine Disease: What the Surgeon Should Know and Practice." *Global Spine Journal* 9 (1_suppl):98S-107S. doi: 10.1177/2192568219830323.

Barzilai, Ori, Ilya Laufer, Adam Robin, Ran Xu, Yoshiya Yamada, and Mark H Bilsky. 2018. "Hybrid Therapy for Metastatic Epidural Spinal Cord Compression: Technique for Separation Surgery and Spine Radiosurgery." *Operative Neurosurgery* 16 (3):310-318. doi: 10.1093/ons/opy137.

Batson, Oscar V. 1942. "The role of the vertebral veins in metastatic processes." *Annals of Internal Medicine* 16 (1):38-45.

Bousset, L., A. Rambur, A. Fouache, J. Bunay, L. Morel, J. A. Lobaccaro, S. Baron, A. Trousson, and C. de Joussineau. 2018. "New Insights in Prostate Cancer Development and Tumor Therapy: Modulation of Nuclear Receptors and the Specific Role of Liver X Receptors." *Int. J. Mol. Sci.* 19 (9). doi: 10.3390/ijms19092545.

Cofano, Fabio, Matteo Monticelli, Marco Ajello, Francesco Zenga, Nicola Marengo, Giuseppe Di Perna, Roberto Altieri, Paola Cassoni, Luca Bertero, Antonio Melcarne, Fulvio Tartara, Alessandro Ducati, and Diego Garbossa. 2019. "The Targeted Therapies Era Beyond the Surgical Point of View: What Spine Surgeons Should Know Before Approaching Spinal Metastases." *Cancer control : journal of the Moffitt Cancer Center* 26 (1):1073274819870549-1073274819870549. doi: 10.1177/1073274819870549.

de Bono, J. S., S. Oudard, M. Ozguroglu, S. Hansen, J. P. Machiels, I. Kocak, G. Gravis, I. Bodrogi, M. J. Mackenzie, L. Shen, M. Roessner, S. Gupta, and A. O. Sartor. 2010. "Prednisone plus cabazitaxel or mitoxantrone for metastatic castration-resistant prostate cancer progressing after docetaxel treatment: a randomised open-label trial." *Lancet* 376 (9747):1147-54. doi: 10.1016/s0140-6736(10)61389-x.

Di Perna, Giuseppe, Fabio Cofano, Cristina Mantovani, Serena Badellino, Nicola Marengo, Marco Ajello, Ludovico Maria Comite, Giuseppe Palmieri, Fulvio Tartara, Francesco Zenga, Umberto Ricardi, and Diego Garbossa. 2020. "Separation surgery for metastatic epidural spinal cord compression: A qualitative review." *Journal of Bone Oncology* 25:100320. doi: https://doi.org/10.1016/j.jbo.2020.100320.

Escudier, B., T. Eisen, W. M. Stadler, C. Szczylik, S. Oudard, M. Siebels, S. Negrier, C. Chevreau, E. Solska, A. A. Desai, F. Rolland, T. Demkow, T. E. Hutson, M. Gore, S. Freeman, B. Schwartz, M. Shan, R. Simantov, and R. M. Bukowski. 2007. "Sorafenib in advanced clear-cell renal-cell carcinoma." *N. Engl. J. Med.* 356 (2):125-34. doi: 10.1056/NEJMoa060655.

Escudier, B., A. Pluzanska, P. Koralewski, A. Ravaud, S. Bracarda, C. Szczylik, C. Chevreau, M. Filipek, B. Melichar, E. Bajetta, V. Gorbunova, J. O. Bay, I. Bodrogi, A. Jagiello-Gruszfeld, and N. Moore. 2007. "Bevacizumab plus interferon alfa-2a for treatment of metastatic renal cell carcinoma: a randomised, double-blind phase III trial." *Lancet* 370 (9605):2103-11. doi: 10.1016/s0140-6736(07)61904-7.

Fisher, C. G., C. P. DiPaola, T. C. Ryken, M. H. Bilsky, C. I. Shaffrey, S. H. Berven, J. S. Harrop, M. G. Fehlings, S. Boriani, D. Chou, M. H. Schmidt, D. W. Polly, R. Biagini, S. Burch, M. B. Dekutoski, A. Ganju, P. C. Gerszten, Z. L. Gokaslan, M. W. Groff, N. J. Liebsch, E. Mendel, S. H. Okuno, S. Patel, L. D. Rhines, P. S. Rose, D. M. Sciubba, N. Sundaresan, K. Tomita, P. P. Varga, L. R. Vialle, F. D. Vrionis, Y. Yamada, and D. R. Fourney. 2010. "A novel classification system for spinal instability in neoplastic disease: an evidence-based approach and expert consensus from the Spine Oncology Study Group." *Spine (Phila Pa 1976)* 35 (22):E1221-9. doi: 10.1097/BRS.0b013e3181e16ae2.

Fisk, B., T. L. Blevins, J. T. Wharton, and C. G. Ioannides. 1995. "Identification of an immunodominant peptide of HER-2/neu protooncogene recognized by ovarian tumor-specific cytotoxic T lymphocyte lines." *J. Exp. Med.* 181 (6):2109-17. doi: 10.1084/jem.181.6.2109.

Fleege, Christoph, Marcus Makowski, Michael Rauschmann, Katharina Luise Fraunhoffer, Peter Fennema, Mohammad Arabmotlagh, and Marcus Rickert. 2020. "Carbon fiber-reinforced pedicle screws reduce artifacts in magnetic resonance imaging of patients with lumbar spondylodesis." *Scientific Reports* 10 (1):16094. doi: 10.1038/s41598-020-73386-5.

Gerszten, P. C., E. Mendel, and Y. Yamada. 2009. "Radiotherapy and radiosurgery for metastatic spine disease: what are the options, indications, and outcomes?" *Spine (Phila Pa 1976)* 34 (22 Suppl):S78-92. doi: 10.1097/BRS.0b013e3181b8b6f5.

Goodwin, C. R., N. Abu-Bonsrah, L. D. Rhines, J. J. Verlaan, M. H. Bilsky, I. Laufer, S. Boriani, D. M. Sciubba, and C. Bettegowda. 2016. "Molecular Markers and Targeted Therapeutics in Metastatic Tumors of the Spine: Changing the Treatment Paradigms." *Spine (Phila Pa 1976)* 41 Suppl 20:S218-s223. doi: 10.1097/brs.0000000000001833.

Helissey, C., S. Champiat, and J. C. Soria. 2015. "Immune checkpoint inhibitors in advanced nonsmall cell lung cancer." *Curr. Opin. Oncol.* 27 (2):108-17. doi: 10.1097/cco.0000000000000167.

Junghans, R. P., Q. Ma, R. Rathore, E. M. Gomes, A. J. Bais, A. S. Lo, M. Abedi, R. A. Davies, H. J. Cabral, A. S. Al-Homsi, and S. I. Cohen. 2016. "Phase I Trial of Anti-PSMA Designer CAR-T Cells in Prostate Cancer: Possible Role for Interacting Interleukin 2-T Cell Pharmacodynamics as a Determinant of Clinical Response." *Prostate* 76 (14):1257-70. doi: 10.1002/pros.23214.

Karhade, Aditya V., John H. Shin, and Joseph H. Schwab. 2019. "Prognostic models for spinal metastatic disease: evolution of methodologies, limitations, and future opportunities." *Annals of translational medicine* 7 (10):219-219. doi: 10.21037/atm.2019.04.87.

Klotz, L., L. Boccon-Gibod, N. D. Shore, C. Andreou, B. E. Persson, P. Cantor, J. K. Jensen, T. K. Olesen, and F. H. Schröder. 2008. "The efficacy and safety of degarelix: a 12-month, comparative, randomized, open-label, parallel-group phase III study in patients with prostate cancer." *BJU Int.* 102 (11):1531-8. doi: 10.1111/j.1464-410X.2008.08183.x.

Lauro, S., C. E. Onesti, R. Righini, and P. Marchetti. 2014. "The use of bevacizumab in non-small cell lung cancer: an update." *Anticancer Res* 34 (4):1537-45.

Lindtner, R. A., R. Schmid, T. Nydegger, M. Konschake, and W. Schmoelz. 2018. "Pedicle screw anchorage of carbon fiber-reinforced PEEK screws under cyclic loading." *Eur Spine J* 27 (8):1775-1784. doi: 10.1007/s00586-018-5538-8.

Maccauro, Giulio, Maria Silvia Spinelli, Sigismondo Mauro, Carlo Perisano, Calogero Graci, and Michele Attilio Rosa. 2011. "Physiopathology of spine metastasis." *International journal of surgical oncology* 2011:107969-107969. doi: 10.1155/2011/107969.

Mesbahi, Asghar, and Farshad Seyed Nejad. 2007. "Monte Carlo study on the impact of spinal fixation rods on dose distribution in photon beams." *Reports of Practical Oncology & Radiotherapy* 12 (5):261-266.

Mian, T A, M C Van Putten Jr, D C Kramer, R F Jacob, and A L Boyer. 1987. "Backscatter radiation at bone-titanium interface from high-energy X and gamma rays." *International Journal of Radiation Oncology* Biology* Physics* 13 (12):1943-1947.

Mok, T. S., Y. L. Wu, M. J. Ahn, M. C. Garassino, H. R. Kim, S. S. Ramalingam, F. A. Shepherd, Y. He, H. Akamatsu, W. S. Theelen, C. K. Lee, M. Sebastian, A. Templeton, H. Mann, M. Marotti, S. Ghiorghiu, and V. A. Papadimitrakopoulou. 2017. "Osimertinib or Platinum-Pemetrexed in EGFR T790M-Positive Lung Cancer." *N. Engl. J. Med.* 376 (7):629-640. doi: 10.1056/NEJMoa1612674.

Nevelsky, Alexander, Egor Borzov, Shahar Daniel, and Raquel Bar-Deroma. 2017. "Perturbation effects of the carbon fiber-PEEK screws on radiotherapy dose distribution." *Journal of applied clinical medical physics* 18 (2):62-68. doi: 10.1002/acm2.12046.

Pirker, R., and M. Filipits. 2009. "Targeted therapies in lung cancer." *Curr. Pharm. Des* 15 (2):188-206. doi: 10.2174/138161209787002915.

Priceman, S. J., E. A. Gerdts, D. Tilakawardane, K. T. Kennewick, J. P. Murad, A. K. Park, B. Jeang, Y. Yamaguchi, X. Yang, R. Urak, L. Weng, W. C. Chang, S. Wright, S. Pal, R. E. Reiter, A. M. Wu, C. E. Brown, and S. J. Forman. 2018. "Co-stimulatory signaling determines tumor antigen sensitivity and persistence of CAR T cells targeting PSCA+ metastatic prostate cancer." *Oncoimmunology* 7 (2):e1380764. doi: 10.1080/2162402x.2017.1380764.

Reck, M., D. Rodríguez-Abreu, A. G. Robinson, R. Hui, T. Csőszi, A. Fülöp, M. Gottfried, N. Peled, A. Tafreshi, S. Cuffe, M. O'Brien, S. Rao, K. Hotta, M. A. Leiby, G. M. Lubiniecki, Y. Shentu, R. Rangwala, and J. R. Brahmer. 2016. "Pembrolizumab versus Chemotherapy for PD-L1-Positive Non-Small-Cell Lung Cancer." *N Engl J Med* 375 (19):1823-1833. doi: 10.1056/NEJMoa1606774.

Redman, J. M., J. L. Gulley, and R. A. Madan. 2017. "Combining immunotherapies for the treatment of prostate cancer." *Urol. Oncol.* 35 (12):694-700. doi: 10.1016/j.urolonc.2017.09.024.

Savas, P., B. Hughes, and B. Solomon. 2013. "Targeted therapy in lung cancer: IPASS and beyond, keeping abreast of the explosion of targeted therapies for lung cancer." *J Thorac Dis* 5 Suppl 5 (Suppl 5):S579-92. doi: 10.3978/j.issn.2072-1439.2013.08.52.

Shah, A. N., and M. Cristofanilli. 2017. "The Growing Role of CDK4/6 Inhibitors in Treating Hormone Receptor-Positive Advanced Breast Cancer." *Curr. Treat Options Oncol.* 18 (1):6. doi: 10.1007/s11864-017-0443-7.

Sledge, G. W., Jr., M. Toi, P. Neven, J. Sohn, K. Inoue, X. Pivot, O. Burdaeva, M. Okera, N. Masuda, P. A. Kaufman, H. Koh, E. M. Grischke, M. Frenzel, Y. Lin, S. Barriga, I. C. Smith, N. Bourayou, and A. Llombart-Cussac. 2017. "MONARCH 2: Abemaciclib in Combination With Fulvestrant in Women With HR+/HER2- Advanced Breast Cancer Who Had Progressed While Receiving Endocrine Therapy." *J. Clin. Oncol.* 35 (25):2875-2884. doi: 10.1200/jco.2017.73.7585.

Smith, M. R., F. Saad, R. Coleman, N. Shore, K. Fizazi, B. Tombal, K. Miller, P. Sieber, L. Karsh, R. Damião, T. L. Tammela, B. Egerdie, H. Van Poppel, J. Chin, J. Morote, F. Gómez-Veiga, T. Borkowski, Z. Ye, A. Kupic, R. Dansey, and C. Goessl. 2012. "Denosumab and bone-metastasis-free survival in men with castration-resistant prostate cancer: results of a phase 3, randomised, placebo-controlled trial." *Lancet* 379 (9810):39-46. doi: 10.1016/s0140-6736(11)61226-9.

Sundaresan, N., G. V. Digiacinto, J. E. Hughes, M. Cafferty, and A. Vallejo. 1991. "Treatment of neoplastic spinal cord compression: results of a prospective study." *Neurosurgery* 29 (5):645-50. doi: 10.1097/00006123-199111000-00001.

Togawa, D, and KU Lewandrowsky. 2006. The pathophysiology of spinal metastases. Cancer in the Spine. *Current Clinical Oncology*, Humana Press, Totowa, NJ.

Tokuhashi, Yasuaki, Hiroshi Uei, and Masashi Oshima. 2017. "Classification and scoring systems for metastatic spine tumors: a literature review." *Spine surgery and related research* 1 (2):44-55. doi: 10.22603/ssrr.1.2016-0021.

Tong, C. W. S., M. Wu, W. C. S. Cho, and K. K. W. To. 2018. "Recent Advances in the Treatment of Breast Cancer." *Front Oncol.* 8:227. doi: 10.3389/fonc.2018.00227.

Uei, Hiroshi, and Yasuaki Tokuhashi. 2018. "Prognostic factors in patients with metastatic spine tumors derived from lung cancer-a novel scoring system for predicting life expectancy." *World journal of surgical oncology* 16 (1):131-131. doi: 10.1186/s12957-018-1439-x.

Ziu, E., V. K. Viswanathan, and F. B. Mesfin. 2021. "Spinal Metastasis." In *StatPearls*. Treasure Island (FL): StatPearls Publishing Copyright © 2021, StatPearls Publishing LLC.

Chapter 3

Spinal Trauma Surgery

Orlin Pavlov, MD
Department of Neurosurgery, Helios Klinikum Krefeld, Germany

Abstract

The spinal cord injury (SCI) is a permanent or transient loss of spinal motor, sensory and autonomic functions. SCI is often due to direct trauma to the spinal cord or compression due to traumatic disc herniation, fracture or epidural hematoma. The advances in the spinal trauma surgery could be divided into two groups: 1. Advances in non-surgical treatment of SCI and 2. Advances in the surgical treatment of SCI. The application of neuroprotective and neuroregenerative pharmacological agents has been object of interest for many decades now, where methylprednisolone took a central role. The current guidelines recommend the treatment with methylprednisolone within 8 hours of injury considering the possible complications, associated with the treatment. Some new agents, such as Minocycline, Riluzole, GM-1 ganglioside (Sygen), Cethrin, Anti-NOGO and olfactory ensheathing cells have shown promising results. Many of these pharmacological agents are still in phase I/II clinical trials. The advances in the perioperative management of SCI have also improved the outcome after trauma. The introduction of new subdural electrodes for measure of intraspinal pressure and computing the spinal cord perfusion pressure is a new viable method to ensure a better neurological outcome. The recent guidelines recommend an early surgery (<8) after the trauma.

In: Neurosurgery Research
Editors: Amit Agrawal, Pradeep Chouksey, Adesh Shrivastava et al.
ISBN: 978-1-68507-837-9

Spinal Trauma Surgery

Timeline of Spinal Cord Injury

The spinal cord injury (SCI) is a permanent or transient loss of spinal motor, sensory and autonomic functions. SCI is often due to direct trauma to the spinal cord or compression due to traumatic disc herniation, fracture or epidural hematoma. Pathophysiologically the SCI could be divided into primary and secondary SCI. The primary SCI occurs due to distribution of the mechanical forces onto the nerve tissue. This could occur through a direct compression or through a secondary compression due to fractures, traumatic disc herniation, epidural hematoma or fracture.

Advances in the Non-Surgical Treatment

Pharmacological Agents Used in SCI

In this group two types of agents are going to be considered: neuroprotective drugs and neuroregenerative drugs.

Table 1. Types of pharmacological agents used in the treatment of SCI

Neuroprotective	Neuroregenerative
Methylprednisolone	GM-1 ganglioside (Sygen)
Naloxone	Cethrin
Tirilazad	Anti-Nogo
Nimodipine	Chondroitinase ABC (ChABC)
Riluzole	Olfactory ensheathing cells (OECs)
Minocyclin	Mesenchymal stem cell
Fibroblast growth factor	

Neuroprotective Pharmacological Agents

Methylprednisolone is a well-known medicament and one of the first drugs ever used in the treatment of SCI. The mechanism of action relays on the decrease of peroxidation of membrane lipids and posttraumatic inflammation

(Wilson, Forgione, and Fehlings 2013). The clinical usage of methylprednisolone remains controversial despite its preclinical effects. A study from Cochrane Injuries Group assessed the usage of high-dose 24 h infusion of methylprednisolone to assess the motor function improvement at 6-months after the injury. This study failed to demonstrate any significant improvement after the treatment with methylprednisolone (Bracken 2002). The study showed that if the treatment has begun within 8 hours of the injury, an additional 4-point improvement in National Acute SCI Study (NASCIS) motor score was observed. The current guidelines recommend the treatment with methylprednisolone within 8 hours of injury, considering the possible complications associated with the treatment (Wilson, Forgione, and Fehlings 2013).

Naloxone, tirilazad, and nimodipine have undergone Phase 3 randomized controlled trials, which failed to demonstrate any significant improvement in NASCIS motor score recovery or in the American Spinal Injury Association (ASIA) motor score between treatment and placebo groups (Bracken et al., 1997, Pointillart et al., 2000).

Riluzole is a new and very promising pharmacological agent. It belongs to the group of the sodium channel blockers. Currently Riluzole is used for the treatment of amyotrophic lateral sclerosis. The mechanism of action is based on the blocking of sodium channels and blocking the release of neuronal glutamate and thus preventing secondary injury (Schwartz and Fehlings 2002). Phase I/II trials have shown very promising results. An improvement of the motor score at 180 days after the injury was reported by some studies (Grossman et al., 2014). Phase IIB/III double-blinded randomized controlled trial was started in 2014, and it expected to be finished by 2025.

Minocycline is a modified form of tetracycline, which has shown promising results in animal models with SCI. The mechanism of action is based on decrease in the apoptosis of oligodendrocytes and activation of the microglia (Festoff et al., 2006). The randomized controlled Phase II clinical trials in cervical SCI showed an improvement in pinprick and motor function in the minocycline group compared to placebo (Grossman et al., 2014). A Phase III study is completed in 2018. However, the data is still not published.

Neuroregenerative Pharmacological Agents

GM-1 Ganglioside (Sygen)

The laboratory studies have shown that Sygen would enhance the axonal regeneration. However, a randomized placebo-controlled clinical trial failed to demonstrate any clinical benefit from the treatment with Sygen (Geisler et al., 2001).

Fibroblast growth factor reduces glutamate-mediated excitotoxicity and thus has neuroprotective effects. There are several Phase I/II ongoing clinical trials, which will further investigate the efficacy of this agent.

Cethrin is a permeable paste, which could be directly applied on the dura during surgery. This pharmacological agent inhibits the Rho pathway, and promotes axonal growth *in vitro* (Wilson, Forgione, and Fehlings 2013, Shah et al., 2020). Several Phase I/IIa studies have shown that this pharmacological agent improved the motor function on the ASIA scale after cervical spinal cord injury.

Anti-NOGO

Bioengineered monoclonal NOGO-A antibodies also inhibit the Rho-ROCK pathway. These antibodies are applied intrathecally and currently a Phase II clinical trial is in preparation (Zörner and Schwab 2010). The primary results showed promising results on the motor function in rats and macaque monkeys.

Chondroitinase ABC (ChABC) is an enzyme, which degrades CSPGs (chondroitin sulfate proteoglycans) in the glial scar to effectively remove initiators of Rho-ROCK pathway (Ahuja, Martin, and Fehlings 2016). *Zhang* et al. conducted a study on the effect of the treatment with ChABC in rats, after intrathecal injection (Zhang et al., 2013). The authors conclude that the ChABC is a potent neuroregenerative pharmacological agent. Numerous preclinical trials have confirmed this data.

Olfactory ensheathing cells (OEC) cover the olfactory neurons, having potent phagocytic capabilities, secreting neurotrophic support factors (Ekberg and St John 2015). These cells have shown to improve the axonal regeneration and remyelination in animal models (Liu et al., 2014). So far, a couple of clinical trials have been conducted with OEC and a recent meta-analysis of this data showed no increase in the serious adverse effects. The assessment of the efficacy of OEC remains difficult because of the lower quality of the clinical trials (Li et al., 2015).

The cells-based therapies are a very promising treatment for the patients with chronic SCI. Embryonic stem cells (ESCs) and induced pluripotent stem cells (iPSCs) are capable of remyelinating denuded axons, modulating inflammatory response, restoring lost neuronal circuits and improving the microenvironment (Arriola et al., 2010, Okamura et al., 2007, Ahuja, Martin, and Fehlings 2016). There are several clinical trials, which investigate the effect of iPSCs on the motor and sensory function recovery in cervical and thoracic trauma. The results remain difficult to interpret due to competing interest and significant publication bias (Deinsberger, Reisinger, and Weber 2020).

Advances in Surgical Treatment of Spinal Trauma

1. Timing

The timing of surgery after spinal cord injury remains a controversial topic. In order to prevent secondary spinal cord damage, an early (less than 24 hours) intervention is required. At the moment level 2 evidence supports an early surgical decompression, however there are not any guidelines, suggesting that an early surgery is safe and effective (Fehlings, Vaccaro, Wilson, Singh, W Cadotte, et al., 2012). This level 2 evidence is based on the STATICS (Surgical Timing in Acute Spinal Cord Injury Study). It was shown that decompression prior to 24 hours after SCI can be performed safely and is associated with improved neurologic outcome, defined as at least two grades improvement on the AIS scale at 6 months follow-up (Fehlings, Vaccaro, Wilson, Singh, D, et al., 2012). The recruitment for one of the largest studies-SCI-POEM (Spinal Cord Injury: A Prospective, Observational European Multicentre Study) was completed in 2019. The results are yet to be published, but the primary data suggests that early surgery (less than 12 hours) was associated with a better neurological outcome (van Middendorp et al., 2012).

The newest recommendation of WFNS Spine committee, after performing meta-analysis of the current literature, states that the decompression of the spinal cord needs to be done prior to 8 hours after the trauma. When no decompression is possible within 8 hours, a decompressive surgery within 24 hours is aimed. Also, not only the incomplete lesions but also the complete lesions are amenable for treatment (Sánchez et al., 2020).

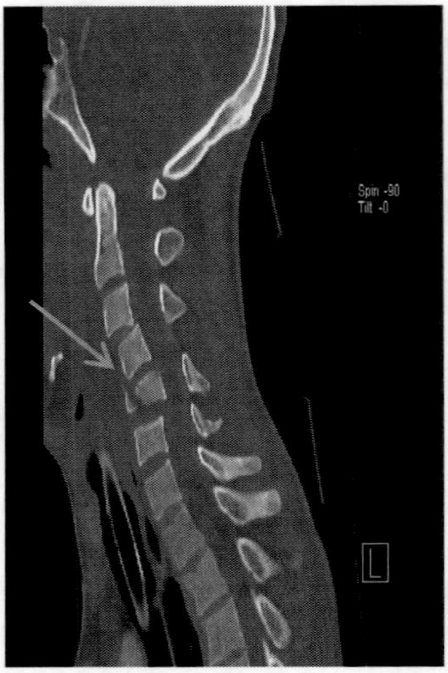

Figure 1.

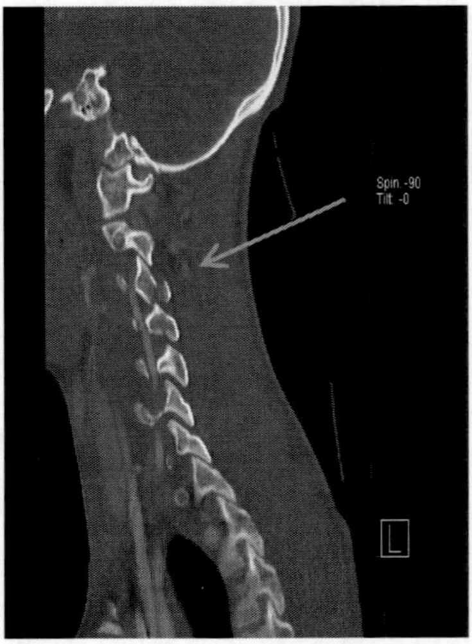

Figure 2.

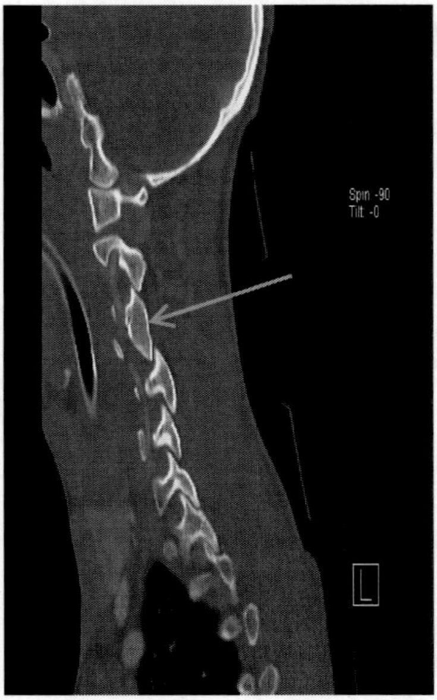

Figure 3.

Figures 1 to 3 depict a CT scan of a 22-years old patient with ASIA A after motorbike incident with A3 fracture of C4 and fracture of the facets C3/C4. The surgery was performed within 3 hours of admission. ** Author's archive.

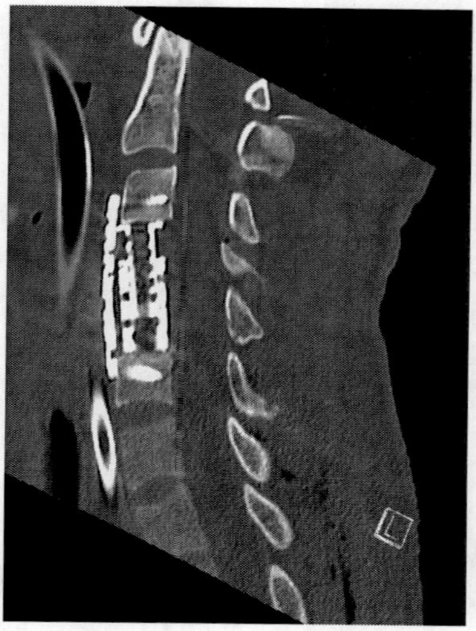

Figure 4.

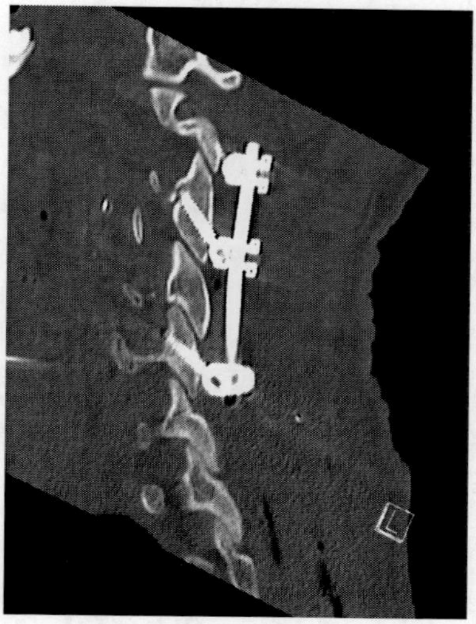

Figure 5.

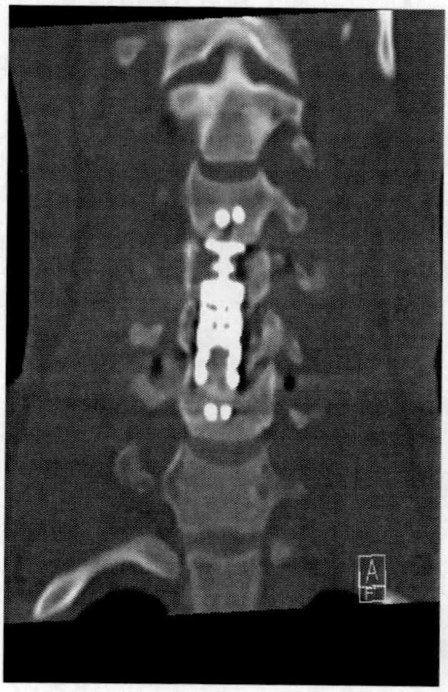

Figure 6.

Figures 4 to 6 depicting the postoperative CT of the cervical spine after circumferential reconstruction. The surgery was performed firstly with ventral approach and then the patient was placed in Concord position for the dorsal fixation. Despite the timing of the surgery, the patient didn't improve neurologically. ** Author's archive.

2. Perioperative Management

Mean arterial pressure (MAP) is a major factor for achieving a good neurological outcome. It is recommended to augment the MAP up to 85-90mmHg. The MAP is strongly connected to the spinal cord perfusion pressure (SCPP) and intraspinal pressure, similar to intracranial pressure and cerebral perfusion pressure. The SCPP can be calculated reliably, using the following formula: SCPP = MAP-ISP (Saadoun and Papadopoulos 2016). A new subdural probe for monitoring of ISP has been developed. At the moment there are no randomized trials with this new technology. The main theoretical advantage is that through the increased perfusion pressure, the intraspinal penumbra could be salvaged.

Some of the already established protocols for traumatic brain injury (TBI) could be implemented for SCI. For this instance, performing a duroplasty during decompression of the spinal cord, reduces ISP and increases SCPP. It is interesting to point out, that the increase of SCPP by 10 mmHg increases significantly the levels of methylprednisolone at the site of injury (Saadoun, Chen, and Papadopoulos 2017). This could lead to a reconsideration of some of the neuroprotective pharmacological agents, which were abandoned due to lack of positive neurological effect.

The MAP control is one of the key recommendations in the management of SCI, according to WFNS Spine committee. MAP above 85 for 7 days improves neurological deficit. Correction of hypotension and avoiding systolic blood pressure (SBP) < 90mmHg is associated with a better neurological outcome (Sánchez et al., 2020).

3. Surgical Techniques

The aims of spinal surgery in trauma patients are to achieve decompression, stabilization and correction of the segment. The early benefits of surgery are based on decompression of the spinal canal and thus neurological improvement of the patients. The late benefits are achieved through the stabilization. It is necessary to mention here, that all spine surgeons are in a different training level, when they come across a patient with traumatic lesion. It is mandatory to say, that not all young trainees in spine surgery are capable of performing stabilization of the craniocervical junction or in the cervico-thoracic junction. As mentioned above, the first goal of the surgery is to achieve decompression of the spinal canal within 8 hours after the trauma. Stabilization of the segment via ventral/dorsal or circumferential reconstruction could be performed later as a two-staged surgery.

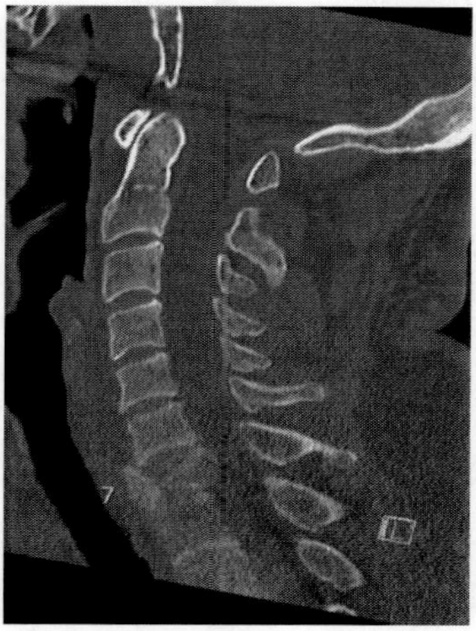

Figure 7.

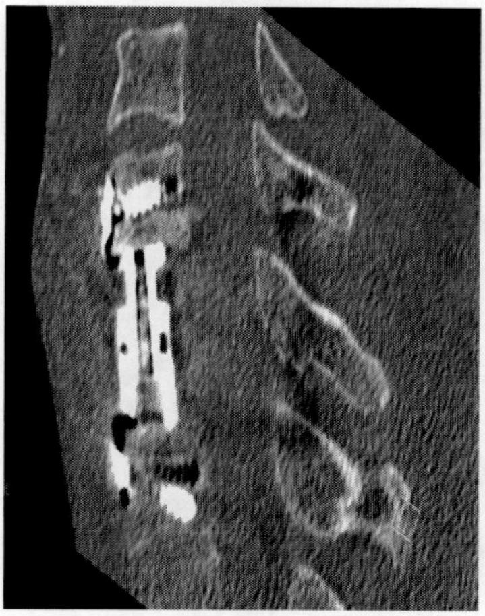

Figure 8.

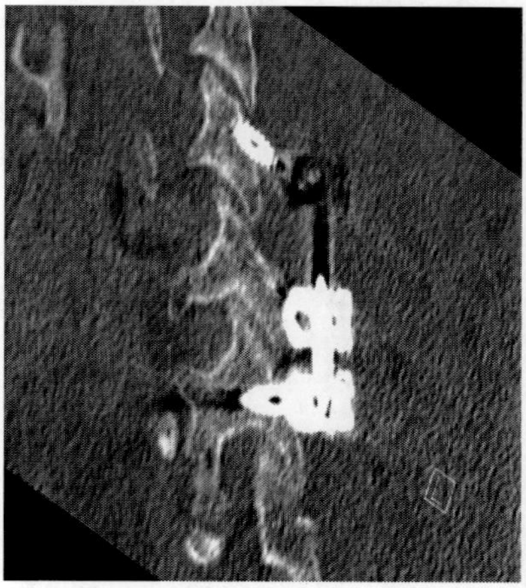

Figure 9.

Figure 7 to 9 depicting a CT of a patient after motorbike incident On Figure 7 A4 fracture of C7. Fig 8 and 9 depict the postoperative CT. The surgery was double staged. Firstly a ventral corpectomy was performed with expandable cage and then 7 days later a dorsal fixation. ** Author's archive.

World Federation of Neurosurgery (WFNS Spine committee) published in 2020 its newest recommendations, regarding the subaxial spine. One of the most interesting recommendations is the use of SLICS (Subaxial Cervical Spine Injury Classification) classification system over AO Spine classification system due to better reliability and validity (Kepler et al., 2016, Sharif et al.,

2020). The choice of anterior versus posterior approach should be based on the pathology of the injury pattern (Sharif et al., 2020). The anterior approaches have several advantages over the posterior approaches, including less blood loss, minimal surgical trauma, etc. The decompression could be achieved through corpectomy or discectomy. However, these approaches are best avoided in the setting of locked facet joints or clinically relevant dural leaks. The treatment of posterior injuries (masa lateralis, facets and ligament injuries) is best managed with posterior approaches. In the cases of complex fractures, a circumferential reconstruction of the segment may be required. The WFNS recommends an MRI in patients with locked facet joint to help in the decision-making process. Most of the locked facet joints could be managed with an anterior approach.

WFNS Spine Committee published in 2020their recommendations regarding thoracolumbar spine trauma. Both AO Spine and TLICS are recommended for clinical application. In contrast with cervical spine, the AO Spine classification has an advantage, regarding the indications for surgical treatment. According to these recommendations, a CT scan and MRI scans need to be performed prior to surgery. In the setting of acute trauma and severe neurological deficit, a CT scan is sufficient. Depending on logistics at the institution, it could be difficult obtaining an MRI scan. Here, it is up to the spine surgeon to decide, how much more important information an MRI scan would hold. According to these recommendations, all type C and B fractures have to undergo a surgical treatment. Type A2, 3 and 4 fractures could be treatment conservatively, if no significant vertebral body collapse or significant angulation is observed. These fractures need to be treated surgically, if neurological deficit is present. Interestingly, burst fractures without neurological deficit could be treated either surgically or conservatively. There are no hard evidence supporting, which strategy is better, but most of spine surgeons prefer a surgical treatment to avoid the risk of late complications, such as kyphotic deformity. The surgical strategy in burst fractures is a short-segment stabilization, however if the burst fracture affects the thoracolumbar junction, a short-segment stabilization, incorporating the fracture level or long-segment stabilization is preferred. There is level 3 evidence suggesting that the minimally invasive procedures for stabilization deliver the same outcome as open procedures.

Several patients-related factors are associated with worsened surgical outcome - obesity, increasing age and smoking. Anterior vertebral body height loss more than 50% may lead to progression of kyphotic deformity, requiring a circumferential reconstruction of the segment. It is mandatory after the initial ventral decompression to obtain an MRI, if it is not obtained preoperatively, in order to assess the posterior ligaments. Such injuries have a negative impact on the biomechanical stability.

Conclusion

In the settings of traumatic spine lesion with neurologic deficit, a surgical decompression is recommended within 8 hours after spinal trauma. Sometimes, one has to work with limited diagnostic tools, in order to achieve decompression in timely fashion. Since all trauma departments are organized differently, several factors play important role in securing the best neurological outcome of the patient:

1. Time from accident place to hospital
2. Time from CT/MRI to operating room
3. Time for decompression

Sometimes even simple decompressive surgery could be successful, when the settings for stabilization are not met. The best results after spinal trauma surgery are expected when the decompression is done in timely manner. Some of the novel pharmacological agents, such as Minocycline, could lead to a further improvement in the neurological outcome.

References

Ahuja, Christopher S., Allan R. Martin, and Michael Fehlings. 2016. "Recent advances in managing a spinal cord injury secondary to trauma." *F1000 Research* 5:F1000 Faculty Rev-1017. doi: 10.12688/f1000research.7586.1.

Arriola, A., M. E. Kiel, Y. Shi, and R. D. McKinnon. 2010. "Adjunctive MSCs enhance myelin formation by xenogenic oligodendrocyte precursors transplanted in the retina." *Cell Res.* 20 (6):728-31. doi: 10.1038/cr.2010.63.

Bracken, M. B. 2002. "Steroids for acute spinal cord injury." *Cochrane Database Syst. Rev.* (3):Cd001046. doi: 10.1002/14651858.cd001046.

Bracken, M. B., M. J. Shepard, T. R. Holford, L. Leo-Summers, E. F. Aldrich, M. Fazl, M. Fehlings, D. L. Herr, P. W. Hitchon, L. F. Marshall, R. P. Nockels, V. Pascale, P. L. Perot, Jr., J. Piepmeier, V. K. Sonntag, F. Wagner, J. E. Wilberger, H. R. Winn, and W. Young. 1997. "Administration of methylprednisolone for 24 or 48 hours or tirilazad mesylate for 48 hours in the treatment of acute spinal cord injury. Results of the Third National Acute Spinal Cord Injury Randomized Controlled Trial. National Acute Spinal Cord Injury Study." *Jama* 277 (20):1597-604.

Deinsberger, Julia, David Reisinger, and Benedikt Weber. 2020. "Global trends in clinical trials involving pluripotent stem cells: a systematic multi-database analysis." *npj Regenerative Medicine* 5 (1):15. doi: 10.1038/s41536-020-00100-4.

Ekberg, J. A., and J. A. St John. 2015. "Olfactory ensheathing cells for spinal cord repair: crucial differences between subpopulations of the glia." *Neural Regen. Res.* 10 (9):1395-6. doi: 10.4103/1673-5374.165504.

Fehlings, M. G., A. Vaccaro, J. R. Wilson, A. Singh, W. Cadotte D, J. S. Harrop, B. Aarabi, C. Shaffrey, M. Dvorak, C. Fisher, P. Arnold, E. M. Massicotte, S. Lewis, and R. Rampersaud. 2012. "Early versus delayed decompression for traumatic cervical spinal cord injury: results of the Surgical Timing in Acute Spinal Cord Injury Study (STASCIS)." *PLoS One* 7 (2):e32037. doi: 10.1371/journal.pone.0032037.

Fehlings, Michael G., Alexander Vaccaro, Jefferson R. Wilson, Anoushka Singh, David W Cadotte, James S. Harrop, Bizhan Aarabi, Christopher Shaffrey, Marcel Dvorak, Charles Fisher, Paul Arnold, Eric M. Massicotte, Stephen Lewis, and Raja Rampersaud. 2012. "Early versus delayed decompression for traumatic cervical spinal cord injury: results of the Surgical Timing in Acute Spinal Cord Injury Study (STASCIS)." *PloS one* 7 (2):e32037-e32037. doi: 10.1371/journal.pone.0032037.

Festoff, B. W., S. Ameenuddin, P. M. Arnold, A. Wong, K. S. Santacruz, and B. A. Citron. 2006. "Minocycline neuroprotects, reduces microgliosis, and inhibits caspase protease expression early after spinal cord injury." *J. Neurochem.* 97 (5):1314-26. doi: 10.1111/j.1471-4159.2006.03799.x.

Geisler, F. H., W. P. Coleman, G. Grieco, and D. Poonian. 2001. "The Sygen multicenter acute spinal cord injury study." *Spine (Phila Pa 1976)* 26 (24 Suppl):S87-98. doi: 10.1097/00007632-200112151-00015.

Grossman, R. G., M. G. Fehlings, R. F. Frankowski, K. D. Burau, D. S. Chow, C. Tator, A. Teng, E. G. Toups, J. S. Harrop, B. Aarabi, C. I. Shaffrey, M. M. Johnson, S. J. Harkema, M. Boakye, J. D. Guest, and J. R. Wilson. 2014. "A prospective, multicenter, phase I matched-comparison group trial of safety, pharmacokinetics, and preliminary efficacy of riluzole in patients with traumatic spinal cord injury." *J. Neurotrauma* 31 (3):239-55. doi: 10.1089/neu.2013.2969.

Kepler, C. K., A. R. Vaccaro, J. D. Koerner, M. F. Dvorak, F. Kandziora, S. Rajasekaran, B. Aarabi, L. R. Vialle, M. G. Fehlings, G. D. Schroeder, M. Reinhold, K. J. Schnake, C. Bellabarba, and F. Cumhur Öner. 2016. "Reliability analysis of the AOSpine thoracolumbar spine injury classification system by a worldwide group of naïve spinal surgeons." *Eur. Spine J* 25 (4):1082-6. doi: 10.1007/s00586-015-3765-9.

Li, L., H. Adnan, B. Xu, J. Wang, C. Wang, F. Li, and K. Tang. 2015. "Effects of transplantation of olfactory ensheathing cells in chronic spinal cord injury: a systematic review and meta-analysis." *Eur. Spine J.* 24 (5):919-30. doi: 10.1007/s00586-014-3416-6.

Liu, J., P. Chen, Q. Wang, Y. Chen, H. Yu, J. Ma, M. Guo, M. Piao, W. Ren, and L. Xiang. 2014. "Meta analysis of olfactory ensheathing cell transplantation promoting functional recovery of motor nerves in rats with complete spinal cord transection." *Neural Regen. Res.* 9 (20):1850-8. doi: 10.4103/1673-5374.143434.

Okamura, R. M., J. Lebkowski, M. Au, C. A. Priest, J. Denham, and A. S. Majumdar. 2007. "Immunological properties of human embryonic stem cell-derived oligodendrocyte progenitor cells." *J. Neuroimmunol.* 192 (1-2):134-44. doi: 10.1016 /j.jneuroim.2007.09.030.

Pointillart, V., M. E. Petitjean, L. Wiart, J. M. Vital, P. Lassié, M. Thicoipé, and P. Dabadie. 2000. "Pharmacological therapy of spinal cord injury during the acute phase." *Spinal Cord* 38 (2):71-6. doi: 10.1038/sj.sc.3100962.

Saadoun, S., S. Chen, and M. C. Papadopoulos. 2017. "Intraspinal pressure and spinal cord perfusion pressure predict neurological outcome after traumatic spinal cord injury." *J. Neurol. Neurosurg. Psychiatry* 88 (5):452-453. doi: 10.1136/jnnp-2016-314600.

Saadoun, Samira, and Marios C. Papadopoulos. 2016. Spinal cord injury: is monitoring from the injury site the future? *Critical care (London, England)* 20 (1): 308. Accessed 2016/10//. doi:10.1186/s13054-016-1490-3.

Sánchez, J. A. S., S. Sharif, F. Costa, Jair Rangel, C. D. Anania, and M. Zileli. 2020. "Early Management of Spinal Cord Injury: WFNS Spine Committee Recommendations." *Neurospine* 17 (4):759-784. doi: 10.14245/ns.2040366.183.

Schwartz, G., and M. G. Fehlings. 2002. "Secondary injury mechanisms of spinal cord trauma: a novel therapeutic approach for the management of secondary pathophysiology with the sodium channel blocker riluzole." *Prog. Brain Res.* 137:177-90. doi: 10.1016/s0079-6123(02)37016-x.

Shah, Manan, Catherine Peterson, Emre Yilmaz, Dia Radi Halalmeh, and Marc Moisi. 2020. "Current advancements in the management of spinal cord injury: A comprehensive review of literature." *Surgical neurology international* 11:2-2. doi: 10.25259/SNI_568_2019.

Sharif, Salman, Muhammad Yassar Jazaib Ali, Ibet Marie Y. Sih, Jutty Parthiban, and Óscar L. Alves. 2020. "Subaxial Cervical Spine Injuries: WFNS Spine Committee Recommendations." *Neurospine* 17 (4):737-758. doi: 10.14245/ns.2040368.184.

van Middendorp, J. J., G. Barbagallo, M. Schuetz, and A. J. Hosman. 2012. "Design and rationale of a Prospective, Observational European Multicenter study on the efficacy of acute surgical decompression after traumatic Spinal Cord Injury: the SCI-POEM study." *Spinal Cord* 50 (9):686-94. doi: 10.1038/sc.2012.34.

Wilson, J. R., N. Forgione, and M. G. Fehlings. 2013. "Emerging therapies for acute traumatic spinal cord injury." *Cmaj* 185 (6):485-92. doi: 10.1503/cmaj.121206.

Zhang, T., Y. Shen, L. Lu, Z. Fan, and W. Huo. 2013. "[Effect of chondroitinase ABC on axonal myelination and glial scar after spinal cord injury in rats]." *Zhongguo Xiu Fu Chong Jian Wai Ke Za Zhi* 27 (2):145-50.

Zörner, B., and M. E. Schwab. 2010. "Anti-Nogo on the go: from animal models to a clinical trial." *Ann. N. Y. Acad. Sci.* 1198 Suppl 1:E22-34. doi: 10.1111/j.1749-6632.2010.05566.x.

Chapter 4

Foramen Magnum Meningioma

Kuntal Kanti Das, Kamlesh Rangari, Ashish Sharma and Priyadarshi Dikshit
Department of Neurosurgery, Sanjay Gandhi Postgraduate Institute of Medical Sciences, Lucknow, India

Abstract

Foramen magnum (FM), also called the cranio-cervical junction, is a critical area from a neurosurgical point of view. Its deep location and important neurovascular relationships pose special challenges during surgery. Meningiomas are one of the commonest lesions at the FM, accounting for 70% of all FM tumors. However, FMMs, as such, account for only 1.8-3.2% of all meningiomas of the central nervous system. These tumors often assume very large dimensions at presentation posing significant clinical as well as surgical dilemmas. Based on their dural attachment, the neuraxial structures get displaced variably providing certain corridors that can be exploited during their surgical resection. Over the years, an ideal approach to FMMs has been a matter of intense debate, particularly for the anterior/anterolateral tumors. In this chapter, we provide a brief overview of these tumors in general, with a special emphasis on surgical approaches and results with a review of literature.

Keywords: foramen magnum, far lateral, extreme lateral, condylar resection, myelopathy, endoscopy

In: Neurosurgery Research
Editors: Amit Agrawal, Pradeep Chouksey, Adesh Shrivastava et al.
ISBN: 978-1-68507-837-9

Introduction

Meningiomas are the most common benign intracranial tumours, comprising 14.3-19% of all intracranial tumors. The foramen magnum meningiomas (FMM) constitutes around 1.8-3.2% of all cases which indicates their rarity (Arnautović et al. 2000). This anatomical location has a complex bony anatomy, contain important intradural structures like the lower brainstem, upper cervical spinal cord, vertebral artery (VA), accessory nerve and a capacious subarachnoid space. A combination of all these anatomical attributes, coupled with the well-known insidious growth of meningiomas, result in often very large tumors, late and non-specific symptoms, critical involvement/displacement of the VAs and finally a dilemma with respect to selection of surgical approaches (MR Boulton, 2003). Therefore, FMMs have come to assume a very unique challenge in neurosurgery. The advent of stereotactic radiosurgery, refinements in surgical techniques and better understanding of the disease in general have improved the overall outcomes of FMM. This chapter aims to discuss the FMMs in general with a special emphasis on surgical approaches and results with a review of literature.

Definition

FMMs arise from arachnoid cells from the duramater of the craniovertebral junction. According to George et al. (Bruneau & George, 2010; GEORGE & B, 2000), it is defined by the attachment of meningiomas in the region of FM, which they defined as an area bound by: (1) anterior; lower third of clivus to superior edge of C2 vertebral body, (2) Posterior; anterior border of squamous occipital bone to C2 vertebral spinous process, and (3) Lateral; bounded to jugular tubercles to the C2 laminae.

Bruneau and George (Bruneau & George, 2010) provided a comprehensive classification for the FMMs. It was based on the preoperative radiological features to guide preoperative surgical planning. They used three key radiological findings to classify these tumors as shown below:

A. Based on compartment involvement:

- Intradural
- Extradural, and

- intra and extra dural meningiomas

Approximately 90% of FMMs are intradural, rest are either extradural or both intra and extradural. They noted that extradural meningiomas were infiltrative to the soft tissues and VA, invaded the bones more frequently and hence these tumors are less likely to be completely resected.

B. Based on Dural attachment

Based on the preoperative finding of dural base (on MRI), they classified these tumors into: Anterior (on either side of midline), lateral (between midline and denticulate ligament), and posterior compartment (behind the denticulate ligament).

This classification is important because it gives an idea about the surgical corridor likely to be available during surgery. In anteriorly based tumors, the neuraxis is pushed posteriorly, thereby only marginally increasing the working space between the lateral FM bone and the neuraxis, particularly if the tumor is small. Such cases may require an additional bony work (condylar resection) to adequately expose the tumor. The lateral tumors, on the other hand, push the neuraxis posteromedially creating a natural surgical working window. In such cases, one may do away with the need for condylar resection. The posterior meningiomas push the neuraxis anteriorly or anteromedially, thus, may be approached directly from behind.

C. Depending on the relationship with the VA entry into the duramater:

Tumor below the VA: These represent easier cases as the lower cranial nerves (LCNs) are displaced superiorly and posteriorly. It is only during the removal of the upper pole that the LCNs are encountered.

Tumor above the VA: These tumors have unpredictable relationship with the LCNs and these tumors are surgically challenging. It is only after some intratumoral decompression that the neurovascular relationships become clearer.

Tumor on either side of VA: These are similarly difficult due to an unpredictable LCN involvement by the upper part of the tumor and possible invasion of the dural entry zone along with adventitia of the intradural VA.

Surgical Anatomy

The most important prerequisite for the performance of surgery at the FM in general and FMM is to know the anatomy of the of this region as thoroughly as possible.

FMMs have important relationships with the LCNs, brain stem, and VA. It is thus paramount to have a clear understanding of the anatomy of this region discussed under following headings:

Bony Anatomy and Definition

From a pure bony anatomy point of view, we know the FM to be a circular window in the occipital bone, anterior rim being formed by the clivus while occipital squama forms the posterior rim. From a surgical viewpoint, the definition of FM is more liberal. George and George defined FM as an area bound by: (George B et al. 1997)

- Anterior border: From the lower third of the clivus to the upper edge of the body of C2
- Lateral borders: From the jugular tubercles to the upper aspect of the C2 laminae
- Posterior border: From the anterior edge of the squamous occipital bone (posterior rim of FM) to the C2 spinous process.

Detailed anatomy of FM can be found elsewhere (Rhoton, 2000), here we focus on the bony anatomy relevant to the surgical approaches commonly employed. The three bones that participate in the formation of FM are occipital bone, atlas and the axis. In addition, three other processes need to be understood namely the atlanto-occipital condylar joint, the occipital condyles and jugular tubercle.

The anatomical foramen magnum is oval in shape, being wider posteriorly to lodge the medulla oblongata (Figure 1). The anterior narrow part provides space for the odontoid process. The posterior rim is formed by occipital squama while the anterior part is formed by basi-occiput, a part that forms clivus. The anterior rim is thus thick and has a pharyngeal tubercle for anterior pharyngeal raphe to attach. Occipital condyles are located on the anterior half. They are oval in shape, convex inferiorly and oriented with their long axis directed anteriorly and laterally. Therefore, it is apparent that condyles pose minimal hindrance, barring the posterior part, in accessing ventral lesions from a posterolateral aspect. The condyle lodges hypoglossal nerve in a bony tunnel, called hypoglossal canal. It courses through the upper part of the condyle, directed posterior to anterior. The hypoglossal canal represents the limit of condyle drilling in motion sparing trans condylar approaches, roughly corresponding to the junction of anterior 2/3rd and posterior 1/3rd. Any more drilling needs to be supplemented with cranio-cervical fixation.

Condylar fossa is a bony depression on the external aspect of the condyle. It is an important bony landmark during surgical exposure. Generally, a brisk venous bleeding is encountered while approaching this area. This bleeding is due to injury to an emissary vein that traverses through the condylar canal to connect to sigmoid sinus inside.

Jugular foramen is located lateral and superior to the anterior half of the condyle (Figure 1). Jugular tubercle is an oval elevation on top of the condyle (on the intracranial side), just above the hypoglossal canal. The caudal part of the jugular tubercle has a furrow for the lower cranial nerves.

The relevant anatomy of atlas involves the groove/course of V3 segment of the VA and the atlanto-axial joint. The atlas bone is like a ring, having two lateral masses, one on each side with anterior and posterior arches. The posterior arch has a groove on its superior surface on the lateral 3rd, called sulcus arteriosus. It can sometimes be converted into a tunnel by an additional bone coming from the occipital squama. It lodges the horizontal segment of the V3 segment of the VA. A periosteal layer and venous plexus generally surround this part of the VA which can be exploited during surgery in mobilizing this artery.

The atlanto-axial joint is a highly mobile joint, predominantly allowing a rotational movement. The joint is only supported by the joint capsule, which is stronger medially. This joint is characterised by its incomplete neural foramen so that the traversing nerve root (C2 root) is visible from behind. Of note, the VA traversing between C2 and C1 foramen transversarium always lies anterior to the C2 nerve root.

Neural Anatomy (Spinal Cord/Brainstem and Cranial Nerves)

The distinction between medulla oblongata and cervical spinal cord is the origin of the first cervical nerve. Since the dorsal root of this nerve is less consistent than the ventral one, the distinction is sometimes difficult from a posterior aspect. Nevertheless, it is the medulla oblongata that occupies the anatomical FM. The LCNs leave the cranium through jugular foramen, located lateral to the condyles. However, the spinal component of the accessory nerve ascends through the FM, often wraps on the surface of an anteriorly based FMM and it is visible just below the denticulate ligaments.

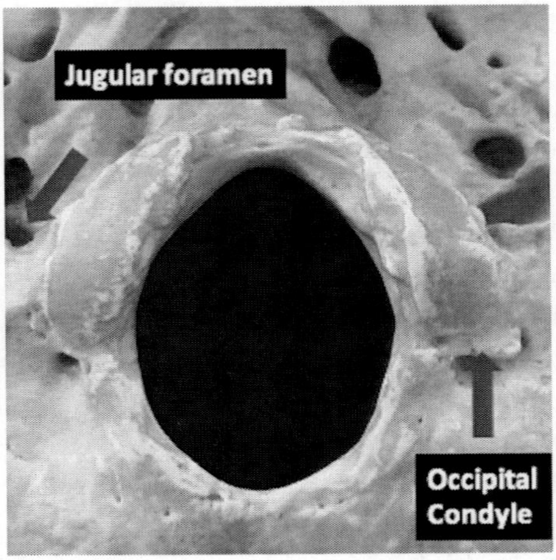

Figure 1. Inferior view of the FM. It is oval, being narrow anteriorly. Occipital condyles are located lateral to the anterior half of FM. Jugular foramen lies just lateral to the condyles.

The denticulate ligaments are fibrous bands attaching pia on the lateral aspect of the spinal cord to the duramater, in between the ventral and the dorsal spinal roots. The first denticulate ligament attaches at the level of the bony FM. The second denticulate ligament attaches to the dura just below and behind the intradural vertebral artery. During surgery, division of the denticulate ligaments not only widens the exposure but also allows slight rotation of the neuraxis.

Anatomy of the V3 and V4 Segments of VA

The VA segment between C2 transverse foramen and entry into the cervical duramater lies in close relationship with the FM. This segment is called the V3 segment (Figure 2). V3 segment has 3 parts again:

- A vertical part between C2 and C1 foramen transversarium.

- A horizontal part on the sulcus arteriosus of the atlas, having turned horizontal after leaving C1 transverse foramen.
- An oblique ascending part after leaving the sulcus arteriosus of atlas till penetration of the duramater.

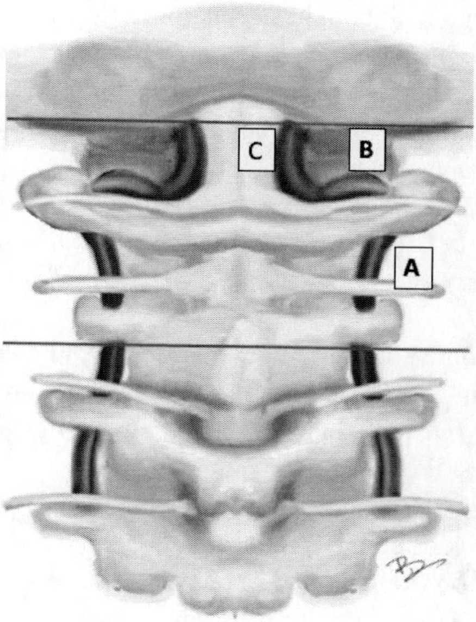

Figure 2. Anatomy of V3 segment of VA (between entry into foramen transversorium of C2 until dural entry above the C1 posterior arch, marked with red horizontal lines). It has a vertical segment (A) between C2 and C1, a horizontal segment (B) on the superior surface of the lateral 3rd of C1 posterior arch and finally an oblique ascending third part (C) before it enters the dural opening.

The dural entry of vertebral artery is just below the anatomical FM, laterally on the cervico-cranial dural junction. This part of the dura is very thick, adherent to the arterial adventitia, akin to the distal dural ring of the internal carotid artery and has a course of around 3-4 mm. The first cervical nerve and posterior spinal artery also traverse through this dural opening. This dural entry point tethers an otherwise highly mobile V3 segment.

This segment of VA generally has a few muscular and meningeal branches. in the middle of the posterolateral aspect of the C1–C2 portion, corresponding to the C2 radicular artery, a small muscular branch coursing posteriorly at the upper exit of the C1 transverse foramen, the posterior meningeal artery, and the posterior spinal artery, just before its dural penetration (E Oliveira, 1985; Rhoton, 2000). Sometimes, the posterior spinal artery and posterior inferior cerebellar artery will have an extradural origin before entering the dura and one must be mindful of these anatomical variations.

It is important to be cognisant of the fact that the anatomical orientation of the VA can change with both head rotation, as well as surgical positioning. In the neutral position, the vertical and horizontal portions of the V3 segment are nearly perpendicular. However, with head rotation, both segments are stretched and run parallel, only separated by the posterior arch of the atlas (Rhoton, 2000) (Bruneau et al. 2006).

Muscular Anatomy

During surgery from a posterolateral aspect, a number of muscles need elevation/division in order to expose the surgical structures of interest i.e., the bone and VA. The relevant anatomy is of the posterior triangle, bounded by the sternocleidomastoid and the trapezius. This actually forms the first layer of muscles that are exposed surgically. Beneath this lie 3 more muscles which arise from the cervico-thoracic spinous process and attach on the occipital and adjoining temporal bone and include: splenius capitis, semispinalis capitis and longissmus capitis. Division and reflection of these muscles laterally lead to the final layer of muscles which form the so called sub occipital triangle (Figure 3). Three muscles forming this triangle are:

- *Superior oblique:* attaches between C1 transverse process and the occipital bone between the nuchal lines, lateral to the insertion point of semispinalis capitis.
- *Inferior oblique:* Attaches between C2 spinous process and lamina to the C1 transverse process.
- *Rectus capitis major and minor:* While major attaches between C2 spinous process and lateral part of the inferior nuchal line, minor attaches C1 posterior tubercle to the medial end of the inferior nuchal line, lying below the major muscle.

The floor of this triangle is formed by posterior occipito-cervical membrane and contains the horizontal segment of the V3 segment of vertebral artery and the first cervical nerve.

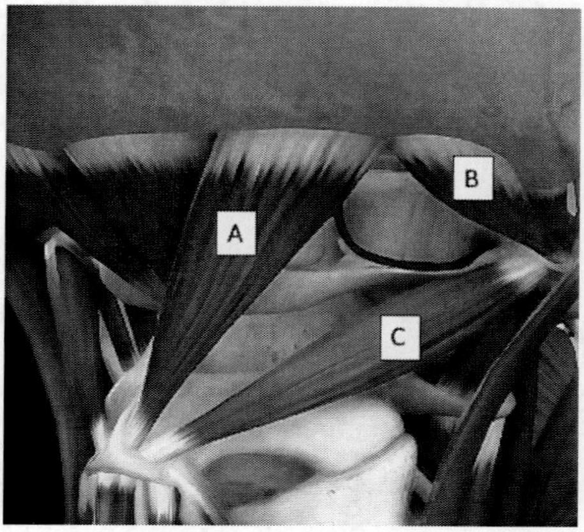

Figure 3. The suboccipital triangle is formed by rectus capitis major and minor medially, superior oblique muscle superolaterally and inferior oblique muscle inferolaterally. This triangle houses the horizontal segment of the V3 segment of VA.

Clinical Symptoms

A combination of the wider sagittal diameters of the first two cervical vertebrae and decreased girth of the spinal cord compared to the subaxial cervical cord enlargement, accounts for a generous buffer subarachnoid space in this area (Crockard & Sen, 1991).

The clinical features are mainly dependent on the size and location of the tumour, and symptoms generally develop as a result of compression of the adjacent neurovascular structures. As they slowly grows, they have a long insidious course, and they are usually diagnosed until they attains a large size. It has been reported that the clinical diagnosis may be as delayed as 30.8 months on average even in this era of MRI diagnosis. Their initial presentation is occipital and posterior cervical pain and hyperesthesia in the C2 dermatome. Pain may be unilateral and exacerbated by extension, lateral flexion of the neck, even on coughing, sneezing and straining. Different combinations of limb motor and sensory deficits, may even advance to spastic quadriplegia and marked loss of sensations and various presentations of compressive myelopathy. Most common neurologic deficit is hyperreflexia, followed by weakness of the limbs. LCNs (CN IX, X, XI, XII) palsies are usually present in half of the patients. One third patients shows dissociated sensory loss, loss of coordination in hands, down beat nystagmus, nuchal rigidity. Rarely presents with papilledema, Horner's syndrome and dysarthria.

Classic foramen magnum syndrome, although rarely observed, is characterised by the development of unilateral arm sensory and motor deficits, which progress to the ipsilateral leg, then the contralateral leg, and finally contralateral upper extremity. Long tract findings may paradoxically accompany atrophy in the intrinsic muscles of the hands. LCN palsies, hypoglossal weakness, and atrophy of trapezius, sternocleidomastoid may be evident in very late presentations. Close attention to sensory testing of the C-2 dermatome generally helps establish the diagnosis. Terminal event is generally secondary to an inability to maintain airway protection with secondary pneumonitis, and ultimately respiratory arrest.

Preoperative Radiologic Assessment

A comprehensive imaging workup with computed tomography (CT) and magnetic resonance imaging (MRI) with an angiography are essential before undertaking this procedure. The very aim is to confirm the diagnosis and plan a surgical treatment.

A gadolinium-based MRI shows tumour extension in various planes and their relationships to the adjoining structures. The direction of tumour growth and the side shift of the neuraxis in the axial plane are crucial information required for choosing the side of surgical approach. MRI Angiography not only shows the vertebral artery (VA) encasement but also illustrates the dominance of the vessels. Simultaneous encasement and luminal narrowing indicate adventitial infiltration by the tumor and such a finding helps decide the surgical plan beforehand (a sub total resection vis-à-vis a complete tumor resection with arterial reconstruction). In case of a strictly midline tumour, side of nondominant VA is usually chosen (Das et al, 2014). This ensures the dominant VA intactness, in case of injury, dissection, or thrombosis of VA. A MR venogram helps to identify the anatomy of the transverse and sigmoid sinuses, including the side of dominance and position of the jugular bulb.

Despite a good anatomy delineation, T1WI are not very helpful. T2WI are most informative, particularly in estimating the tumor consistency and arachnoid plane surrounding the tumor. A lack of arachnoid plane with cord edema indicates a possible pial transgression and such cases are surgically high-risk scenarios. Thus, one can plan a conservative resection beforehand. Post gadolinium contrast imaging delineates the tumor more clearly and gives an idea of the tumor origin based on the dural tail sign.

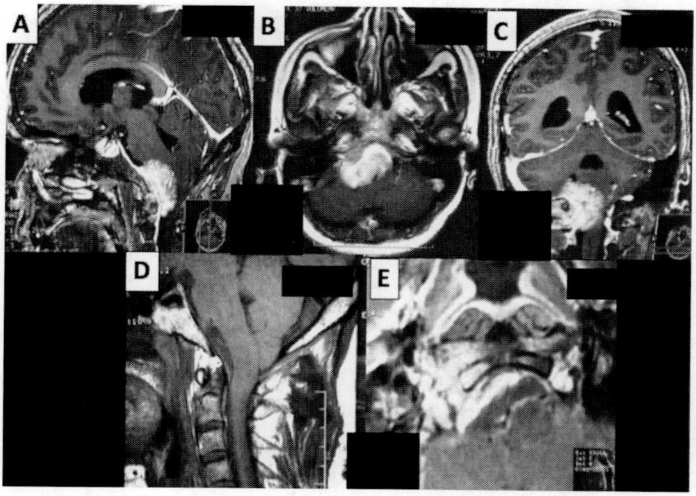

Figure 4. Shows pre and postoperative images of a case of FMM operated using FLA. On sagittal postcontrast MRI, the mass is globular, homogenously enhancing, extending from lower clivus to C2 (A). It is located anterolaterally on the right side and the neuraxis is shifted posteriorly and to the left (B). Coronal sections show some infiltrative extradural part (C). Postoperative MRI after a FLA shows complete resection of the intradural part (D) while the extradural part was still in situ (E).

A preoperative CT scan provides information about intratumoral calcification, hyperostotic changes and the available surgical corridor. Assessment by MRI and CT scan helps to determine the size of the surgical corridor, i.e., the distance between the posteromedial margin of the occipital condyle and the outer margin of cord in the axial plane. CT scan is better in this regard as MRI tends to over-estimate the surgical corridor available (Flores et al. 2013).

Although less commonly applied, an intraarterial angiogram may delineate the vascular supply of the meningioma, normally drawn from the meningeal branches of VA, ascending pharyngeal and occipital arteries. Sometimes, if the feeding artery is amenable, preoperative embolization may also be performed. There are two specific situations where a preoperative angiogram may be useful: (Flores et al. 2013; George & Lot, 2008).

1. If a highly vascularized tumor is suspected and embolization is contemplated.

2. To perform a balloon occlusion test in case of VA encasement (extradural or recurrent meningioma and meningioma inserted around the VA).

Figure 4 shows the imaging findings in a typical case of FMM operated using a far lateral approach.

Preoperative Decision Making

A proper preoperative discussion with the patient is of paramount importance. Surgery for FMM is a major undertaking and therefore, multiple sessions of counselling and discussion with the patient and relatives go a long way. A careful historical evaluation may give an indication of the tempo of the disease, patients' expectations particularly, quality of life expectations and alternate treatment options. Also, the likelihood of residual tumor must also be discussed clearly.

Preoperative clinical evaluation must try to screen out the established neurological deficits like hypoglossal palsy, LCN deficits which not only tend to worsen but also show very little chances of recovery. Particular attention needs to be paid to LCN deficits as postoperatively these patients may require assisted feeding and tracheostomy for airway protection.

As stated earlier, a combination of MRI and CT scan must be thoroughly evaluated preoperatively, once a decision for surgery has been finalised. Epicentre of the lesion, direction of displacement of the spinal cord and available corridor between the spinal cord and the condyle must be evaluated to decide the approach. Also, a history of previous surgery must be taken into account in the selection of surgical approach. A decision has to be made preoperatively whether condylar resection would be necessary and arrangements for the same will have to be made. Possibility of spinal fixation may also have to be considered in specific cases where large condylar resections may be deemed necessary.

Another important consideration is the status of the VA. Generally, the side of approach to a pure ventral lesion is from the side of the non-dominant VA. Therefore, it is important to determine the calibre of VA bilaterally including the pattern of dominance. Also, careful study is necessary to determine the origin of the PICA to avoid an intraoperative surprise. Encasement of vertebral artery, as evident from location of the VA flow void within the tumor with luminal narrowing, mandates exposure of the VA more proximally, if needed by releasing the VA from the C1 transverse foramen. Also, if a radical resection with arterial repair is planned then arrangements need to be made accordingly.

Intraoperative monitoring has evolved tremendously in the recent years. From an ancillary tool to an indispensable adjunct, intraoperative neurophysiological monitoring is equally useful in the surgery of the FMM (Arnautović et al. 2000; MR Boulton, 2003). While a combination of motor evoked potential (MEP) and somato-sensory evoked potential (SSEP) is employed to monitor long tracts of the neuraxis, triggered electromyogram of LCNs and hypoglossal nerve are frequently employed for their intraoperative preservation. The associated anaesthetic considerations need to be discussed with the anaesthesia team.

Surgical Approaches

The surgical approaches to the foramen magnum include:

a) Anterior approach: Transoral-transpharyngeal approach
b) Anterolateral or the extreme lateral approach
c) Posterolateral or Far lateral approach
d) Posterior midline approach

Anterior approach is seldom applied for these tumors, although recent emergence of endoscopic extended endonasal approaches have regenerated interest (discussed separately) (Khattar et al. 2018). The major obstacles to an anterior approach are limited working space, inadequate tumor visualisation particularly those extending laterally, chances of CSF leak and infection as well as iatrogenic instability if transverse ligament or total odontoid removal is performed.

Posterior approach includes a posterior midline approach where laminectomy of C1 and C2 (if needed) is combined with variable removal of the occipital bone and posterior margin of anatomical foramen magnum. This approach is applicable to the posterior and posterolateral meningiomas located behind the denticulate ligaments and provide good resection rates. In these tumors, the neuraxis is shifted anteriorly and thus neuraxial handling/retraction are not big concerns. Since this approach is one of the more common neurosurgical approaches, the learning curve and results are much better. In 2009, Kandenwein et al. reported 87.5% Simpson grade 1 /2 excision in foramen magnum meningioma through posterior sub-occipital approach while in 12.5% of cases subtotal resection was done as tumor was adherent at transit point of vertebral artery through the dura.

Some authors have advocated posterior approach to anterolateral foramen magnum tumors.(Goel et al. 2001; Gupta et al. 2009) They argue that large foramen magnum tumors displace the neuraxis in such a way that sufficient working space may be obtained with only a few minor modifications to the posterior approach which include: larger bony opening on the side of the tumor, division of denticulate ligaments, if needed division of the C2 nerve root, contralateral tilting of the operating table and appropriate angulation of the operating microscope.

Gupta et al. reported posterior midline approaches for anterior and anterolateral foramen magnum lesions in 2004. A total 27 patients were operated in which 13 patients were operated through the standard midline approach. Total excision was possible in 11 patients. In 2 patients, the lesion was adherent to the VA or its branches. They reported complete recovery in 8 patients and no patient had deterioration in neurological status in the post-operative period. In 2001, Goel et al. reported conventional sub-occipital approaches for anterior FMM. In this report, out of the 17 patients, they able to achieve complete tumor resection in 14 patients while in 1 patient tumor was missed inadvertently and in 2 patients, a part of tumor was left behind due to attachment at VA and PICA. Only 1 patient had permeant lower cranial nerve palsy. Rest all patients had neurological improvement (Goel et al. 2001).

However, it is generally agreed that a posterior approach may be a too simplistic answer for the more daunting anterior and antero-lateral tumors, that constitute nearly 90% of all FMMs. Not only an increased risk of neurological deficits but also inferior rates of extent of resections have been reported.

Lateral Approaches

The lateral approaches are the most commonly employed approaches for anterior and anterolateral FMMs. Two types of approaches are popular with specific indications and include:

1. Posterolateral or Far lateral approach (FLA)
2. Anterolateral of Extreme lateral approach (ELA)

While there are a number of confusions with respect to the nomenclature, anterolateral approach is conducted in front of the sternomastoid (SCM). It is a direct lateral route to this area and involved a more extensive bony drilling. The bony drilling mandates a more extensive VA mobilization and a subsequent fusion. On the other hand, FLA is performed from behind the SCM, it is a posterolateral rather than a direct lateral approach and bone drilling is more conservative with a limited VA mobilisation. Condylar drilling can be performed in both, and this point is not a differentiating point between the two approaches (A Nanda, 2002; G Lanzino, 2005; Kratimenos & Crockard, 2009, Behari et al. 2016, Behari et al. 2021).

Far Lateral Approach (FLA)

The far-lateral approach is nothing but a lateral extension of the retrosigmoid approach. It is intended to improve visualization of the ventral portion of the FM. Originally described by Heros (Heros, 1986) for VA aneurysms, it was modified for the removal of anterior FM benign tumors by George et al. *(B George, 1988; Bruneau & George, 2007; George & Lot, 2000, 2008) and has undergone subsequent modifications over the years. While the details of the surgical steps may be obtained from previous publications, we present the key elements of the approach below:

Skin Incision and Muscular Dissection

The patient can be positioned in different ways like sitting, prone, lateral or supine positions. Some degree of head flexion improves the opening of the FM while minimising head rotation maintains normal alignment and course of the V3 segment of VA. However, head flexion may cause compression of the neuraxis by the tumor and hence this manoeuvre requires judgement on the part of the surgeon. There are two commonly used variations for skin incision. The first is a C-shaped incision starting 2 finger breaths above the pinna and extending down well below the mastoid. The other is a more traditional "hockey-stick" midline incision extending from approximately the fourth cervical vertebra to the occipital protuberance and then extending laterally towards the mastoid process on the affected side. The opening of the musculature proceeds systematically beginning with the first layer (sternocleidomastoid and trapezius), then the second layer (spinalis capitis, semispinalis capitis and longissmus capitis). These are divided close to their occipital attachments and reflected laterally. The suboccipital triangle is thus exposed. The superior and the inferior oblique are reflected laterally while the rectus capitis is reflected medially. This exposes the occipital bone, C1 lamina and posterior arch, and, if necessary, the C2 lamina.

VA Control

The VA courses within a periosteal sheath along the sulcus arteriosus on the posterior arch of C1. Within this periosteal sheath exists a venous plexus that surrounds the VA. Gaining control of the VA in the anterior FM is essential. It improves exposure of the ventral FMM, allows a proximal control and provides an opportunity to repair arterial injuries if any (Hasegawa et al. 1983, Sekhar and Qazi, 2019). Methodological differences exist in the literature on this point. Most authors report coagulation of the venous plexus that surrounds the VA (Hasegawa et al. 1983; Kratimenos & Crockard, 2009). However, George, et al. emphasize the importance of exposing the VA and its venous plexus by dissecting in the subperiosteal plane of the posterior arch of C1 from medial to lateral and inferior to superior. In this way, the VA and venous plexus are naturally protected by the periosteal sheath and unnecessary bleeding from the venous plexus is avoided (Ibrahim et al. 1986; Ingraham, 1938). This also obviates the concerns related to inadvertent injuries to the aberrant vessels coming off from this portion of the VA like extradural posterior inferior cerebellar artery (PICA). Exposure of the horizontal portion of the VA may be more difficult if the sulcus arteriosus is converted into a tunnel. Once exposed, the VA is displaced superiorly to expose the lateral part of the C1 posterior arch and the lateral mass of.

Bony Opening

Typically, the posterior arch of atlas is resected towards the transverse process ipsilaterally while the contralateral side undergoes resection about halfway from the midline. Elevation of the VA from the sulcus arteriosus helps in extending C1 posterior arch removal more laterally.

There is controversy in the need and extent of condylar resection in approaching anterolateral FMMs. Bruneau and George mention that laterally located FMM do not require any lateral FM drilling as the natural corridor is sufficient for tumor removal. For ventral tumors, they suggest lateral bony resection (either C1 lateral mass for tumors below the VA or medial part of the occipital condyle in tumors above the VA). They also suggest lateral bone removal if the VA is encased. This philosophy was echoed by many other authors as well. Others describe more aggressive approaches such as routine drilling of one-third to one half of the condyle in order to create a better working space, without any reports of cranio-cervical instability or need for occipito-cervical (OC) fusion (Goel et al. 1997; Kratimenos & Crockard, 2009). Nanda et al. noted that condylar drilling is needed in cases where the tumor is purely ventral, in large tumors with bony invasion and in patients with VA encasement. Therefore, one can assume that resection of medial 30-50% condyle/C1 lateral mass is needed only in a specific few situations in FMM and if the resection is more than that then simultaneous occipito-cervical fusion must be added (A Nanda, 2002).

Intradural Tumor Removal

A C-shaped dural incision, from superolateral to the inferolateral corners of the bony exposure is recommended. It is imperative to take a dural cuff around the VA for allowing lateral mobilization of the VA as well as to allow a tight dural closure later (Bruneau & George, 2008; George & Lot, 2008). The medial dural leaf is left over the cerebellum and the spinal cord for protection.

The first recommended step before starting tumor resection is to visualise all the structures exposed and release the neuraxis. In order to further expand the surgical field anterior to the spinal cord, the first two attachments of the dentate ligament must be sectioned. The most rostral attachment of the dentate ligament is located just ventral to the dural incision above the VA as it enters the dura and behind the spinal accessory nerve while the second attachment of the dentate ligament occurs just below and behind the intradural portion of the VA (Bruneau et al. 2006; Bruneau & George, 2008; George & Lot, 2008). VA can be traced from V3 segment, then dural entry and then the V4 segment. The first cervical nerve can also be sectioned distal to its connection with the spinal accessory nerve with minimal clinical consequence and provides better surgical access (Hasegawa et al. 1983).

Care must be taken to protect the LCNs during tumor removal. George et al. originally described an approach based on the location of the FM meningioma relative to the position of the VA (Kowada et al. 1972). For example, most tumors are located below the VA, therefore pushing the LCNs superiorly and can be reliably located when resecting the superior border of the tumor. Tumors located above the VA or above and below the VA, however, displace the lower cranial nerves in an unpredictable manner and the position of the lower cranial nerves cannot be anticipated. In this case, the cranial nerve rootlets must be identified and followed along their course towards the meningioma. As the tumor is progressively debulked, the rootlets can be visualized and separated from the tumor capsule. Finally, a watertight dural closure is required to prevent a postoperative CSF leakage.

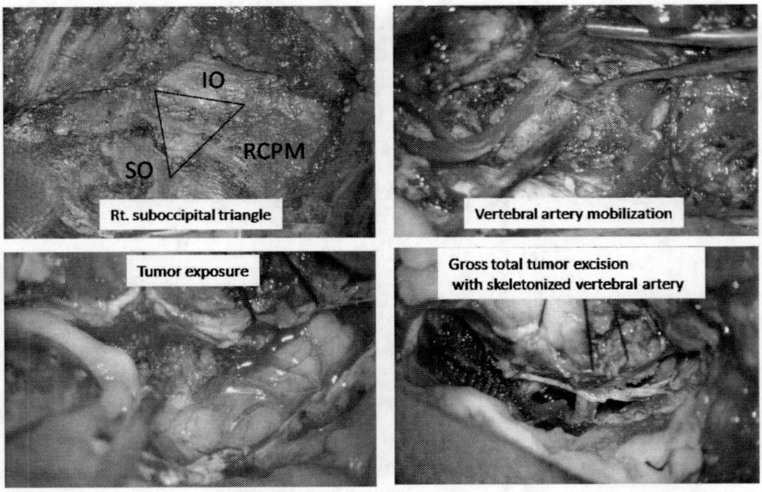

Figure 5. Shows the intraoperative images of FMM resection using FLA. Suboccipital triangle is exposed as the last layer of muscle (bounded by IO=inferior oblique, SO=superior oblique and RCPM=rectus capitis posterior major and minor). The V3 segment of VA is found here (A). By subperiosteal dissection, VA was elevated off the sulcus arteriosus and retracted with a loop laterally to allow a lateral resection of the C1 posterior arch (B). The first step after dural opening is thorough release of the neuraxis and tumor decompression (C) which allows vital structures to be protected. Final image shows completed tumor resection with an intact intradural VA (D).

Figure 5 shows the surgical steps in a representative case of FLA.

Extreme Lateral Approach: ELA

This approach was first described by Sen and Sekhar in 1990. As the name suggests, in this approach, the line of vision is more lateral and involves a more aggressive bone removal and VA mobilisation. Therefore, chances of VA injury, CSF leak and uniform requirement of O-C fusion are the drawbacks of this approach. There has been a steady decrease in the use of this approach for FMMs but used more frequently for extradural lesions like chordoma with lateral extension. Only those FMMs which are extradural or involve the lateral bones more extensively are subjected to this approach now a days (Sen & Sekhar, 1990, Sekhar and Qazi, 2019).

The salient technical aspects of this approach are:

1. A slight head extension and contralateral head rotation is required. Therefore, the VA loops become parallel above and below the C1 arch and one must be aware of that.
2. Incision is more extensive and the lateral limb drops below the mastoid tip.
3. VA needs to be released from C1 transverse foramen and the segment between C2 and dural entry must be retracted medially to expose the C1 lateral mass and occipital condyle. Depending on the tumor extension, VA may have to be released from the C2 foramen as well.
4. Bony removal is tailored to the exposure needed.
5. Dural opening is needed if the FMM is both intra and extra dural. This can be more difficult.
6. Interposition strut graft/bone filled cage between Occiput and C2 with O-C2 fixation is necessary after completion of the procedure.

Six variations of the ELA have been described (Komotar et al, 2010). All variations except for the retrocondylar approach involve at least partial occipital condyle drilling and removal.

Surgical Morbidity and Mortality Using the Far Lateral, Extreme Lateral and Posterior Midline Approaches

Komotar et al. reviewed the surgical morbidity and mortality in 2010. They noted that surgical mortality ranged from 0-13% with an average of 5.2%. The permanent morbidities ranged from 0-31% with a mean of 7.8%. These included lower cranial nerve deficits, paralysis, and infarcts resulting from VA injury. As would be expected, temporary morbidities are seen more frequently (24.8%) with typical complications including transient lower CN palsies, transient hemiparesis, and CSF leaks.

Salas et al. have published the largest series to date using anterolateral approach and advocate variations of its use depending on the type of lesion present (Salas et al. 1999). In total, 161 cases of a version of the extreme lateral approach to treat an FM lesion have been reported since Sen and Sekhar's original report in 1990 [Sen and Sekhar, 1990]. Mortality in these cases was 5.6%, comparable to the 5.3% seen using the far lateral approach. Morbidity is reported in 151 of these cases resulting in 41.7% temporary morbidity and a 14.6% permanent morbidity rate. This compares to a 21.8% temporary morbidity and 7.5% permanent morbidity rate seen using the far lateral approach. Given the small number of cases, no conclusions can be drawn regarding the morbidity and mortality rates.

Resection rates using the FLA are quite good, although authors have used varying definitions for ascertaining the degree of resection. Some authors report resection rate using the Simpson grading scale, while others merely report "total" or "subtotal" resections. Most authors define "total" resections as Simpson grades 1 and 2, "subtotal" resections as Simpsons grade 3, and "partial" resections as grade 4. Using this definition for all studies that report FM tumor resection rates (n = 149), Komotar et al. (2010) found that the FLA achieved gross total resection in 93.2% of all cases, subtotal resection in 5.4%, and partial resection in 1.3% of all cases.

For the ELA, they found that gross total resection rates were 74.7%, and subtotal resection rates were 25.3%. While resection rates were rarely reported for most of the older studies using the posterior midline approach, the French Cooperative Study (n = 103) did report their results, showing 77.7% total, 15.5% subtotal and 6.8% partial resection rates (as defined above).(Mizukami et al. 1972) Factors leading to subtotal removal were similar for all approaches with firm consistency, neovascularity, adherence to surrounding structures, large overall size, and prior radiation therapy being the most common causes of subtotal removal. Given the high degree of variability and paucity of data, it is difficult to draw conclusions regarding resection rates. As far as the postoperative clinical recovery is concerned, there was no difference between the two approaches (B et al. 1997; Pamir et al. 2004).

Finally, for posterior midline approaches in all studies that reported data for FM lesions (n = 246), 72% of patients improved or had good results, 6.9% of patients were unchanged or had fair results, and 17.5% worsened or had poor results compared to 80.6%, 6.7% and 9%, respectively in the far lateral group. Again, it seems likely that the more modern approaches offer significant benefit in terms of postoperative recovery but comparison is difficult given the different measures of recovery and the improvements in peri-operative care mentioned earlier would certainly impact postoperative recovery status as well. FM tumor recurrence rates have been variably reported throughout the history of these studies. The review by Komotar et al. (2010) found that there were large inconsistencies in the reporting of recurrences in FLA vs ELA. They concluded that it was features like adherence to surrounding structures, size of tumor, and prior radiation therapy or surgery rather than an approach that determines tumor recurrence.

Endoscopy in FMM Resection

The horizon of endonasal endoscopic surgery is ever expanding. Thus, reports on EES for ventral FMM are also increasing. The advantages of such an approach, like the trans oral approach, are direct access to the tumor, minimal or no handling of the brainstem and the opportunity to ensure Simpson grade I resection (A et al. 2015; Wang et al. 2016). The risk of direct infection is lesser compared to the transoral approach. Recent reports suggested that the endoscopic endonasal approach is useful for ventral FMMs (Khattar et al. 2018; Revuelta Barbero et al. 2019; Wang et al. 2016). Even medial condylectomy is possible in EES using a line extending inferiorly from the proximal part of the petroclival fissure and the hypoglossal canal. Lateral extension enables direct access to the lateral dural attachment of the meningioma. Additionally, the V4 segment of the VA could be visualized in its entirety. The operative corridor can be extended inferiorly by resection of the upper aspects of the C1 anterior arch and the odontoid tip. A wide exposure obtained in this fashion requires minimal condyle resection on each side. Although this procedure does not lead to any craniocervical instability, it is not widely practiced yet, and further cases and longer follow-up data are required to confirm its effectiveness. Recently, Khattar et al. (Khattar et al. 2018) reported their experience of EES with ventral FMM and compared that with their experience of FLA. They noted that EES could be useful in tumors with more rostral extension when compared with FLA which would otherwise require a cerebellar retraction and manipulation of 5th to 8th cranial nerves, in addition to the LCNs which anyway come in the way. They also highlighted a high chance of grade I resection which is practically impossible with FLA. They however noted certain limitations of EES like lack of caudal exposure below C1 ring/tip of odontoid without endangering CCJ stability and limitation is laterally extending the exposure beyond the jugular tubercle. CSF leak remained the most important complication of EES, despite recent improvement in leak rates. The authors also showed one case where endoscopy was added to FLA to obtain a grade I resection. Therefore, the authors concluded that both techniques were complimentary and the scope of EES in FMM may expand further in the future.

Stereotactic Radiosurgery in FMM

Stereotactic radiosurgery (SRS) using gamma knife platform has been in use for FMMs. Studies have shown control rates of up to 80% but with small size of the studies and insufficient follow-up durations, their role has remained somewhat less defined (Muthukumar et al. 1999). Generally, this is utilized in recurrent cases or in small postoperative residuals as a repeat surgery in such situations is quite hazardous. GKS has also been used as an upfront treatment in small to medium FMMs. Mehta et al. (Mehta et al. 2017) recently reported a multicentre study with 57 patients, the largest study so far on GK for FMM. They reported a 92% progression free survival at 10 years, which was quite impressive. The typical dosage leading to tumor regression was > 12 Gy and more than 50% patients showed symptomatic improvement. The cranial nerve deficits, however, did not improve. Therefore, GKS remains an option in surgically unfit patients (elderly with co-morbidities) with small to moderate FMMs and in recurrent/residual cases.

Conclusion

FMM are rare, technically demanding tumors occupying the junction between the head and the spinal column. Often these tumors reach a significant size at presentation due to a naturally wider subarachnoid space, slow growth of meningiomas and very non-specific symptoms. More than 90% of such tumors are located anterior or anterolateral to the neuraxis. It is important to determine the tumour's dural base, location with respect to the cross section of the spinal column and in relation to the VA. While very small tumors in medically unfit or unwilling patients may be treated by stereotactic radiosurgery (SRS), microsurgical resection remains the main treatment option in most of the cases. Posterior approach and posterolateral approaches are most widely used, with the latter being almost uniformly used in anterior tumors. Condylar resection is needed in a limited number of patients. Residual or recurrent tumors are best treated using SRS. A sound anatomical knowledge, technical prowess with these surgical approaches and wisdom gained from experience of own and others ensure satisfactory postoperative outcomes in the contemporary era. A select group of patients may be operated using endonasal endoscopic route.

References

A, B. F., EA, V., L, B., & AC, S. (2015). Endoscopic Endonasal Approach to Ventral Posterior Fossa Meningiomas: From Case Selection to Surgical Management. *Neurosurgery Clinics of North America*, *26*(3), 413–426. https://doi.org/10.1016/J.NEC.2015.03.006.

Arnautović, K. I., Al-Mefty, O., & Husain, M. (2000). Ventral foramen magnum meningiomas. *Journal of Neurosurgery: Spine*, *92*(1), 71–80. https://doi.org/10.3171/SPI.2000.92.1.0071.

B, G., G, L., & H, B. (1997). Meningioma of the foramen magnum: a series of 40 cases. *Surgical Neurology*, *47*(4), 371–379. https://doi.org/10.1016/S0090-3019(96)00204-2.

Behari S, Das KK, Bhaisora KS (2016) *Extreme lateral transcondylar approache to the foramen magnum, in atlas of neurotology and skullbase surgery*, Thieme.

Behari S, Sharma A, Das KK, Bhaisora KS (2021) *Far and extreme lateral approaches to the foramen magnum, in 360 degree atlas of skullbase surgery*, Thieme.

Boulton, MR, M. C. (2003). Foramen magnum meningiomas: concepts, classifications and nuances. *Neurosurg Focus*, *14*(6), e10.

Bruneau, M., & George, B. (2007). Foramen magnum meningiomas: detailed surgical approaches and technical aspects at Lariboisière Hospital and review of the literature. *Neurosurgical Review 2007 31:1*, *31*(1), 19–33. https://doi.org/10.1007/ S10143-007-0097-1.

Bruneau, M., & George, B. (2008). Foramen magnum meningiomas: Detailed surgical approaches and technical aspects at Lariboisière Hospital and review of the literature. *Neurosurgical Review*, *31*(1), 19–33.

Bruneau, M., & George, B. (2010). Classification system of foramen magnum meningiomas. *Journal of Craniovertebral Junction and Spine*, *1*(1), 10. https://doi.org/10.4103/0974-8237.65476.

Bruneau, M., Cornelius, J. F., & George, B. (2006). Antero-Lateral Approach To The V3 Segment Of The Vertebral Artery. *Operative Neurosurgery*, *58*(suppl_1), ONS-29. https://doi.org/10.1227/01.NEU.0000193930.74183.42.

Crockard, A. H., & Sen, C. N. (1991). The Transoral Approach for the Management of Intradural Lesions at the Craniovertebral Junction: Review of 7 Cases. *Neurosurgery*, *28*(1), 88–98. https://doi.org/10.1227/00006123-199101000-00014.

Das KK, Kumar R, Ashish K, Bettaswamy G, Mehrotra A, Jaiswal S, Sahu RN, Jaiswal AK, Behari S. Extramedullary foramen magnum tumors and their surgical management: An experience with 29 cases. *Asian J Neurosurg*. 2014 Oct-Dec;9(4):223-32. doi: 10.4103/1793-5482.146616.

Flores, B. C., Boudreaux, B. P., Klinger, D. R., Mickey, B. E., & Barnett, S. L. (2013). The far-lateral approach for foramen magnum meningiomas. *Neurosurgical Focus*, *35*(6), E12. https://doi.org/10.3171/2013.10.FOCUS13332.

George, & B. (2000). Surgical approach to the foramen magnum. *Cranial Base Surgery*. https://ci.nii.ac.jp/naid/10017239807.

George, B, C. D. J. C. (1988). Lateral approach to the anterior portion of the foramen magnum. *Surg Neurol*, *29*(6), 484–490. https://doi.org/10.1016/0090-3019(88)90145-0.

George, B., & Lot, G. (2000). *Surgical approaches to the foramen magnum* (pp. 259–279). Churchill Livingstone.

George, B., & Lot, G. (2008). Anterolateral and Posterolateral Approaches to the Foramen Magnum: Technical Description and Experience from 97 Cases. *Skull Base Surgery*, *5*(01), 9–19. https://doi.org/10.1055/S-2008-1058945.

Goel, A., Desai, K., & Muzumdar, D. (2001). Surgery on anterior foramen magnum meningiomas using a conventional posterior suboccipital approach: A report on an experience with 17 cases. *Neurosurgery*, *49*(1), 102–107.

Goel, A., Nitta, J., & Kobayashi, S. (1997). *Supracondylar infrajugular bulb keyhole approach to anterior medullary lesions* (pp. 201–203). Churchill Livingstone.

Gupta, S., Khosla, V., Chhabra, R., & Mukherjee, K. (2009). Posterior midline approach for large anterior/anterolateral foramen magnum tumours. *Http://Dx.Doi.Org/10.1080/02688690410001681028*, *18*(2), 164–167. https://doi.org/10.1080/02688690410001681028.

Hasegawa, T., Kubota, T., Ito, H., & Yamamoto, S. (1983). Symptomatic duplication of the vertebral artery. *Surgical Neurology*, *20*(3), 244–248. https://doi.org/10.1016/0090-3019(83)90061-7.

Heros, R. C. (1986). Lateral suboccipital approach for vertebral and vertebrobasilar artery lesions. *Journal of Neurosurgery*, *64*(4), 559–562. https://doi.org/10.3171/JNS.1986.64.4.0559.

Ibrahim, A. W., Satti, M. B., & Ibrahim, E. M. (1986). Extraspinal meningioma: Case report. *Journal of Neurosurgery*, *64*(2), 328–330. https://doi.org/10.3171/JNS.1986.64.2.0328.

Ingraham, F. D. (1938). Intraspinal tumors in infancy and childhood. *The American Journal of Surgery*, *39*(2), 342–376. https://doi.org/10.1016/S0002-9610(38)91252-8.

Khattar, N., Koutourousiou, M., Chabot, J. D., Wang, E. W., Cohen-Gadol, A. A., Snyderman, C. H., Fernandez-Miranda, J. C., & Gardner, P. A. (2018). Endoscopic Endonasal and Transcranial Surgery for Microsurgical Resection of Ventral Foramen Magnum Meningiomas: A Preliminary Experience. *Operative Neurosurgery*, *14*(5), 503–514. https://doi.org/10.1093/ONS/OPX160.

Komotar RJ, Zacharia BE, McGovern RA, Sisti MB, Bruce JN, D'Ambrosio AL. Approaches to anterior and anterolateral foramen magnum lesions: A critical review. *J Craniovertebr Junction Spine*. 2010 Jul;1(2):86-99. doi: 10.4103/0974-8237. 77672.

Kowada, M., Yamaguchi, K., & Takahashi, H. (1972). *Fenestration of the Vertebral Artery with a Review of 23 Cases in Japan1*. *Https://Doi.Org/10.1148/103.2.343*, *103*(2), 343–346. https://doi.org/10.1148/103.2.343.

Kratimenos, G. P., & Crockard, H. A. (2009a). The far lateral approach for ventrally placed foramen magnum and upper cervical spine tumours. *Http://Dx.Doi.Org/10.3109/02688699309103469*, *7*(2), 129–140. https://doi.org/10.3109/02688699309103469.

Kratimenos, G. P., & Crockard, H. A. (2009b). The far lateral approach for ventrally placed foramen magnum and upper cervical spine tumours. *Http://Dx.Doi.Org/10.3109/02688699309103469*, *7*(2), 129–140. https://doi.org/10.3109/02688699309103469.

Lanzino, G, S. P. R. S. (2005). Far-lateral approach to the craniocervical junction. *Neurosurgery*, *57*(4 SUPPL.), 367–371. https://doi.org/10.1227/01.neu.0000176848.05925.80.

Mehta, G. U., Zenonos, G., Patibandla, M. R., Lin, C. J., Wolf, A., Grills, I., Mathieu, D., McShane, B., Lee, J. Y., Blas, K., Kondziolka, D., Lee, C. C., Lunsford, L. D., & Sheehan, J. P. (2017). Outcomes of stereotactic radiosurgery for foramen magnum meningiomas: an international multicenter study. *Journal of Neurosurgery*, *129*(2), 383–389. https://doi.org/10.3171/2017.3.JNS163008.

Mizukami, M., Tomita, T., Mine, T., & Mihara, H. (1972). Bypass anomaly of the vertebral artery associated with cerebral aneurysm and arteriovenous malformation. *Journal of Neurosurgery*, *37*(2), 204–209. https://doi.org/10.3171/JNS.1972.37. 2.0204.

Muthukumar, N., Kondziolka, D., Lunsford, L. D., & Flickinger, J. C. (1999). Stereotactic radiosurgery for anterior foramen magnum meningiomas. *Surgical Neurology*, *51*(3), 268–273. https://doi.org/10.1016/S0090-3019(98)00099-8.

Nanda, A, D. V. P. V. M. B. A. C. (2002). Far-lateral approach to intradural lesions of the foramen magnum without resection of the occipital condyle. *J Neurosurg*, *96*, 302–309.

Oliveira, E, A. R. D. P. (1985). Microsurgical anatomy of the region of the foramen magnum. *Surg Neurol*, *24*(3), 293–352. https://doi.org/10.1016/0090-3019(85)90042-4.

Pamir, M. N., Kılıç, T., Özduman, K., & Türe, U. (2004). Experience of a single institution treating foramen magnum meningiomas. *Journal of Clinical Neuroscience*, *11*(8), 863–867. https://doi.org/10.1016/J.JOCN.2004.02.007.

Revuelta Barbero, J. M., Montaser, A. S., Shahein, M., Beer-Furlan, A., Otto, B. A., Carrau, R. L., & Prevedello, D. M. (2019). Endoscopic Endonasal Focal Transclival-Medial Condylectomy Approach for Resection of a Foramen Magnum Meningioma: 2-Dimensional Operative Video. *Operative Neurosurgery*, *16*(2), 271–271. https://doi.org/10.1093/ONS/OPY145.

Rhoton, A. (2000). The foramen magnum. *Neurosurgery*, *47*(suppl_3), S155–S193. https://doi.org/10.1097/00006123-200009001-00017.

Salas E, Sekhar LN, Ziyal IM, Caputy AJ, Wright DC. Variations of the extreme-lateral craniocervical approach: anatomical study and clinical analysis of 69 patients. *J Neurosurg*. 1999 Apr;90(2 Suppl):206-19. doi: 10.3171/spi.1999.90.2.0206.

Sekhar L, Zeeshan Q. Far lateral approach to anterior foramen magnum meningiomas – When should condyle be drilled? *Neurol India* 2019;67:59-60.

Sen, C. N., & Sekhar, L. N. (1990). An Extreme Lateral Approach to Intradural Lesions of the Cervical Spine and Foramen Magnum. *Neurosurgery*, *27*(2), 197–204. https://doi.org/10.1227/00006123-199008000-00004.

Wang, W.-H., Abhinav, K., Wang, E., Snyderman, C., Gardner, P. A., & Fernandez-Miranda, J. C. (2016). Endoscopic Endonasal Transclival Transcondylar Approach for Foramen Magnum MeningiomasSurgical Anatomy and Technical Note. *Operative Neurosurgery*, *12*(2), 153–162. https://doi.org/10.1227/NEU.00000 00000001102.

Chapter 5

Advances in CVJ Surgery

Orlin Pavlov, MD
Department of Neurosurgery, Klinikum Fulda, University Medicine Marburg, Marburg, Germany

Abstract

The advances in craniovertebral junction (CVJ) are based on the improved intraoperative imaging, surgical techniques and development of new implants. The intraoperative imaging modalities, such as combined iCT (intraoperative CT) plus angiography allow an intraoperative imaging of the vertebral artery and its close relation to the pathologies, affecting CVJ. This technique could be used in the cases of trauma with vertebral artery injury on one side, tumours affecting the CVJ, etc. Achieving a gross total resection of tumours, with a close relation to the vertebral artery, leads to improved survival of the patient. This combined technique uses the advantages of neuronavigation and angiography, depicting not only the osseous anatomy of the CVJ but also the vascular anatomy in real-time. The introduction of new techniques for fusion in the CVJ, such as the recently reported *Goe'sl Spacer,* offers new salvage methods to achieve a solid stabilization. Since the development of 3D-Printing in 1986, this process has undergone a tremendous improvement, in terms of techniques, materials, precision and reliability, making it safe in medicine. This process allows the construction of patient-specific devices and prosthetics, even in the areas with complex osseous anatomy. 3D printing allows the construction of highly complex constructs, even in the preoperative setting, using the data from CT and MRI. Such implants used after corpectomy of C2 offer a viable option for reconstruction, achieving a solid fusion.

In: Neurosurgery Research
Editors: Amit Agrawal, Pradeep Chouksey, Adesh Shrivastava et al.
ISBN: 978-1-68507-837-9

Introduction

The craniovertebral junction (CVJ) is the most mobile part of the spine. The junction could be divided in the following areas: 1. Occipitoatlantal Segment, 2. Atlantoaxial Segment. This topological classification is important for the understanding of the biomechanics of the segment. The CVJ could be affected by tumour (primary, secondary), trauma, degenerative and inflammatory diseases. These pathological processes could lead to biomechanical instability and neurologic deficit. Some pathological processes require a fixation of the CVJ in order to relieve the symptoms. One of the main factors for a good surgical outcome is the preservation of the vertebral artery. Two major anatomical variations need to be considered when performing a fusion in the CVJ: High riding vertebral artery (HRVA), as an anatomical variant and narrow pedicle of the C2 vertebrae (Wajanavisit et al., 2016, Wang et al., 2013). The presence of additional pathology – tumour, trauma, degenerative or inflammatory process – could make the fusion in CVJ extremely difficult due to the distorted anatomy.

Advances in Understanding of CVJ

Goel is currently reshaping the current understandings of the craniovertebral junction. Regarding the atlantoaxial facetal instability, in 2014 *Goel* proposed a novel classification system and later expanded even further the horizon in craniovertebral surgery. The author defines 3 types of atlantoaxial facetal instability, where type 1 is anterior dislocation of the facet of the atlas to the facet of axis. Type 2 atlantoaxial facet instability indicates that the facet of atlas is dislocated posterior to the facet of axis and type 3 atlantoaxial facet instability is where the facets are in alignment and instability was diagnosed on the basis of tell-tale clinical and radiological evidences and confirmed by manual manipulation of bones during the surgical procedure (Goel, 2019b). In type 2 and 3, there could be a normal atlanto-dental interval (ADI) and compression of neural structures could be absent. The author labels type 2 and 3 together as CAAD (central atlantoaxial instability). The presence of CAAD is associated with many entities affecting the CVJ and subaxial spine, including basilar invagination, multisegmental cervical spondylotic disease, Chiari- formation and syringomyelia, ossification of the posterior longitudinal ligament (OPLL) and deformity of the CVJ and subaxial spine (Torticollis, cervical kyphosis and dorsal kyphoscoliosis). The current understanding is that all patients with basilar invagination require dorsal fusion because of atlanto-axial instability (Goel, Jain, and Shah, 2018). CAAD is present in cases where the conventional and validated parameters of identification of atlantoaxial instability are absent (Goel, 2016). Identifying CAAD and applying the appropriate treatment with dorsal stabilization leads to a successful surgery. *Goel* stated that in those cases the decompression of foramen magnum has no clinical relevance (Goel, 2015a). Regarding the multisegmental cervical spondylotic disease (MCSS), the concept of CAAD leads to ground-breaking changes in the operative strategy. CAAD is often seen in the cases where MCSS and stenosis are located in the upper cervical spine and in patients with severe neurological deficits. The presence of retro-odontoid 'pseudotumor' has been identified to be similar to subaxial osteophyte. This 'pseudotumor' is an additional indicator for the presence of CAAD (Goel, 2015b, Goel, 2019b). Abnormally open atlantoaxial joints can be also an indicator for CAAD. In those cases, besides the stabilization of the subaxial spine, atlantoaxial stabilization has to be carried out as well. *Goel et al.* identified the pathogenesis of OPLL, being similar to the pathogenesis of spinal degenerative spondylosis. The authors state that the primary problem is instability and thus stabilization of the segment is aimed, leaving out the decompression (Goel et al., 2015). In the cases of OPLL, CAAD has to be identified and if so, the atlantoaxial region has to be included in the stabilization. Adopting this protocol for treatment, the authors report so far excellent preliminary results (Goel et al., 2015, Goel, 2019a), however so far, no clinical trials have been carried out to test this promising technique. The deformities of the CVJ and upper cervical spine, including torticollis, cervical kyphosis and dorsal kyphoscoliosis are often accompanied by CAAD. For instance, the presence of Chiari-formation with dorsal kyphoscoliosis is a primary indicator for CAAD and thus the operative strategy should be atlantoaxial fixation (Goel et al., 2019a). In their series with 11 patients, atlantoaxial stabilization was performed alone, without decompression of foramen magnum or dura opening. Despite the absence of decompression of the neural structures, the authors report improvement in the neurological deficit, more particularly in breathing capability and voice volume restoration (Goel et al., 2019b).

CAAD in Chiari-malformation will be reviewed in Chapter: Current concepts in management of Chiari I malformation.

Advances in Diagnostic

The incidence of fractures in the upper cervical spine in elderly patients (>65 years) after trauma lies between 1,26% and 3% (Squarza et al., 2019), but the true incidence could be a lot higher, since it depends on the trauma standards in each country and each hospital and the adopted protocols for trauma scan. It is reported in the literature that an increase in the incidence of C2 fractures from 3 to 6 per 100 000 from 1997 to 2014 was observed, mostly due to extended life-expectancy of the people in good health (Robinson, Olerud, and Robinson, 2017). The second factor, which contributes to the increase in the incidence, is the development of strict protocols for emergency CT of cervical spine in elderly population. CT has turned to be the golden standard for detection of fractures of the upper cervical spine with ability to detect up to 99% of the fractures (Acheson et al., 1987). Due to the degenerative alternations in the upper cervical spine, including reduced bone density and increased rigidity, upper cervical spine is more susceptible to flexion, extension, rotation traumas.

The incidence of VAI after trauma is reported to be between 0, 5% and 88% (Fassett, Dailey, and Vaccaro, 2008, Mueller et al., 2011, Willis et al., 1994, Gleizes et al., 2000). The neurological symptomatic from VAI could vary from asymptomatic to severe stroke and death. The mortality rate following VAI reported in literature varies from 8% to 18% (Fusco and Harrigan, 2011). Up to 70% of the traumatic VAI have an associated cervical spine fracture (Miller et al., 2001). These facts make the intraoperative preservation of the vascular structures of utter importance.

Advances in Surgical Techniques

The treatment options for upper cervical spine/CVJ pathologies vary from a conservative treatment (halo-fixation, hard collar, soft collar immobilisation) to surgery, including fixation with hooks and rods, wiring (Gallie Technique), plate and screw fixation (Laheri Technique), transarticular screws fixation (Magerl Technique), C1 lateral mass screws and C2 pedicle or pars screws (Harms and Melcher Technique in 2001) lateral mass screw fixation in subaxial spine (Roy-Camille, Magerl) or ventral fusion (Vergara et al., 2012). When aiming for stabilization in the CVJ, the lateral screw fixation (Goel/Harms technique) and the transarticular screw fixation (Magerl technique) have shown a superior fusion rate, compared to the other techniques (wiring, hooks, etc.), thus gaining more acceptances among the spine surgeons. These techniques could be performed in free-hands technique, with fluoroscopy or with the aid of neuronavigation, including O-Arm (Medtronic), Robotic Guidance System for Spinal Surgery (Mazor) or with integrated navigation fluoroscopy The postoperative complications rate in Goel/Harms technique is reported up to 10,6% and in Magerl technique up to 21% (Neo et al., 2005). The risk for vertebral artery injury, when performing either of those techniques lies between 8% and 9, 5% (Yeom et al., 2013, Pavlov, Mirchev, and Behr, 2020a) when using C-Arm fluoroscopy. To our knowledge, the incidence of vertebral injury (VAI) for stabilization in CVJ with O-Arm navigation or free-hands is unknown. One of the newest techniques for stabilization in the craniovertebral junction was introduced by Goel in 2013. In this technique, debridement of facetal articular cartilage and distraction of the facets is aimed. Afterwards, *Goel Spacer* is inserted in the articular cavity and fortification by lateral mass plate and screw fixation follows (Goel, 2013). This technique was employed in the cases, where transarticular/intraarticular screw placement was not possible. The author reports 3 cases so far with follow-up between 30 and 36 months. This technique has the potential of becoming a salvage method for stabilization, when the conventional methods fail.

Advances in Intraoperative Imaging

One of the key factors for a successful surgery in the CVJ is intraoperative imaging. One of the newest techniques, developed at our institution, is the intraoperative iCT (intraoperative CT) plus CT-Angiography. After the development of the theoretical basis of this technique in 2020, the description of this technique was published (Pavlov, Mirchev, and Behr, 2020b). To conduct this technique, we used our experience with O-Arm (Medtronic) and implemented intravenously contrast, prior to first intraoperative scan. In that way, we suggested that the vascular anatomy of the CVJ would be transferred to the navigation monitor and thus respected in surgery. Because of tumour lesions and fractures, the normal anatomy could be distorted and thus the risk for vascular injuries remains high. In 2021, we began using this technique in the cases of VAI, tumours, which encompass the vertebral artery on one side or previous VAI and dislocation fractures. The first paper with the first three case series is scheduled to be published at the end of 2021. On Figure 1 this intraoperative hybrid technique for intraoperative imaging of the vertebral artery is illustrated.

Leng et al. were the first to describe the fusion between intraoperative three-dimensional rotational angiography and flat panel detector computed tomography, in their case series it was used for cerebrovascular navigation (Leng et al., 2013).

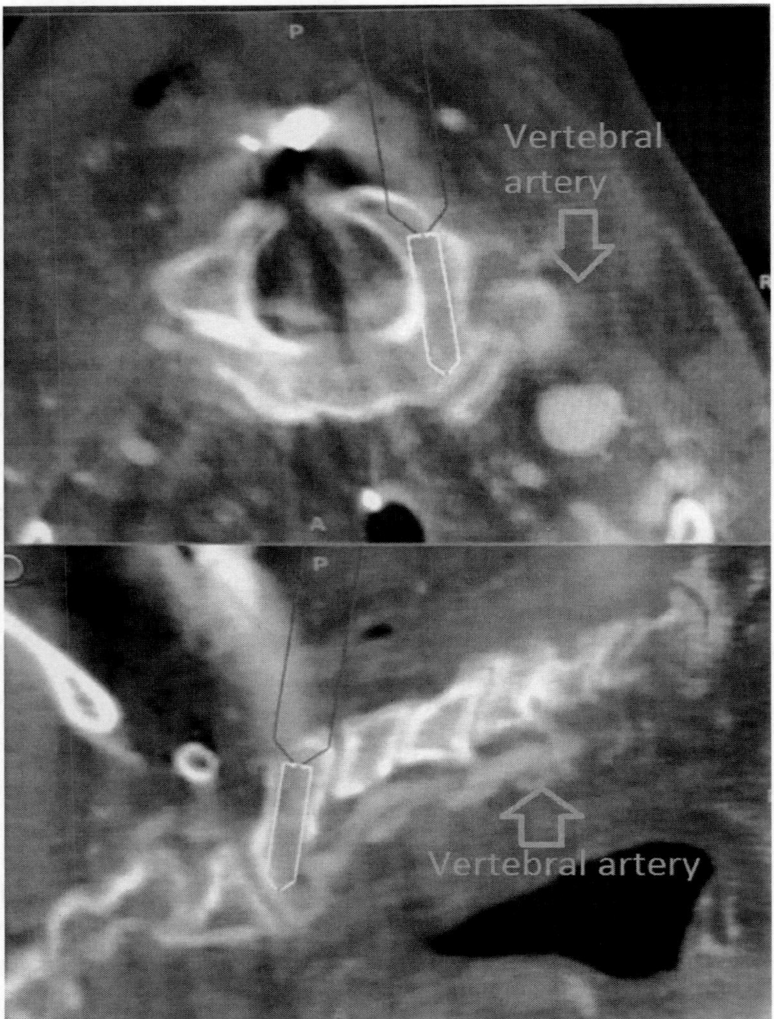

Figure 1. Intraoperative imaging of the vertebral artery (All rights reserved to the author (Author's archive)).

The authors stated that the success of the surgery was not because of this fusion method, but it adds up to the arsenal of techniques, available for the surgeon. Tumours of the craniovertebral junction (CVJ) represent a challenging entity for the neurosurgeon (Bydon et al., 2014). Bydon et al. showed that the rate of vertebral artery involvement significantly affects the rate of radical resections of the tumours, located in the CVJ. The patients without involvement of the artery had a total resection, statistically significant to those with involvement of the vertebral artery (Bydon et al., 2014). This changes the paradigm of treatment of the tumours in this location. The surgeon needs additional support for orientation during tumour removal. Pirotte et al. and Talacchi et al. showed that aiming for a total resection of the tumours in CCJ, which involve the vertebral artery, is related to many postoperative complications, including lateromedullary infarction, respiratory failure, cranial nerve palsy, etc. (Pirotte, Brotchi, and DeWitte, 2010, Talacchi et al., 2012). Kern et al. were the first to use O-Arm navigation in 2014 for resection of a chordoma in CVJ. The authors did not use however the combination of angiography and O-Arm navigation (Kern, Indro, and Amit, 2014). Because of the altered anatomy, due to tumour growth and invasion, the intraoperative landmarks can't be appreciated in some cases. The aid of O-Arm navigation is proven to be effective and accurate in both processes: tumour removal and stabilization of the CVJ. Sciubba et al. developed in John Hopkins University algorithm (Sciubba et al., 2006), for the treatment of hemangioblastomas in the cervical spine. 3D digital subtraction angiography provides high-resolution images of the vascular structures, however often it does not provide reliable anatomical information about the nearby osseous structures, or in the cases, when it does, resolution of the vascular anatomy in the immediate vicinity of bone sacrificed (Sciubba et al., 2006). So far only two case reports have been published with this new technique. *Su et al.* used the O-Arm navigation plus on-table angiography for the resection of tumour in the CVJ in 10/2020 (Su et al., 2020, Pavlov, Mirchev, and Behr, 2020a). This technique, also similar to the already published from us in 02/2020, offers a new perspective about the intraoperative mapping of highly vascular tumours, located in difficult to access areas.

Advances in the Implants

In 2020, *Ji et al.* presented the first biomechanical study on clivus plate for stabilization of the CVJ (Ji et al., 2016). The study was conducted in the cadavers and compared the clivus plate against conventional mesh cage fixation for ventral defects caused by lesions involving the upper cervical spine. After the insertion of the clivus and mesh cage, the specimens were subjected to 1,5Nm pure movement in extension, flexion, axial rotation and lateral bending. The authors conclude that- the clivus plate system fixation is biomechanically superior to the conventional fashioned mesh cage fixation in flexion, lateral bending and axial rotation, but equivalent in extension (Ji et al., 2016).

Since the development of 3D-Printing in 1986, the process has undergone a tremendous improvement, in terms of techniques, materials, precision and reliability, making it safe in medicine. This process allows the construction of patient-specific devices and prosthetics, even in the areas with complex osseous anatomy. 3D printing allows the construction of highly complex constructs, even in the preoperative setting, using the data from CT and MRI. The 3D-priting has been recently used in the reconstruction of C2, after corpectomy. *Wei et al.* managed to use this technique in 9 patients, and they published their results in 2020 (Wei et al., 2020). The authors performed a 1mm thin-layer CT scan of the target spine was performed, prior to surgery. The MIMICS 15.0 software (Materialise, Leuven, Belgium) was used for the implant design, after the importation of the data. After processing of the implant for 7 days, in order to match the set parameters for the trabecular structure and size of the micro-pores, the implant was ready to use. Since the authors performed this technique only for primary tumours of the spine, affecting the C2, the implantation of the cage was performed, after the dorsal fixation (double-staged surgery).

Achieving a complete removal of the tumour in C2, knowing that you can reconstruct the segment without any problems, is most beneficial for the patient since the overall prognosis is dependent on the amount of tumour resection. The 3D-printed cages provide larger contact area and a superior match to the adjacent bony surfaces, reducing the risk for cage subsistence, endplate fracture or implant failure. Another advantage of this system is the porous bone-contacting surface of the implant, allowing a better bone growth throughout the bone and better healing. The authors showed, yet another, positive effect of 3D-implants.

Since all of the 9 patients underwent radiotherapy, where the risk for instrumentation failure is higher, the authors observed in serial CT scans, that bone growth through the pores did not stop. In the author's opinion, this is going to be the future of implantology. The further improvement of the materials, used for the construction of the implants, tailoring the specific postoperative treatment is one of the key future concepts. *Wei et al.* used melted titanium alloy powder (Ti6Al4V, particle size, 45–100μm) in their ground-braking case series.

Conclusion

With the recent advances in understanding the CVJ, intraoperative neuroimaging and the surgical techniques, there is a progressing interest in the surgical therapy as definitive treatment. One can see the changing paradigm towards a more aggressive type of treatment in pathologies, involving the CVJ.

References

Acheson MB, Livingston RR, Richardson ML and Stimac GK. 1987. "High-resolution CT scanning in the evaluation of cervical spine fractures: Comparison with plain film examinations". *American Journal of Roentgenology,* 148 (6):1179-1185. doi: 10.2214/ajr.148.6.1179.

Bydon, Mohamad, Ting Martin Ma, Xu Risheng, Weingart Jon, Olivi Alessandro, Gokaslan Ziya L, Tamargo Rafael J, Brem Henry and Bydon Ali. 2014. "Surgical outcomes of craniocervial junction meningiomas: A series of 22 consecutive patients". *Clinical neurology and neurosurgery,* 117:71-79. doi:10.1016/j.clineuro.2013.11.023.

Fassett DR, Dailey AT and Vaccaro AR. 2008. "Vertebral artery injuries associated with cervical spine injuries: a review of the literature". *J Spinal Disord Tech,* 21 (4):252-8. doi: 10.1097/BSD.0b013e3180cab162.

Fusco MR and Harrigan MR. 2011. "Cerebrovascular dissections: A review. Part II: blunt cerebrovascular injury". *Neurosurgery,* 68 (2):517-30; discussion 530. doi: 10.1227/NEU.0b013e3181fe2fda.

Gleizes V, Jacquot FP, Signoret F and Feron JM. 2000. "Combined injuries in the upper cervical spine: Clinical and epidemiological data over a 14-year period". *European Spine Journal: Official Publication of the European Spine Society, the European Spinal Deformity Society, and the European Section of the Cervical Spine Research Society,* 9 (5):386-392. doi: 10.1007/ s005860000153.

Goel A. 2015a. "Can foramen magnum decompression surgery become historical?" *J Craniovertebr Junction Spine,* 6 (2):49-50. doi: 10.4103/0974-8237.156037.

Goel A. 2015b. "Retro-odontoid mass: An evidence of craniovertebral instability". *J Craniovertebr Junction Spine,* 6 (1):6-7. doi: 10.4103/0974-8237.151578.

Goel A. 2016. "Central or axial atlantoaxial instability: Expanding understanding of craniovertebral junction". *J Craniovertebr Junction Spine,* 7 (1):1-3. doi:10.4103/ 0974-8237.176602.

Goel A. 2019a. "Ossification of the Posterior Longitudinal Ligament: Analysis of the Role of Craniovertebral and Spinal Instability". *Acta Neurochir Suppl,* 125:63-70. doi: 10.1007/978-3-319-62515-7_10.

Goel A, Jain S and Shah A. 2018. "Radiological Evaluation of 510 Cases of Basilar Invagination with Evidence of Atlantoaxial Instability (Group A Basilar Invagination)". *World Neurosurg,* 110:533-543. doi: 10.1016/ j.wneu.2017.07.007.

Goel A, Nadkarni T, Shah A, Rai S, Rangarajan V and Kulkarni A. 2015. "Is Only Stabilization the Ideal Treatment for Ossified Posterior Longitudinal Ligament? Report of Early Results with a Preliminary Experience in 14 Patients". *World Neurosurg,* 84 (3):813-9. doi: 10.1016/j.wneu.2015.05.017.

Goel A, Vutha R, Shah A, Dharurkar P, Jadhav N and Jadhav D. 2019a. "Spinal Kyphoscoliosis Associated with Chiari Formation and Syringomyelia 'Recovery' Following Atlantoaxial Fixation: A Preliminary Report and Early Results Based on Experience with 11 Surgically Treated Cases". *World Neurosurg,* 125:e937-e946. doi: 10.1016/j.wneu.2019.01.212.

Goel Atul. 2013. "Alternative technique of cervical spinal stabilization employing lateral mass plate and screw and intra-articular spacer fixation". *Journal of craniovertebral junction & spine,* 4 (2):56-58. doi: 10.4103/0974-8237.128527.

Goel Atul. 2019b. "A Review of a New Clinical Entity of 'Central Atlantoaxial Instability': Expanding Horizons of Craniovertebral Junction Surgery". *Neurospine,* 16 (2):186-194. doi: 10.14245/ns.1938138.069.

Goel Atul, Vutha Ravikiran, Shah Abhidha, Dharurkar Pralhad, Jadhav Neha and Jadhav Dikpal. 2019b. "Spinal Kyphoscoliosis Associated with Chiari Formation and Syringomyelia 'Recovery' Following Atlantoaxial Fixation: A Preliminary Report and Early Results Based on Experience with 11 Surgically Treated Cases". *World Neurosurgery,* 125:e937-e946. doi: https://doi.org/10.1016/j.wneu.2019.01.212.

Ji Wei, Jie Tong, Zhiping Huang, Minghui Zheng, Xiuhua Wu, Jianting Chen and Qingan Zhu. 2016. "Stabilization of the Craniovertebral Junction with Clivus Plate Constructs: Biomechanical Comparison with Conventional Technique". *World Neurosurgery,* 94:42-49. doi: https://doi.org/10.1016/ j.wneu.2016.06.104.

Kern H Guppy, Chakrabarti Indro and Banerjee Amit. 2014. "The use of intraoperative navigation for complex upper cervical spine surgery". *Neurosurgical Focus FOC,* 36 (3):E5. doi: 10.3171/2014.1.FOCUS13514.

Leng LZ, Rubin DG, Patsalides A and Riina HA. 2013. "Fusion of intraoperative three-dimensional rotational angiography and flat-panel detector computed tomography for cerebrovascular neuronavigation". *World Neurosurg,* 79 (3-4):504-9. doi:10.1016/ j.wneu.2011.09.008.

Miller PR, Fabian TC, Bee TK, Timmons S, Chamsuddin A, Finkle R and Croce MA. 2001. "Blunt cerebrovascular injuries: Diagnosis and treatment". *J Trauma,* 51 (2):279-85; discussion 285-6. doi: 10.1097/00005373-200108000-00009.

Mueller Christian-Andreas, Peters Inga, Podlogar Martin, Kovacs Attila, Urbach Horst, Schaller Karl, Schramm Johannes and Kral Thomas. 2011. "Vertebral artery injuries following cervical spine trauma: A prospective observational study". *European Spine Journal: Official Publication of the European Spine Society, the European Spinal Deformity Society, and the European Section of the Cervical Spine Research Society,* 20 (12):2202-2209. doi: 10.1007/ s00586-011-1887-2.

Neo M, Sakamoto T, Fujibayashi S and Nakamura T. 2005. "The clinical risk of vertebral artery injury from cervical pedicle screws inserted in degenerative vertebrae". *Spine,* (Phila Pa 1976) 30 (24):2800-5. doi: 10.1097/ 01.brs.0000192297.07709.5d.

Pavlov O, Mirchev N and Behr R. 2020a. "A possible novel technique for intraoperative imaging of the vertebral artery during arthrodesis of the upper cervical spine". *Medical hypotheses,* 140:109641. doi: 10.1016/ j.mehy.2020.109641.

Pavlov O, Mirchev N and Behr R. 2020b. "A possible novel technique for intraoperative imaging of the vertebral artery during arthrodesis of the upper cervical spine". *Med Hypotheses,* 140:109641. doi: 10.1016/ j.mehy.2020.109641.

Pirotte BJ, Brotchi J and DeWitte O. 2010. "Management of anterolateral foramen magnum meningiomas: Surgical vs conservative decision making". *Neurosurgery,* 67 (3 Suppl. Operative):ons58-70; discussion ons70. doi: 10.1227/01.neu.0000382971.63877.dd.

Robinson Anna-Lena, Claes Olerud and Yohan Robinson. 2017. "Epidemiology of C2 Fractures in the 21st Century: A National Registry Cohort Study of 6,370 Patients from 1997 to 2014". *Advances in Orthopedics,* 2017:6516893. doi:10.1155/ 2017/6516893.

Sciubba DM, Mavinkurve GG, Gailloud P, Garonzik IM, Recinos PF, McGirt MJ, Woodworth GF, Witham T, Khavkin Y, Gokaslan ZL and Wolinsky JP. 2006. "Preoperative imaging of cervical spine hemangioblastomas using three-dimensional fusion digital subtraction angiography. Report of two cases". *J Neurosurg Spine,* 5 (1):96-100. doi: 10.3171/spi.2006.5.1.96.

Squarza S, Uggetti CL, Politi MA, Pescatori, LC, Bisogno R, Campi A, Reganati P and Cariati M. 2019. "C1-C2 fractures in asymptomatic elderly patients with minor head trauma: Evaluation with a dedicated head CT protocol". *Radiol Bras,* 52 (1):17-23. doi: 10.1590/0100-3984.2017.0154.

Su Zhangjie, Prezerakos Georgios Shiraz Sabah K and Rezajooi Kia. 2020. "Novel use of intraoperative cone-beam imaging with on-table angiography for excision of an occipitocervical tumour: A technical note and its feasibility". *Interdisciplinary Neurosurgery,* 22:100784. doi: https://doi.org/10.1016/ j.inat.2020.100784.

Talacchi A, Biroli A, Soda C, Masotto B and Bricolo A. 2012. "Surgical management of ventral and ventrolateral foramen magnum meningiomas: Report on a 64-case series and review of the literature". *Neurosurg Rev,* 35 (3):359-67; discussion 367-8. doi: 10.1007/s10143-012-0381-6.

Vergara P, Bal JS, Hickman Casey AT, Crockard HA and Choi D. 2012. "C1-C2 posterior fixation: Are 4 screws better than 2?" *Neurosurgery,* 71 (1 Suppl. Operative): 86-95. doi: 10.1227/NEU.0b013e318243180a.

Wajanavisit Wiwat, Thamrong Lertudomphonwanit, Praman Fuangfa, Pongsthorn Chanplakorn, Chaiwat Kraiwattanapong and Supaneewan Jaovisidha. 2016. "Prevalence of High-Riding Vertebral Artery and Morphometry of C2 Pedicles Using a Novel Computed Tomography Reconstruction Technique". *Asian spine journal,* 10 (6):1141-1148. doi: 10.4184/asj.2016.10.6.1141.

Wang Janhua, Hong Xia, Qingshui Ying, Yang Lu, Zenghui Wu, Fzhi Ai and Xiangyang Ma. 2013. "An anatomic consideration of C2 vertebrae artery groove variation for individual screw implantation in axis". *European Spine Journal: Official Publication of the European Spine Society, the European Spinal Deformity Society, and the European Section of the Cervical Spine Research Society,* 22 (7):1547-1552. doi: 10.1007/s00586-013-2779-4.

Wei Feng, Zhehuang Li, Zhongjun Liu, Xiaoguang Liu, Liang Jiang, Miao Yu, Nanfang Xu, Fengliang Wu, Lei Dang, Hua Zhou, Zihe Li and Hong Cai. 2020. "Upper cervical spine reconstruction using customized 3D-printed vertebral body in 9 patients with primary tumors involving C2". *Annals of Translational Medicine,* 8 (6):332-332. doi: 10.21037/atm.2020.03.32.

Willis BK, Greiner F, Orrison WW and Benzel EC. 1994. "The incidence of vertebral artery injury after midcervical spine fracture or subluxation". *Neurosurgery,* 34 (3):435-41; discussion 441-2. doi: 10.1227/00006123-199403000-00008.

Yeom JS, Buchowski JM, Kim HJ, Chang BS, Lee CK and Riew KD. 2013. "Risk of vertebral artery injury: Comparison between C1-C2 transarticular and C2 pedicle screws". *Spine J,* 13 (7):775-85. doi: 10.1016/j.spinee.2013.04.005.

Chapter 6

3D Printing in Cranio-Vertebral Junction (CVJ) Surgery

Rashim Kataria* **and Mudit Mehrotra**
Department of Neurosurgery, SMS Medical College, Jaipur, Rajasthan, India

Abstract

CV Junction region is an unforgiving location because of the presence of the Brain stem, Vertebral arteries & cranial nerves etc.,to make things worse, the vertebral arteries often have an anomalous course in this region. Hence the surgery in this area is associated with high mortality & morbidity, especially during the initial learning curve.

The customized 3D printed models provide the same anatomy as that of the patient & hence can be used to study the surgical anatomy in detail before the actual operation. This includes knowing in detail the orientation of the joints, abnormal course of vertebral arteries, size of the lateral masses, pars, pedicle & lamina, etc.

It also allows performing a rehearsal of the actual surgery and thus a plan B can be thought of beforehand in case the proposed plans doesn't work, thus reducing the duration of surgery & avoiding preventable complications. It makes a relatively difficult operation safe. In addition, the 3D printed models are a very important teaching/simulation tool for the residents & young surgeons.

The chapter discusses in detail the author's personal experience of more than 50 patients of CV Junction surgeries (For Congenital anomalies & Traumatic cases) and also describes the current utility of 3D printed models & their limitations and how can these be overcome.

---

*Corresponding Author's Email: rashim_kat@yahoo.com.

In: Neurosurgery Research
Editors: Amit Agrawal, Pradeep Chouksey, Adesh Shrivastava et al.
ISBN: 978-1-68507-837-9

Introduction

The complex anatomy of the Cranio-Vertebral junction (CVJ) and its surrounding structures has made surgery in this region a very challenging task, and so the preoperative information regarding the osseous deformities, course of the vertebral arteries (VA), pedicle size, and location of the transverse foramina is instrumental to surgeons operating on these challenging cases. Given this complex anatomy of CVJ and the delicate nature of surrounding structures, three-dimensional printing, also known as rapid prototyping, has the potential to aid surgical planning and procedural accuracy.

Normal & Variant Anatomical Aspects at the CVJ

The Occipitoatlantal joint provides more stability in comparison to mobility & the reverse is true for the atlantoaxial joint, which offers more mobility leading to higher chances of injury and dislocation at this joint [1]. The patients with C1-C2 instability (atlantoaxial dislocation, AAD) present with a plethora of symptoms ranging from neck pain and restricted neck movements to numbness and weakness in upper and lower limbs [2-5]. The treatment of AAD is aimed at correcting mal-alignment of bilateral C1-C2 joints in all planes, followed by stabilization of these joints [6-11]. The surgical management of AAD primarily consists of posterior approaches using the screw-rod system [12], which includes pedicle screw system; lateral mass screws system, transarticular screws system, and laminar screws system. Of these, the transarticular screw system is the strongest, but the most commonly used method of internal fixation for posterior cervical surgery is the pedicle screw system because of its excellent biomechanical property and the ease of surgery [13].

CVJ is one of the most complex regions of the body to operate because of the limited space available as surgical corridor, unforgiving structures in the surrounding (such as the brain stem, VA) and to add to the complexity the course of the VA is often anomalous, especially in congenital CVJ anomalies. The VA can be anomalous in 2-3% of the normal population and 20% of congenital CVJ anomalies [14-15]. The patient-to-patient variability in the size, angulation, and orientation of the joints, facets, and pedicle of axis and atlas vertebra also add to the complexity of this region. The use of sharp instruments and screws, as well as high-speed drills in this space-constrained environment, makes the surgery difficult, especially for a naive surgeon in this field. Surgery may lead to complications such as limb paralysis, VA Injury leading to catastrophic haemorrhage causing life-threatening emergencies. The anatomy is further complicated by the presence of congenital osseous anomalies in this region. Occipitalisation of the atlas is seen in 0.1–0.8% of the normal population [16] while it is considerably higher in patients with AAD [17-19]. Sardhara et al. [20] in their study found occipitalisation of the atlas in 72% of their enrolled CVJ anomaly patients. It has been seen that occipitalisation of atlas and C2–C3 fusion is frequently associated with lateral joint asymmetry due to their common embryological development [20]. This frequently leads to facetal instability and consequently AAD [21]. C2 bony anomalies include segmentation defects of the odontoid process such as os odontoideum etc., and uncommonly absence of C2 posterior elements leading to C2-C3 spondyloptosis (Figure 1) [22].

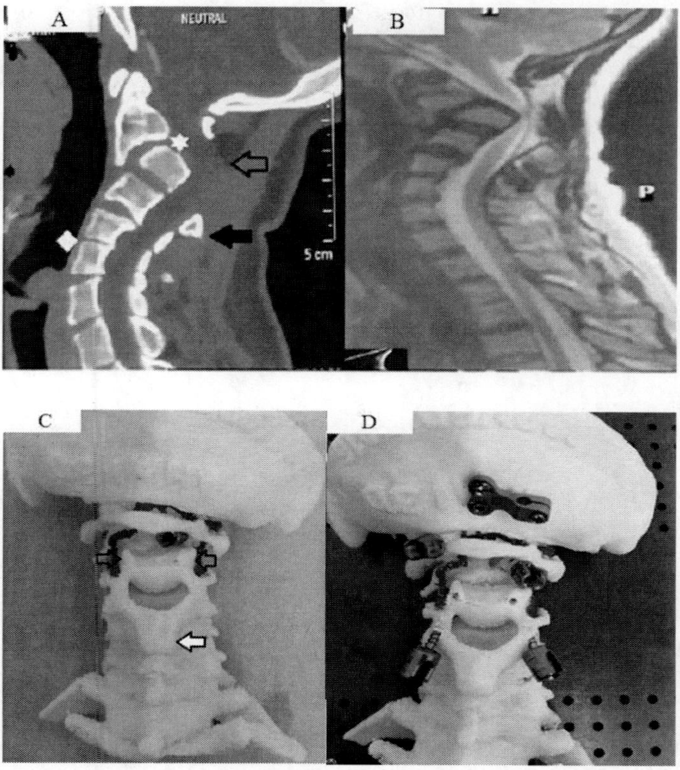

Figure 1. (Continued)

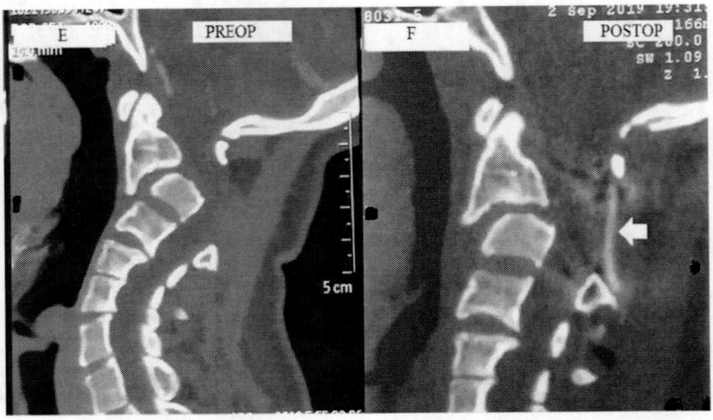

Figure 1. Uncommon case of absent C2 posterior elements with C2-C3 Spondyloptosis. A) Preop CT scan (mid sagittal section) showing absent C2 lamina (hollow arrow), C2-C3 spondyloptosis (asterisk), hypertrophied spinous process of C3 (solid arrow), C5-C6 block vertebra (diamond). B) MRI T2W image, Mid Saggital section showing severe cord compression by retropulsed C3body. C) 3D model of the CV junction of the patient showing the posterior view with absent C2 lamina, well developed Uncinate process of C3 (hollow arrow), hypertrophied spinous process of C3 (solid arrow). D) Showing hands-on practice on the model preoperatively. E) and F) shows a comparison between the preoperative and postoperative CT scan (mid sagittal section) of the patient showing acceptable reduction and realignment of the C2-C3 body with increased canal diameter at the level of C3, iliac bone graft between C1 Posterior Arch and C3 spinous process in situ (solid arrow). The model helped us in better understanding the complex anatomy and planning preoperatively.

Importance of 3D Anatomical Knowledge

A sound 3D anatomical knowledge of any region of surgical interest is desirable to execute a surgical operation free of complications. There is a natural tendency of forming a 3D image in one's mind by looking at the 2D CT or MRI films. Only an experienced & excellent surgeon can form a near-identical 3D image of the problem in his mind by looking at to the 2D pictures.

3D reconstructed computed tomography (CT) images are better than the 2D pictures & can help in understanding the complex anatomy, but they are of limited use intra-operatively as they can be viewed only on a CT film and provide only a 2D perspective of the region concerned. The newer neuro-navigation devices like CT 3D navigation system, G-arm, O-arm can serve the purpose of providing a 3D perspective of the region intra-operatively. The practical applications of these devices are limited by factors such as a lack of equipment, insufficient training, and high costs [23-26].

Recently 3D printing technology has been introduced in the field of neurosurgery for assisting surgeons in better understanding the complex anatomy of different regions and pathologies of the patients. Even though in its infancy, the 3D printing technology is proving to be of immense help in understanding the complex anatomy of the CVJ, studying the course of the vertebral artery, evaluate the dimensions of the bones and their orientation for identifying the best possible trajectory of screw implantation in posterior fixation surgeries. The 3D model can be used to practice the operation before the actual surgery, the size of the plates and screws to be used and the angle of insertion of the screws can be calculated preoperatively from these 3D models. The model also provides information about the overriding joints angulation, the size of the screw able structures such as pars, pedicle, lateral masses, lamina, etc. The entry points of the screws can be selected & the screws can be inserted into the model. This saves the operative time during the actual operation and also reduces blood loss [27]. If the surgeon discovers that, say the pedicle of C2 (Axis) is small to accommodate the screws he can decide to insert the screws in the pars or the lamina of the Axis (C2). Hence a plan B can be decided before the actual operation. The rehearsal minimizes the surprises encountered during the actual operation. Repeated attempts of screw insertion in the model reduce the chances of screw malposition during the operation on the patient. A naive surgeon is more comfortable operating on a patient after rehearsing the same anatomy provided by the 3D model. He has a sense of familiarity with the anatomy during the actual surgery [28]. Last but not least these 3D models can also be used as teaching tools for the residents in institutions and act as aids for patient education and counseling preoperatively [27-29].

History

3D printing was invented by Charles Hull in the early 1980s and was called Stereolithography [30]. This process is also referred to as additive manufacturing (AM), rapid prototyping (RP), or solid free-form technology (SFF). Hull later founded the company 3D Systems, which developed the first 3D printer, called a "stereolithography apparatus." In 1988, 3D Systems introduced the first commercially available 3D printer, the SLA-250 [23]. Since then 3D printing has affected many aspects of day-to-day life and now has made its way into the field of medical science. Newer 3D printers available for use specifically in medical fields are FORMIGA P 110 Velocis, EOS P 770/500, HBD-1000, etc.

Currently, many companies like Helisys, Ultimateker, and Organovo, Adler Ortho group have started using 3D printing for commercial medical applications like using 3D printing to fabricate living human tissue, orthopaedic implants, personalised anatomical surgical models, enhanced surgical tools, and medical and dental devices like prosthetics, braces, dentures. According to a report by market research firm, SmarTech Analysis, the market for medical 3D printing is currently estimated to be worth $1.25 billion. By 2027, the market value is set to grow to $6.08 billion. The potential for 3D printing is rising exponentially within the healthcare system [30].

The 3D printer selected for bioprinting depends firstly on the materials to be used and secondly on how the layers in the finished product are bonded. The three most commonly used 3D printer technologies in medical applications are selective laser sintering (SLS), thermal inkjet (TIJ) printing, and fused deposition modelling (FDM) [30].

The powdered material is used as a substrate for 3D printing in the SLS printer. A laser draws the shape of the object in the powder and lays it down layer by layer fusing it to ultimately form the object. This type of 3D printing can be used to create metal, plastic, and ceramic objects. 3D printed models with intricate details and precision can be made using this method [31].

Inkjet printing uses thermal, electromagnetic, or piezoelectric technology to deposit tiny droplets of "ink" onto a substrate according to digital instructions. These 3D printers have shown promise in the field of tissue engineering, regenerative medicine, and drug delivery & gene transfection during tissue construction. This printing has shown high precision, great versatility, and control in printing simple 2D and 3D tissues and organs, known as bio-printing [31].

FDM printers are much more commonly used and inexpensive than the other printer types. These FDM printers use a technique similar to an inkjet printer but they use beads of heated plastic in place of ink. The beads of heated plastic are released from the print-head as it moves, building the object in thin layers. This process is repeated over and over, allowing for a detailed and precise construction of the object. FDM printers can use a variety of plastics [31].

Out of all the raw materials for 3D printing in use today, plastic is the most common. The most common varieties used for 3D printing are Polylactic acid (PLA), Acrylonitrile butadiene styrene (ABS), Polyvinyl Alcohol Plastic

(PVA), Polycarbonate (PC). Of these ABS and PLA are most common and inexpensive. But the brittleness and stiffness of plastic have led to the use of more malleable materials like powders, the most popular are Polyamide (Nylon) and Alumide. The second-most-popular material in the industry of 3D printing is metal, which is used through a process known as direct metal laser sintering or DMLS. The most popular metals in 3D printing for medical purposes are titanium and stainless steel. Other metals used are bronze, gold, nickel, and aluminum, but have limited utilization in the medical field. Resins are also used as a material for 3D printing but are less popular due to their limited strength and flexibility. Graphite, Graphene, and Carbon fiber are also being used for 3D printing. As a common material in medical implants, Nitinol is valued in the 3D printing world for its super-elasticity. Made from a mixture of nickel and titanium, Nitinol can bend to considerable degrees without breaking and has been found as an invaluable base material for bio-printing lastly now the focus of the scientific community has now shifted to living cells for 3D printing of organs, tissues, and blood vessels. Previously single material was being used for 3D printing, that too brittle plastic such as ABS but now multi-material printing is possible making these models much more malleable and elastic.

Even though 3D printing is in its very early stages in the field of neurosurgery it has improved the approach and success rates of various surgeries previously considered difficult due to their complex anatomies, especially in the field of aneurysmal surgery, surgery of deep-seated brain tumours, cranioplasty and spine surgeries, etc. The first report of the use of this technology in the CV junction surgery dates back to 2015-16, from New York University Langone Medical Centre, New York (USA), KEM Medical College, Mumbai(India), and SMS Medical College, Jaipur (India) [27-29], where the authors used customised 3D printed models of the CV junction regions of the patient to be operated upon. They claimed that rehearsing the operation on the model proved to help carry out the actual surgery. Various studies have also given evidence in favor of these 3D printed models [45-47].

Making the Model

The patients underwent a CT scan using Philips 128 slice CT scanner. The scans are obtained from a level extending from the occipital region up to the upper dorsal vertebra. 60 ml of iodinated contrast is injected IV at a rate of 4.5 ml/second. Axial 0.8-mm-thick images are obtained at 0.5-mm intervals. This data is in DICOM format. The angiography images of these patients are used to extract 3D files in STL (Surface Tessellation Language) format. This STL file is then sent electronically to a local lab with a 3 D printer station for the printing of the 3D model. The models are prepared using Acrylonitrile Butadiene Styrene (ABS) polymer by fused dependent modeling (FDM 3D) printer. The FDM 3D printer used is ProtoCentre999 (Figure 2), the printer was introduced in 2013 and it is India's first dual extruder with support material printing. The printer achieves repeatability and reliability at a very cost-effective price, it has 9x9x9 cubic inches build volume and can print with soluble support. Post-processing sanding and printing isdone to ensure a smooth finish. Colouring of vertebral arteries is done for their proper identification. The model requires approximately 5-8 hours to be made depending on the size and the approximate cost of each model ranges from 5000-10000 INR. The model provides a valuable tool to assess the anatomy of the region in a 3D perspective and the model can be grasped and moved in various surgical positions, thereby helping in formulating and rehearsing the entire surgical plan preoperatively. The size of the model matches exactly with the patient's anatomy and makes it possible to evaluate the region and to preoperatively decide on the sizes of the implants. The model is invaluable in assessing the exact size, dominance, and course of the vertebral artery and its relationship with the C1-C2 joints. This information helps in locating the best possible site for screw insertion and helps in avoiding injury to the vertebral artery. The model can be utilised for the identification of alternative sites for screw insertion. The model aided in the identification of the exact location of the facets in a 3D perspective. It helps to decide which region needed to be drilled, it also solidifies the surgical strategy concerning bony abnormalities in this region and thus gives a 3D perspective of the status of facets and their alignment preoperatively. The rotational abnormalities in this region leading to the subsequent changes in the alignment could be visualised directly. The more accessible atlantoaxial joint was identified on the model and that side could be approached first while planning the surgical steps. The model also gives us an idea regarding atypical areas of fusions and bone formation that could cause hindrance in our approach to the atlantoaxial joint. On the whole, the models provide us with a remarkably true picture of the intraoperative bone structures, thus proving to be a significant confidence booster during the drilling and dissection of structures. It also helps reduce surgical time [27-29]. The exact sizes of the screws and plates/rods could be calculated preoperatively along with the angle of insertion.

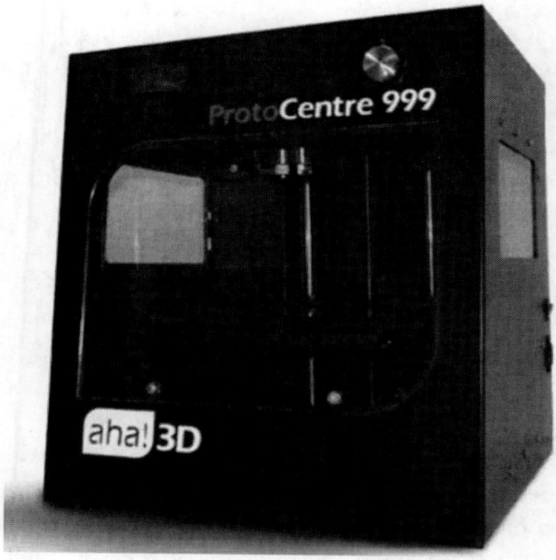

Figure 2. ProtoCentre999 3D printer (type of FDM 3D printer) used for constructing the 3D printed models.

Precision in Screw Insertion

Despite the biomechanical superiority of cervical pedicle screws [32], the placement of cervical pedicle screws has a considerable risk of injury, either to nerves or to the VA. Abumi et al. [33] reported that 45 out of 669 inserted screws (6.7%) were misplaced in their early series. Onishi et al. [34] reported on a patient who suffered cerebral infarction due to brain embolism after the placement of cervical pedicle screws. Having a tangible model of a patient's anatomy available for a surgeon to study or use to simulate surgery is preferable to the costly and not easily available neuro-navigation techniques used for assistance in surgeries in this region. Guo et al. [35] found a greater acceptance rate of screw placement in 94.6% of the patients in which 3D model-based navigation templates were used as compared to a 70.27% satisfactory rate in the control group in which screws were fixed using fluoroscopy. Yang et al. [36] in their study stated that screw positions were incorrect in 32.9% of patients who were treated with conventional free-hand techniques as compared to 11.3% of patients who were treated with screw fixation assisted by 3D-printed models. Wright and Lauryssen [37] reported that VA injury can be as high as 4.1% per patient or 2.2% per screw inserted, which can be drastically reduced by using 3D models based on intraoperative navigation. According to a study by Sugimoto et al. [38], the effectiveness of 3D printing escalates many folds with the complexity of the pathology, as the surgeon can better appreciate the patient's anatomy with the life-size model in his hands as compared to mentally reconstructing the patient's anatomy in his mind during surgery using the preoperative CT scan images. Izatt et al. [39] in his study found that the use of a 3D printed model improved surgical results in 78% of cases, he also stated that these additional costs which were incurred during manufacturing of these 3D printed models were counterbalanced in 59% of cases by the more proficient operative technique and planning afforded by the models, as well as fewer intra-operative complications and higher precision associated with the use of these 3D models. This study was supported by Wang et al. [40], who in his study said that the diminished need for intra-operative navigation reduced the operating costs of the procedure. The benefit provided by 3D printed models in revision surgery was validated by Otsuki et al. [41], in his study he demonstrated their effectiveness as screw insertion is more demanding in revision surgeries due to morphology changes caused by the first operation.

Authors Experience

The senior author has got experience of operating more than 70 patients with the help of 3D printed models. The authors in a recent, unpublished prospective study comprising of 42 patients, compared the radiological correction & clinical improvement in patients where 3D printed models were used with another group where the models were not used. The group allocation was done on a random basis. The posterior internal fixation surgery was done in each patient according to preoperative CT, and MRI findings. In patients with Atlanto-occipital assimilation, internal fixation was performed using an occipital plate and C-2 pedicle screws. C-1 lateral mass screw and C-2 pedicle screw fixation using Goel's and Harm's technique was the procedure of choice in patients without atlanto-occipital assimilation. Intra-articular spacer or autologous bone graft was used in patients in both groups where ever needed. In case the pedicles of the C2 were not of adequate size or in cases of high riding vertebral artery, C2 translaminar or C2 pars interarticularis screws were used. C-3 lateral mass screw fixation (occiput-C2-C3) was added in some traumatic cases to reinforce the construct. They compared the preoperative and the postoperative values of the Atlanto-Dental interval (ADI), the distance of the tip of dens from Wackhenheims clivus canal line (WCCL), and lastly the distance of the tip of dens from the Chamberlain's line (CL). The neurological assessment of patients in the pre-operative and the postoperative period was done by using the modified Japanese Orthopaedic Association score (mJOA) (Figure 3) [42]. Using the modified JOA score the recovery rate [43] was calculated for every patient in each group using the formula

$$Recovery\ rate = \frac{postoperative\ m\,JOAS - preoperative\ m\,JOAS}{total\ m\,JOAS - preoperative\ m\,JOAS}$$

The recovery rate was found to be statistically significant in the study group as compared to the control group (Table 1). Other parameters like ADI, WCCL, and chamberlain's line when compared for both preoperative and postoperative values came out to be significant in both groups (Table 2). Screw malposition was an important parameter compared between the two groups. Criteria are used for deciding screw malposition were based on the radiological findings in postoperative CT scans and on the neurological status of the patient. The radiological criteria were: any cortical breach of pedicle on the medial side, cortical breach on the lateral and inferior side of more than 2 mm, and lastly cortical breach superiorly and anteriorly more than 4 mm. These criteria were established using McGill's scoring system for the revision of pedicle screws [44]. Of the total screws inserted in the cases and controls, screw malposition was found in 2/66 screws in the cases and 11/60 screws in the control group, this was found to be statistically significant (<0.05). The occipital screws were left out of this total screw inserted. The patients were followed up for 1 year. Figure 4 shows a patient who presented with basilar invagination with AAD and was operated on using a 3D printed model, the patient improved neurologically in the post-op period as shown in postoperative CT scan.

They concluded that Posterior internal fixation performed using individualised 3D printed model is realistic and effective in treating CVJ abnormalities. The 3D printed models have found more utility in patients with CVJ congenital abnormalities as compared to patients presenting with traumatic CVJ fractures as the latter have relatively straightforward anatomy of this region. The 3D printed model is clinically advantageous and may have great potential in guiding surgery in this region, even to relatively less experienced neurosurgeons.

Score	Description
Lower extremity motor dysfunction	
0	Unable to walk
1	Able to walk on flat floor with walking aid
2	Able to walk up and/or down stairs with handrail
3	Lack of stability and smooth reciprocation of gait
4	No dysfunction
Lower extremity sensory deficit	
0	Severe sensory loss or pain
1	Mild sensory loss
2	No deficit
Sensory deficit in trunk	
0	Severe sensory loss or pain
1	Mild sensory loss
2	No deficit
Sphincter dysfunction	
0	Unable to void
1	Marked difficulty in micturition
2	Minor difficulty in micturition
3	No dysfunction

Figure 3. Modified Japanese orthopaedic association score (m JOA), the maximum score is 18.

Table 1.

Variable		Study group (n=23) 3D printed models		Control Group (n=19) without 3d models		p value
		Number	Percentage	Number	Percentage	
Recovery Rate	≤25%	3	13.04	9	47.37	X^2= 10.111 p value= 0.023
	26-50%	8	34.78	8	42.11	
	51-75%	9	39.13	1	5.26	
	76-100%	3	13.04	1	5.26	

Table 2.

Variables	Study Group		p value	Control Group		p value
	Pre op	Post op		Pre op	Post op	
Modified JOA score	11.61±3.26	14.43±3.07	<0.001	11.37±2.81	12.26±3.93	0.06
Atlanto-Dental Interval (ADI)	8.58±2.83	4.64±2.51	<0.001	7.34±2.28	4.19±2.73	<0.001
Chamberlain's line (CL)	3.10±8.83	-1.10±5.91	0.005	1.61±7.84	-1.15±5.47	0.004
Wakenheims clivus canal line (WCCL)	4.15±9.24	-0.40±5.45	0.006	1.94±4.64	-1.29±4.88	0.005

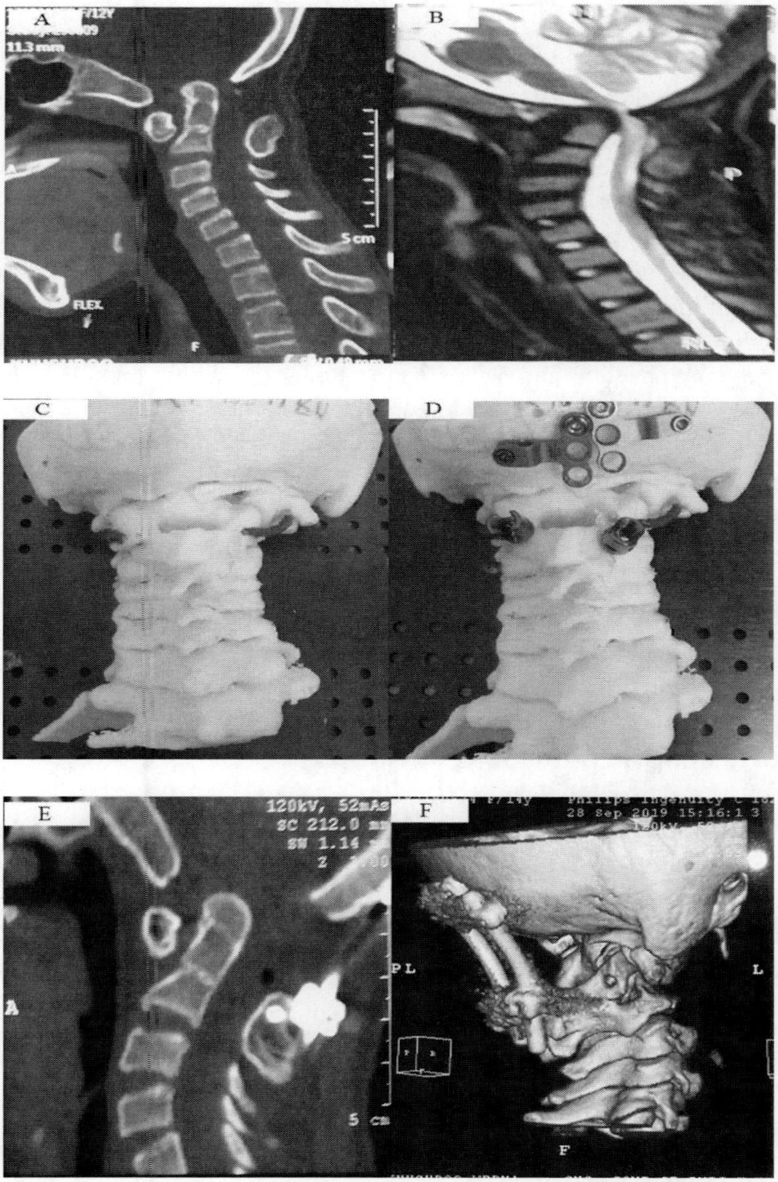

Figure 4. A case of Basilar invagination (BI) and mild AAD. A) Sagittal image of the preop ct showing BI with AAD. B) Sagittal image of the preop MRI showing BI with severe cord compression at cervicomedullary junction. C) 3D model of the patient. D) Hands-on practise before the actual surgery E) & F) Post-operative images showing reduction of BI and AAD after Occiput-C2 fixation.

Shortcomings

Most of the models are made of a single material i.e., plastic (ABS), hence are brittle, they do not yield to the forces & manipulations (e.g., DCER) and break off; hence the targeted correction of the deformity cannot be achieved in the model. The drilling work cannot be done on the models as the plastic melts away with the drilling. The screws are inserted in the patient with intraoperative radiological guidance but the rehearsal on the 3D model is done without radiological support so these two are exactly not comparable procedures. They do not provide us with real-time intraoperative information like the joint positions and facet alignment after the institution of the cervical traction could. The joints in the model are immobile and hence are unable to provide information about the nature of the joint instability and flexibility. No information regarding the venous anatomy and the extent of venous congestion in the region of lateral gutters could be deciphered from the models. The model provides details about the osseous & arterial anatomy only & does not provide information on the strength & integrity of various ligaments & soft tissues. In re-do cases, models with a single material are not able to distinguish between the bones & the implant.

Future of 3D Printing in CVJ Surgery

Multimaterial 3D printing can be used instead of ABS only, so that differential tissue densities, compressibility, and elasticity could be generated representing ligaments, joint capsules, vessels, etc. in this region, allowing the operating surgeon to predict the forces required for deformity correction and to test the limit of permutability of vessels and neural structures in real-time. Appropriate bio-printable, bio-compatible or metallic materials are available in the market & in the times to come these may help in performing as aggressive surgery as the total replacement of the CVJ.

Conclusion

Even though there are few shortcomings with these 3D models, they provide a hands-on approach preoperatively and help immensely in decoding the complex anatomy of the craniovertebral junction which can help us in achieving a complication-free surgery in an otherwise complex region. This is even more relevant in cases of congenital CVJ anomalies where the anatomy is severely deranged and there are more chances of anomalous course of the vertebral artery. A novice surgeon can have an excellent understanding of anatomy by having hands-on experience with the model. With further advances in technology, it can be stated with reasonable surety that the 3D printer will continue to prove itself as an important and highly cost-effective tool in the management of CVJ lesions.

Acknowledgment

Our sincere thanks to Mrs. JP Kaushal and Mr Akash Kaushal of Aha 3D, Jaipur (India)for helping us out in making the 3D models on a priority basis at a very reasonable price.

References

Abumi, K., Y. Shono, M. Ito, H. Taneichi, Y. Kotani, and K. Kaneda. 2000. "Complications of pedicle screw fixation in reconstructive surgery of the cervical spine." *Spine* (Philadelphia Pa 1976). 25, no. 8 (April): 962–969.

Agarwal, Prashant., S. Chopra, V. D. Sinha, and R. Kataria. 2020. "Three- Dimensional-Printed Model-Assisted Management of Craniovertebral Junction Abnormalities: An Institutional Experience with Literature Review." *Asian Spine Journal.* 14, no.2 (April): 204-211.

Aoude, Ahmed., S. Ghadakzadeh, H. Alhamzah, M. Fortin, P. Jarzem, J. A. Ouellet, and M. H. Weber. 2018. "Postoperative Assessment of Pedicle Screws and Management of Breaches: A Survey among Canadian Spine Surgeons and a New Scoring System." *Asian Spine Journal.* 12, no. 1 (February): 37-46.

Behari, Sanjay., M. V. KiranKumar, D. Banerji, D. K. Chhabra and V. K. Jain. 2004. "Atlantoaxial dislocation associated with the maldevelopment of the posterior neural arch of axis causing compressive myelopathy." *Neurology India.* 52, no.4 (December):489-491.

Chhabra, Sachin., S. Chopra, R. Kataria and V. D. Sinha. 2017. "Use of 3D printer model to study vertebral artery anatomy and variations in developmental craniovertebral junction anomalies and as a preoperative tool-an institutional experience." *Journal of spine Surgery.* 3, no. 4 (December): 572-579.

Fielding, J. W., R. J. Hawkins and S. A. Ratzan. 1976. "Spine fusion for atlanto- axial instability." *The Journal of Bone and Joint Surgery. American volume* 58, no. 3 (April): 400-407.

Gao, Fangyou., Q. Wang, C. Liu, B. Xiong, and T. Luo. 2017. "Individualized 3D printed model-assisted posterior screw fixation for the treatment of craniovertebral junction abnormality: a retrospective study." *Journal of Neurosurgery: Spine.* 27, no. 1 (July):29-34.

Goel, Atul. 2014. "Goel's classification of atlantoaxial "facetal" dislocation." *Journal of Craniovertebral Junction & Spine.* 5, no. 1 (January): 3-8.

Goel, Atul., B. Jankharia, A. Shah and P. Sathe. 2016. "Three-dimensional models: an emerging investigational revolution for craniovertebral junction surgery." *Journal of Neurosurgery: Spine.* 25, no. 6 (December): 740-744.

Guo, Fei., J. Dai, J. Zhang, Y. Ma, G. Zhu, J. Shen and G. Niu. 2017. "Individualized 3D printing navigation template for pedicle screw fixation in upper cervical spine." *PLoS One.* 12, no. 2 (February): e0171509.

Hirabayashi, K., J. Miyakawa, K. Satomi, T. Maruyama, and K. Wakano. 1981. "Operative results and postoperative progression of ossification among patients with ossification of cervical posterior longitudinal ligament." *Spine.* (Philadelphia Pa 1976). 6, no. 4 (July-August):354-364.

Hoy, Matthew B. 2013. "3D printing: making things at the library." *Medical Reference Services Quarterly.* 32, no. 1: 94–99.

Izatt, Maree T., P. L. P. J. Thorpe, R. G. Thompson, P. S. D'Urso, C. J. Adam, J. W. S. Earwaker, R. D. Labrom, and G. N. Askin. 2007. "The use of physical biomodelling in complex spinal surgery." *European Spine Journal.* 16, no.9 (September): 1507- 1518.

Jain, V. K. and S. Behari. 2002. "Management of congenital atlanto-axial dislocation: some lessons learnt." *Neurology India.* 50, no. 4(December):386-397.

Jain, V. K., S. Behari, D. Banerji, V. Bhargava and D. K. Chhabra. 1999. "Transoral decompression for craniovertebral osseous anomalies: perioperative management dilemmas." *Neurology India.* 47, no. 3 (September): 188-195.

Kataria, Rashim., K. V. Pawan and V. D. Sinha. 2018. "Increasing the safety of surgical treatment for complex Cranio-vertebral anomalies using customized 3D printed models." *Journal of Clinical Neuroscience.* 48, (February): 203-208.

Kataria, Rashim., M. Mehrotra, D. K. Purohit and N. Dharker. 2020. "Compressive myelopathy due to C2-C3 spondyloptosis as a consequence of absent C2 posterior elements: A rare case/review of literature." *Interdisciplinary Neurosurgery: Advanced Techniques and Case Management.* 24, no. 1 (December): 101069. https://doi.org/10.1016/j.inat.2020.101069.

Lang, J. 1986. "Craniocervical region, osteology and articulations." *Neuro- Orthopedics.* 1: 67-92.

Magklara, E. P., E. T. Pantelia, E. Solia, E. Panagouli, M. Piagkou, A. Mazarakis, P. Skandalakis, T. Troupis and D. Filippou. 2021. "Vertebral artery variations revised: origin, course, branches and embryonic development." *Folia Morphologica* (Warsz). 80, no. 1: 1-12.

Menezes, A. H., J. C. VanGilder, C. J. Graf and D. E. McDonnell. 1980. "Craniocervical abnormalities. A comprehensive surgical approach." *Journal of Neurosurgery* 53, no. 4 (October): 444-455.

Nordt, J. C. and E. S. Stauffer. 1981. "Sequelae of atlantoaxial stabilization in two patients with Down's syndrome." *Spine* (Philadelphia, Pa. 1976) 6, no.5 (September-October): 437-440.

Onishi, Eijiro., Y. Sekimoto, R. Fukumitsu, S. Yamagata and M. Matsushita. 2010. "Cerebral infarction due to an embolism after cervical pedicle screw fixation." *Spine* (Philadelphia Pa 1976). 35, no. 2 (January): E63–66.

Otsuki, Bungo., M. Takemoto, S. Fujibayashi, H. Kimura, K. Masamoto, and S. Matsuda. 2016. "Utility of a custom screw insertion guide and a full-scale, color- coded 3D plaster model for guidingsafe surgical exposure and screw insertion during spine revision surgery." *Journal of Neurosurgery: Spine.* 25, no. 1 (July): 94- 102.

Pacione, Donato., O. Tanweer, P. Berman, and D. H. Harter. 2016. "The utility of a multimaterial 3D printed model for surgical planning of complex deformity of the skull base and craniovertebral junction." *Journal of Neurosurgery.* 125, no. 5 (November):1194-1197.

Park, Jin Hoon., S. W. Roh and S. C. Rhim. 2015. "A single-stage posterior approach with open reduction and pedicle screw fixation in subaxial cervical facet dislocations." *Journal of Neurosurgery: Spine.* 23, no. 1 (April): 35-41.

Passias, P. G., S. Wang, M. Kozanek, S. Wang and C. Wang. 2013. "Relationship between the alignment of the occipitoaxial and subaxial cervical spine in patients with congenital atlantoxial dislocations." *Journal of Spinal Disorders and Techniques* 26, no. 1 (February): 15-21.

Salunke, Pravin., S. Behari, M. V. Kirankumar, M. S. Sharma, A. K. Jaiswal and V. K. Jain. 2006. "Pediatric congenital atlantoaxial dislocation: differences between the irreducible and reducible varieties." *Journal of Neurosurgery* 104, no. 2 (February): 115-122.

Sardhara, Jayesh., S. Behari, B. M. Mohan, A. K. Jaiswal, R. N. Sahu, A. Srivastava, A. Mehrotra and H. Lal. 2015. "Risk stratification of vertebral artery vulnerability during surgery for congenital atlanto-axial dislocation with or without an occipitalized atlas." *Neurology India.* 63, no. 3 (May-June): 382-391.

Sobolewski, Brad A., M. R. Mittiga and J. L. Reed. 2008. "Atlantoaxial rotary subluxation after minor trauma." *Pediatric Emergency Care* 24, no.12 (December): 852-856.

Sugimoto, Yoshihisa., M. Tanaka, R. Nakahara, H. Misawa, T. Kunisada, and T. Ozaki. 2012. "Surgical treatment for congenital kyphosis correction using both spinal navigation and a 3-dimensional model." *Acta Medica Okayama.* 66, no. 6: 499-502.

Tetreault, Lindsay., B. Kopjar, A. Nouri, P. Arnold, G. Barbagallo, R. Bartels, Z. Qiang, A. Singh, M. Zileli, A. Vaccaro, and M. G. Fehlings. 2017. "The modified Japanese Orthopaedic Association scale: establishing criteria for mild, moderate and severe impairment in patients with degenerative cervical myelopathy." *European Spine Journal.* 26, no. 1 (January): 78-84.

Ventola, C. L. 2014. "Medical applications for 3D printing: current and projected uses." *Pharmacy & Therapeutics.* 39, no. 10 (October) :704–711.

Wang, Chao., M. Yan, H. T. Zhou, S. Wang and G. Dang. 2006. "Open reduction of irreducible atlantoaxial dislocation by transoral anterior atlantoaxial release and posterior internal fixation." *Spine* (Philadelphia, Pa. 1976) 31, no. 11 (May): E306-313.

Wang, Chao., M. Yan, H. T. Zhou, S. Wang and G. Dang. 2007. “Atlantoaxial transarticular screw fixation with morselized autograft and without additional internal fixation: technical description and report of 57 cases.” *Spine* (Philadelphia, Pa. 1976) 32, no. 6 (March): 643-646.

Wang, Yi-Tian, X. J. Yang, B. Yan, T. H. Zeng, Y. Y. Qiu and S. J. Chen. 2016. “Clinical application of three-dimensional printing in the personalized treatment of complex spinal disorders.” *Chinese Journal of Traumatology*. 19, no. 1:31-34.

Weng, Chong., W. Tian, Z. Y. Li, B. Liu, Q. Li, Y. Q. Wang and Y. Z. Sun. 2012. “Surgical management of symptomatic os odontoideum with posterior screw fixation performed using the magerl and harms techniques with intraoperative 3- dimensional fluoroscopy-based navigation.” *Spine* (Philadelphia, Pa. 1976). 37, no. 21 (October): 1839–1846.

White III, A. A. and M. M. Panjabi. 1978. “The clinical biomechanics of the occipitoatlantoaxial complex.” *Orthopedic Clinics of North America* 9, no. 4 (October): 867-878.

Wilcox, Ben., R. J. Mobbs, A. M. Wu, and K. Phan. 2017. “Systematic review of 3D printing in spinal surgery: the current state of play.” *Journal of Spine Surgery*. 3, no. 3 (September): 433-443.

Wright, N. M. and C. Lauryssen. 1998. “Vertebral artery injury in C1-2 transarticular screw fixation: results of a survey of the AANS/CNS section on disorders of the spine and peripheral nerves. American Association of Neurological Surgeons/Congress of Neurological Surgeons.” *Journal of Neurosurgery*. 88, no. 4 (April): 634-640.

Yang, Minyi., N. Zhang, H. Shi, H. Li, S. Liu, Z. Song, L. Shan, Q. Wu, and D. Hao. 2018. “Three-dimensional printed model-assisted screw installation in treating posterior atlantoaxial internal fixation.” *Scientific Reports*. 8, no. 1 (July): 11026. https://doi.org/10.1038/s41598-018-29426-2.

Yang, Yong Liang., D. S. Zhou and J. L. He. 2013. “Comparison of isocentric C- arm 3-dimensional navigation and conventional fluoroscopy for C1 lateral mass and C2 pedicle screw placement for atlantoaxial instability.” *Journal of Spinal Disorders and Techniques*. 26, no. 3 (May): 127–134.

Yang, Yong Liang., D. S. Zhou and J. L. He. 2013. “Comparison of isocentric C- arm 3-dimensional navigation and conventional fluoroscopy for C1 lateral mass and C2 pedicle screw placement for atlantoaxial instability.” *Journal of Spinal Disorders and Techniques*. 26, no. 3 (May): 127–134.

Yang, Yongliang., F. Wang, S. Han, Y. Wang, J. Dong, L. Li and D. Zhou. 2015. “Isocentric C-arm three-dimensional navigation versus conventional C-arm assisted C1-C2 transarticular screw fixation for atlantoaxial instability.” *Archives of Orthopaedic and Trauma Surgery*. 135, no. 8 (August): 1083–1092.

Yin, Yi Heng., G. Y. Qiao, X. G. Yu, H. Y. Tong and Y. Z. Zhang. 2013. “Posterior realignment of irreducible atlantoaxial dislocation with C1-C2 screw and rod system: a technique of direct reduction and fixation.” *The Spine Journal* 13, no. 12 (December): 1864- 1871.

Yu, Xinguang., L. Li, P. Wang, Y. Yin, B. Bu and D. Zhou. 2014. "Intraoperative computed tomography with an integrated navigation system in stabilization surgery for complex craniovertebral junction malformation." *Journal of Spinal Disorders and Techniques.* 27, no. 5 (July): 245–252.

Zhang, Kai., J. Xu, Q. Wang, G. Wang, Z. H. Wu, H. Xia and Q. S. Yin. 2012. "Treatment of dens fractures with posterior atlantoaxial dislocation with transoral atlantoaxial reduction plate surgery: case report and introduction of a novel treatment option." *Spine* (Philadelphia, Pa. 1976) 37, no. 7 (April): E451-455.

Zhou, Yi-Jun., A. Yunus, Z. Tian, J. T. Chen, C. Wang, L. L. Xu and X. H. Song. 2016. "The pedicle screw-rod system is an acceptable method of reconstructive surgery after resection of sacroiliac joint tumours." *Contemporary oncology* (Poznan, Poland). 20, no. 1 (March):73-79.

Chapter 7

Current Concepts in the Management of Chiari Malformation

Orlin Pavlov, MD
Department of Neurosurgery, Klinikum Fulda, University Medicine Marburg, Hesse, Germany

Abstract

The treatment of patients with chiari malformation (CM) has to be tailored according to the accompanying pathology, restraining from absolutions. In the cases of atlantoaxial instability, combined with CM, stabilization should be pursued with or without decompression, as suggested by some authors. When no instability is observed, then a decompressive surgery should be the first choice. CM treatment remains a controversial topic, but some things have been already sorted out, including the unnecessity to perform a lysis of the adhesions. Interestingly, when CM is secondary due to lumbar-peritoneal shunt, ventriculoperitoneal should be initial step of treatment and decompression of the craniocervical junction. Regarding the clinical symptomatic, it is recommended to perform a surgical intervention in short period after the onset of symptoms. A surgical treatment is required only in the cases of symptoms or signs of CM, since the natural history of CM remains benign. The performance of an extensive suboccipital craniectomy and the far lateral opening of the foramen magnum does not offer more favourable clinical outcome compared to standard sized suboccipital craniectomy. However, with the better understanding of the biomechanical factors in the development of CM, a unified approach could be achieved in all patients.

In: Neurosurgery Research
Editors: Amit Agrawal, Pradeep Chouksey, Adesh Shrivastava et al.
ISBN: 978-1-68507-837-9

Introduction

For the purpose of better understanding the underlying pathological mechanism of Arnold-Chiari a brief summary of the pathophysiology, classification and clinical presentation will be reviewed. Arnold-Chiari, also known as Chiari malformation, is a group of entities which encompass the deformities of the posterior fossa and hindbrain. The pathoanatomical findings vary from cerebellar tonsillar herniation in foramen magnum to absence of cerebellum. These findings could be associated further with intracranial and extracranial defects, including hydrocephalus, spinal dysraphism, syrinx and encephalocele (de Arruda et al., 2018, Bhimani et al., 2018). The classification of Arnold-Chiari is based solely on the anatomic defects in imaging or post-mortem.

Table 1. Types of Arnold Chiari with pathoanatomical findings

Type	Pathoanatomical findings
Chiari 0	Syringomyelia without hindbrain herniation (Iskandar et al., 1998).
Chiari I	Projection of the cerebellar tonsils more than 5mm (some authors argue about this value- 3mm) below the line connection the basion and opisthion (McRae Line).
Chiari 1,5	Progression of Chiari I with further descend of cerebellar tonsils and involvement of brainstem.
Chiari II	Brainstem herniation and a towering cerebellum in addition to the herniated cerebellar tonsils and vermis due to an open distal spinal dysraphism/myelomeningocele (Hidalgo, Tork, and Varacallo 2021).
Chiari III	Herniation of hindbrain into low occipital or high cervical meningoencephalocele.
Chiari IV	Severe cerebellar hypoplasia, similar to primary cerebellar agenesis. Now it is considered to be obsolete. It was already a very controversial variant due to its rarity.
Chiari V	Cerebellar agenesis with occipital lobe descent and herniation through the foramen magnum. The most severe variant, not compatible with life (Tubbs et al., 2012).

The etiology has been a subject of interest for many decades now. Many theories were proposed, including molecular, hydrodynamic and mechanical.

Mutations of chromosome 1 and 22 have been identified to cause hereditary posterior fossa hypoplasia (Markunas et al., 2014). The open neural tube defect theory, proposed by McClone and Knepper (McLone and Knepper 1989) is gaining popularity since its publication. According to this theory a reduction of the liquor flow to the fourth ventricle occurs, which leads to a collapse of the fourth ventricle. This continued collapse of the fourth ventricle in utero results in a hypoplastic posterior fossa and cerebellar tonsillar herniation (Hidalgo, Tork, and Varacallo 2021). This theory could potentially explain also the finding in Chiari III, where the herniation of hindbrain occurs into low occipital or high cervical meningoencephalocele.

Goel et al., offer a new look in the etiology and development of Chiari malformation (CM). The authors present a new theory in regard to the atlantoaxial instability in form of "central" or "axial" atlantoaxial instability (CAAD) (Goel 2016). Morphometric assessments of the posterior cranial fossa have identified its reduced volume (Goel, Bhatjiwale, and Desai 1998). In 2013, the authors present their hypothesis that Chiari malformation is the nodal point of pathogenesis of Chiari formation (Goel 2015) and precipitates the formation of other associated finding such as basilar invagination and syringomyelia. In their series of patients, they reported that the majority of the patients with Chiari and syringomyelia actually have CAAD. Of course, this theory changes the surgical paradigm from decompression surgery (golden standard) to stabilization of the atlantoaxial segment. In the neurosurgical community, this went not unnoticed. Wagner et al., carried out a literature review and critical analysis about the origin of the Chiari malformation type I being a product of atlantoaxial instability (Wagner et al., 2020). The authors state, that up to this moment, there is insufficient evidence, supporting the theory of Goel et al., seeing the universal his approach with criticism. The atlantoaxial instability theory offers a unified approach towards this pathology and that is what makes it lucrative.

The neurological signs and symptoms in CM are developed on the basis of two pathological mechanisms: 1. direct compression of the neuronal structures to foramen magnum/spinal canal and 2. syringomyelia or syringobulbia. In the second mechanism, the obstruction of CSF outflow leads to the formation of syrinx. With the expansion of the syrinx cavity, the neurological symptoms will present. In CM type I, the most common clinical symptom is suboccipital/neck pain in more than 80% of the patients. When performing Valsalva maneuver, the symptoms aggravate. Among the other common symptoms of CM are: otoneurologic symptoms (mostly vertigo and dizziness), ocular disturbances and gait ataxia. The clinical presentation could be unspecific and numerous case reports regarding the clinical presentation of CM, illustrate symptoms, which were commonly found in CM, including shoulder pain, extremity pain and monoparesis. General fatigue and depression are also findings in CM, but in author's opinion, they would be secondary to the progression of the neurologic deficit (Urbizu et al., 2013). Myelopathy classically presents with "dissociated sensory loss" (loss of pain and temperature sensation, preserved fine touch and proprioception) and motor weakness (Rogers, Savage, and Stoodley 2018). Cerebellar signs, including ataxia, dysmetria, and nystagmus, and lower cranial nerve deficits (IX, X, XI, XII CN) could be observed in the patients with CM. They result either from direct compression of the cerebellum or medulla at the foramen magnum or from syringomyelia. With the compression of brainstem, upper spinal cord and lower cranial nerves, a weakness in the pharyngeal muscles could occur, resulting in sleep apnoea. It is important to note, that some of the patients does not have any symptoms from CM, thus the CM findings are incidental.

To Decompress, To Stabilize or Both?

Because of controversies in the treatment of CM, many possible surgical strategies were developed. Already Fernández et al., published their difficulties and succeeded to achieve a consensus among the specialists about the etiology, treatment strategies (surgical vs. conservative) and the period to follow-up the patients (Fernández et al., 2009). However, there is no consensus about the most accurate surgical approach to these patients. The missing consensus shows that our understanding of CM has not reached its highest point. As summary of the different operative approaches to CM are summarized in Table 2.

Due to the profile of our institution, cases of paediatric CM are not referred to us. Most of the patients are referred to our institution from the general practitioners with MRI of the CVJ. To complete the diagnostic, a head MRI is also needed to exclude hydrocephalus. Routine diagnostics such as X-Ray and functional X-ray are not performed. It is mandatory to indicate surgery only in the patients with symptomatic CM with radiological evidence of hindbrain abnormalities (Nash et al., 2002). When the symptoms are present, then surgery is indicated. The presence of symptoms and signs, such as sleep apnoea, scoliosis, cervical pain and headache are favourable for the prognosis after surgery. Procedure of choice is decompression of the cerebellomedullary junction (CMJ) through opening of the foramen magnum (suboccipital craniotomy) and removal of posterior arch of C1. Afterwards a dura opening is performed with resection of the caudal part of the tonsil with duroplasty. This approach has been validated by many clinical investigators, including Krieger et al., (Krieger, McComb, and Levy 1999), Sindou et al., (Sindou, Chávez-Machuca, and Hashish 2002), Valentini et al., (Valentini et al., 2011), Mottolese et al., (Mottolese et al., 2011), Parker et al., (Parker et al., 2011), etc. Most of the authors report an improvement of the symptoms in up to 95%–97% of the patients (Krieger, McComb, and Levy 1999). Persistent postoperative headache and nausea were present in 26% and 16% of the patients respectively. The size of the syrinx is reduced in most of the cases, but some are going to require shunting. Lysis of arachnoidal adhesion was one of most controversial topics in 2010, but it is becoming less popular since Yundt et al., postulated that in children younger than 2 years old, development of arachnoidal adhesion is extremely rare and thus the lysis does not alter the outcome after surgery (Yundt et al., 1996).

Table 2. Types of surgical procedures in CM

Decompression	Stabilization	Shunting
Suboccipital craniectomy	Atlantoaxial Stabilization	Syringosubarachnoid
Suboccipital craniectomy + cervical laminectomy	Atlantoaxial Stabilization + Suboccipital craniectomy	Ventriculoperitoneal
Suboccipital craniectomy + cervical laminectomy, durotomy + duroplasty	Atlantoaxial Stabilization + Suboccipital craniectomy + cervical laminectomy	
Suboccipital craniectomy + cervical laminectomy, durotomy + duroplasty+ cerebellar tonsils	Atlantoaxial Stabilization + Suboccipital craniectomy + cervical laminectomy, durotomy	
Suboccipital craniectomy + cervical laminectomy, durotomy + duroplasty+ cerebellar tonsils+ lysis of adhesions	Atlantoaxial Stabilization + Suboccipital craniectomy + cervical laminectomy, durotomy duroplasty+/- Resection of the cerebellar tonsils	
Decompression with or without shunt	Atlantoaxial Stabilization +Shunt?	

The amount of removed bone, in order to achieve decompression of CMJ, is yet another very controversial topic in the treatment of CM. Sindou et al., recommends a very extensive decompression, including suboccipital craniectomy with extreme lateral foramen magnum opening, accompanied by removal of posterior arch of C1 and sometimes C2. After the bony decompression, a Y-shaped opening of the dura is performed with duroplasty. The authors reported improvement of the neurological status in all patients with postoperative CSF leakage of 4, 5% and wound infection in 11, 5%. The syrinx improved in 60% of the patients and in 40% it was stable.

The duroplasty itself has been challenged by many authors, including Hankinson et al., (Hankinson, Tubbs, and Wellons 2011). The authors conducted a decompression of CMJ with and without expandable duroplasty. They concluded that suboccipital craniectomy plus removal of the posterior arch of C1 is sufficient for the treatment of patients with CM. However, due to the wide clinical and pathophysiological spectrum of CM, no precise recommendations could be made regarding the surgical approach. Genitori et al., published their results with CM. Only the symptomatic patients were treated and with the same surgical approach: bony decompression of posterior fossa through a suboccipital craniectomy along with removal of the posterior arch of C1 and removal of the outer layer of the dura without actual arachnoidal opening (Siasios, Kapsalaki, and Fountas 2012). The aim of this team was to show, that even with a simple extradural surgical approach, a good clinical outcome could be achieved. In their series, the improvement rate was 97, 2%, whereas syrinx-associated symptoms were resolved or improved in 94.4%. It has to be noted that through this approach, many postoperative complications can be avoided, including postoperative CSF leakage. Duroplasty, on the other hand has a lower rate of reoperation because of persistent compression of the brainstem (Durham and Fjeld-Olenec 2008).

In regards of the CM patients with deformity (scoliosis or kyphosis), Eule et al., published their interesting results in the paediatric population (Eule et al., 2002). 11 of 19 patients underwent a decompression of the CMJ and atlantoaxial stabilization. 8 of the patients did not undergo stabilization and only decompression was carried out. Of these 8 patients, 3 showed progression of the deformity, 1 remained stable and 4 had improvement of the deformity after the posterior fossa decompression. All these patients underwent a surgery before the age of 8 and before the scoliotic curve became severe.

The acquired form of CM requires also a surgical treatment. Payner et al., reported their case series of 10 children with lumbar-peritoneal shunts in whom previous radiographic studies had confirmed a normal hindbrain configuration (Payner et al., 1994, Siasios, Kapsalaki, and Fountas 2012). MRI scan detected *de novo* in 7 of 10 patients a herniation of the cerebellar tonsils and 4 out 7 patients were symptomatic. Two of the four patients underwent removal of the lumbar-peritoneal shunt and conversion into ventriculoperitoneal shunt and the other underwent decompression of the CMJ. Regression of the symptoms was observed immediately after the surgery and all patients became asymptomatic 6 months after the surgery. The authors conclude that lumbar-peritoneal shunts create a negative craniospinal pressure gradient and thus herniation of the cerebellar tonsils. The authors recommend the usage of ventriculoperitoneal shunt in the paediatric population, in order to reduce the risk for complications. Also, they recommend an annual MRI scan of the CMJ in the patients with lumbar-peritoneal shunts. Finally, if a symptomatic tonsillar herniation does occur in patients with lumbar-peritoneal shunts, they recommend the conversion into ventriculoperitoneal shunt before decompression of the CMJ (Payner et al., 1994).

In 2015, Goel et al., presented his novel research in the field of CM, making the hypothesis that CM is secondary to atlantoaxial instability. His unorthodox approach to the topic has brought new understanding of this pathology. He examined 65 patients with CM, where patients with brain and spinal malformations, hydrocephalus, tumour, infection and connective tissue disorder were excluded. All patients had a symptomatic CM. The selected patients underwent atlantoaxial stabilization fortified by plate and screw fixation and clinical and radiological reassessment was obtained 3 months after surgery. CT scan showed a solid bony fusion after the stabilization. The evaluation of syrinx was not possible in all patients, because titanium implants were available after June 2013. Regarding the neurological improvement, 63 out 65 patients showed immediate postoperative improvement and it is sustained at 3 months follow up. One patient had a persistent neuropathic pain after surgery. In the cases with basilar invagination with radiological evidence of instability, including facet distraction and craniovertebral, atlantoaxial, instrumentation of the C1/C2 segment should be the treatment of choice. The authors also raise the question, which is first- the basilar invagination, CM or atlantoaxial instability or are they merely the same -atlantoaxial instability but in different stages, which could coexist all together.

Conclusion

The surgical approach to the patients with CM has to be tailored according to the specific pathology, restraining from absolutions. In the cases of atlantoaxial instability and CM, stabilization should be pursued with or without decompression. When no instability is observed, then a decompressive surgery should be the first choice of treatment. CM remains a controversial topic, but some things have been already sorted out: 1. No lysis of adhesions is required. 2. Despite the presence of duroplasty or not, the authors report similar results in improvement of the neurologic deficit. 3. In the presence of secondary CM due to lumbar-peritoneal shunt, ventriculoperitoneal should be initial step of treatment. 4. In the paediatric population- a shorter duration of the symptoms leads to better clinical outcome. 5. Patients with CM and syringomyelia require posterior fossa decompressive surgery. 6. The surgical treatment is required only in the cases of symptoms or signs of CM, since the natural history of CM remains benign. 7. The performance of an extensive suboccipital craniectomy and the far lateral opening of the foramen magnum does not offer more favourable clinical outcome compared to standard sized suboccipital craniectomy.

References

Bhimani, A. D., D. R. Esfahani, S. Denyer, R. G. Chiu, D. Rosenberg, A. L. Barks, G. D. Arnone, and A. I. Mehta. 2018. "Adult Chiari I Malformations: An Analysis of Surgical Risk Factors and Complications Using an International Database." *World Neurosurg.* 115:e490-e500. doi: 10.1016/j.wneu.2018.04.077.

de Arruda, José-Alcides, Eugênia Figueiredo, João-Luiz Monteiro, Livia-Mirelle Barbosa, Cleomar Rodrigues, and Belmiro Vasconcelos. 2018. "Orofacial clinical features in Arnold Chiari type I malformation: A case series." *Journal of clinical and experimental dentistry* 10 (4):e378-e382. doi: 10.4317/jced.54419.

Durham, S. R., and K. Fjeld-Olenec. 2008. "Comparison of posterior fossa decompression with and without duraplasty for the surgical treatment of Chiari malformation Type I in pediatric patients: a meta-analysis." *J. Neurosurg. Pediatr.* 2 (1):42-9. doi: 10.3171/ped/2008/2/7/042.

Eule, J. M., M. A. Erickson, M. F. O'Brien, and M. Handler. 2002. "Chiari I malformation associated with syringomyelia and scoliosis: a twenty-year review of surgical and nonsurgical treatment in a pediatric population." *Spine (Phila Pa 1976)* 27 (13):1451-5. doi: 10.1097/00007632-200207010-00015.

Fernández, A. A., A. I. Guerrero, M. I. Martínez, M. E. Vázquez, J. B. Fernández, E. Chesa i Octavio, L. Labrado Jde, M. E. Silva, M. F. de Araoz, R. García-Ramos, M. G. Ribes, C. Gómez, J. I. Valdivia, R. N. Valbuena, and J. R. Ramón. 2009. "Malformations of the craniocervical junction (Chiari type I and syringomyelia: classification, diagnosis and treatment)." *BMC Musculoskelet. Disord.* 10 Suppl 1 (Suppl 1):S1. doi: 10.1186/1471-2474-10-s1-s1.

Goel, A. 2015. "Is atlantoaxial instability the cause of Chiari malformation? Outcome analysis of 65 patients treated by atlantoaxial fixation." *J. Neurosurg. Spine* 22 (2):116-27. doi: 10.3171/2014.10.spine14176.

Goel, A. 2016. "Central or axial atlantoaxial instability: Expanding understanding of craniovertebral junction." *J. Craniovertebr. Junction Spine* 7 (1):1-3. doi: 10.4103/0974-8237.176602.

Goel, A., M. Bhatjiwale, and K. Desai. 1998. "Basilar invagination: a study based on 190 surgically treated patients." *J. Neurosurg.* 88 (6):962-8. doi: 10.3171/jns.1998.88.6.0962.

Hankinson, T., R. S. Tubbs, and J. C. Wellons. 2011. "Duraplasty or not? An evidence-based review of the pediatric Chiari I malformation." *Childs Nerv. Syst.* 27 (1):35-40. doi: 10.1007/s00381-010-1295-7.

Hidalgo, J. A., C. A. Tork, and M. Varacallo. 2021. "Arnold Chiari Malformation." In *StatPearls*. Treasure Island (FL): StatPearls Publishing Copyright © 2021, StatPearls Publishing LLC.

Iskandar, B. J., G. L. Hedlund, P. A. Grabb, and W. J. Oakes. 1998. "The resolution of syringohydromyelia without hindbrain herniation after posterior fossa decompression." *J. Neurosurg.* 89 (2):212-6. doi: 10.3171/jns.1998.89.2.0212.

Krieger, Mark D, J Gordon McComb, and Michael L Levy. 1999. "Toward a simpler surgical management of Chiari I malformation in a pediatric population." *Pediatric neurosurgery* 30 (3):113-121.

Markunas, Christina A., David S. Enterline, Kaitlyn Dunlap, Karen Soldano, Heidi Cope, Jeffrey Stajich, Gerald Grant, Herbert Fuchs, Simon G. Gregory, and Allison E. Ashley-Koch. 2014. "Genetic evaluation and application of posterior cranial fossa traits as endophenotypes for Chiari type I malformation." *Annals of human genetics* 78 (1):1-12. doi: 10.1111/ahg.12041.

McLone, D. G., and P. A. Knepper. 1989. "The cause of Chiari II malformation: a unified theory." *Pediatr. Neurosci.* 15 (1):1-12. doi: 10.1159/000120432.

Mottolese, C., A. Szathmari, E. Simon, C. Rousselle, A. C. Ricci-Franchi, and M. Hermier. 2011. "Treatment of Chiari type I malformation in children: the experience of Lyon." *Neurol. Sci.* 32 Suppl 3:S325-30. doi: 10.1007/s10072-011-0685-2.

Nash, J., J. S. Cheng, G. A. Meyer, and B. F. Remler. 2002. "Chiari type I malformation: overview of diagnosis and treatment." *Wmj* 101 (8):35-40.

Parker, S. R., P. Harris, T. J. Cummings, T. George, H. Fuchs, and G. Grant. 2011. "Complications following decompression of Chiari malformation Type I in children: dural graft or sealant?" *J. Neurosurg. Pediatr.* 8 (2):177-83. doi: 10.3171/2011.5.peds10362.

Payner, T. D., E. Prenger, T. S. Berger, and K. R. Crone. 1994. "Acquired Chiari malformations: incidence, diagnosis, and management." *Neurosurgery* 34 (3):429-34; discussion 434. doi: 10.1227/00006123-199403000-00007.

Rogers, J. M., G. Savage, and M. A. Stoodley. 2018. "A Systematic Review of Cognition in Chiari I Malformation." *Neuropsychol. Rev.* 28 (2):176-187. doi: 10.1007/s11065-018-9368-6.

Siasios, John, Eftychia Z. Kapsalaki, and Kostas N. Fountas. 2012. “Surgical management of patients with Chiari I malformation.” *International journal of pediatrics* 2012:640127-640127. doi: 10.1155/2012/640127.

Sindou, M., J. Chávez-Machuca, and H. Hashish. 2002. “Cranio-cervical decompression for Chiari type I-malformation, adding extreme lateral foramen magnum opening and expansile duroplasty with arachnoid preservation. Technique and long-term functional results in 44 consecutive adult cases–comparison with literature data.” *Acta neurochirurgica* 144 (10):1005-1019.

Tubbs, R. S., M. Muhleman, M. Loukas, and W. J. Oakes. 2012. “A new form of herniation: the Chiari V malformation.” *Childs Nerv. Syst.* 28 (2):305-7. doi: 10.1007/s00381-011-1616-5.

Urbizu, Aintzane, Claudio Toma, Maria A. Poca, Juan Sahuquillo, Ester Cuenca-León, Bru Cormand, and Alfons Macaya. 2013. “Chiari malformation type I: a case-control association study of 58 developmental genes.” *PloS one* 8 (2):e57241-e57241. doi: 10.1371/journal.pone.0057241.

Valentini, L., S. Visintini, V. Saletti, L. Chiapparini, M. Estienne, and C. L. Solero. 2011. “Treatment for Chiari 1 malformation (CIM): analysis of a pediatric surgical series.” *Neurol. Sci.* 32 Suppl 3:S321-4. doi: 10.1007/s10072-011-0731-0.

Wagner, Arthur, Lukas Grassner, Nikolaus Kögl, Sebastian Hartmann, Claudius Thomé, Maria Wostrack, and Bernhard Meyer. 2020. “Chiari malformation type I and basilar invagination originating from atlantoaxial instability: a literature review and critical analysis.” *Acta Neurochirurgica* 162 (7):1553-1563. doi: 10.1007/s00701-020-04429-z.

Yundt, Kent D, T. S. Park, Vrijesh S. Tantuwaya, and Bruce A. Kaufman. 1996. “Posterior fossa decompression without duraplasty in infants and young children for treatment of Chiari malformation and achondroplasia.” *Pediatric neurosurgery* 25 (5):221-226.

Chapter 8

Advances in Anterior Approaches to Cervical Disc Diseases

Krishan K. Yadav and MS Sridhar
Professors of Neurosurgery, Command Hospital Air Force Bangalore, Karnataka, India

Abstract

Cervical disc disease affects over 50-60% of middle aged and elderly population. From the ancient times, when people with cervical spine disorders were left alone with no treatment options to the present era when the latest state of art surgical interventions are being carried out, the management of these disorders has come a long way.

Most patients with cervical disc disease are asymptomatic and can be managed conservatively. However, a small but significant group of people are affected with features of myelo-radiculopathy or instability. This in turn leads to a significant load of morbidity in society and intervention is needed to manage them. Anterior approach which was first attempted in the mid-fifties has now become the dominant approach to deal with these conditions since most of the etiological factors causing them are anterior to the spinal cord.

Anterior cervical discectomy and fusion, over the years, has become the gold standard in the management in cervical disc diseases. However, as the time progressed, allograft and xenograft came up. They gained popularity as an extra surgery and morbidity in form of bone harvesting was not required. These were soon to be followed by artificial osteogenetic materials. The next advancement came up in form of artificial spacers which were made initially of titanium and subsequently polymers in various shapes and sizes. As the time passed, it was noted that a significant number of people had degeneration in the adjacent areas

In: Neurosurgery Research
Editors: Amit Agrawal, Pradeep Chouksey, Adesh Shrivastava et al.
ISBN: 978-1-68507-837-9

and some movement restrictions led to the next advance that was meant to preserve motion at the disc. So, the artificial cervical discs came up over the last few decades. These artificial discs have further evolved with newer combination of newer materials such as cobalt-chrome as well as more biocompatible polymers. Finally, the most recent entrant among these anterior advances is the percutaneous endoscopic cervical discectomy but it is still under the process of refinement.

All these advances to the cervical disc disease from anterior approach have not only made the management easier but the results have gradually improved, the complications have reduced, the fusion and decompression are optimal.

Keywords: anterior approach, cervical disc disease, anterior cervical discectomy, bone grafts, spacers, artificial discs and endoscopic discectomy

Introduction

Among various conditions affecting the cervical spine, the cervical disc diseases are a fairly common group of conditions seen across the world. It is seen in 50-60% of the middle-aged and elderly population with no significant sex preponderance [1].

Though the incidence of cervical spondylosis is fairly high, most of them remain asymptomatic. The pathological changes of spondylosis are considered to be a combination of protrusion of nucleus pulposus, associated fibrosis and osteophyte formation. Patients are symptomatic only if there is significant tension in the adjacent ligaments or compressive effects of the neural structures. Radiologically the symptomatic patients would have severe changes such as significantly severe osteophytes, narrowed disc spaces, vertebral plate narrowing and degenerative subluxation. Also, these pathological changes are noted to be commonest at the C5/6, C6/7 and C4/5 respectively

Plain radiographs will show evidence of disc degeneration process but magnetic resonance imaging (MRI) is modality of choice for diagnosis. Management in majority of cases of cervical disc disorders is conservative but a small yet significant number with clinical features of myelo-radiculopathy need intervention. Anterior route is preferred for intervention nowadays.

The anterior approach to cervical disc diseases remains the bulwark for management of cervical disc diseases with features of compression. Anterior cervical discectomy and fusion has been the most common and widely accepted form of management in these conditions. Bone grafts harvested from the patients iliac bone and fixation or stabilisation with plates and screws is part of the above surgical procedure. However, in last 3-4 decades numerous advances in form of spacers of titanium or polyetheretherketone, artificial cervical discs and most recently endoscopic management are becoming more and more acceptable which in turn has led to making anterior approach as the preferred approach in dealing with these conditions.

This chapter present an overview of cervical disc diseases, clinico-radiological features and review the literature on their management with special emphasis on the newer advances with special emphasis on the anterior approaches.

Historical Evolution

Although the ancient Egyptians mentioned it with case discussions in Edwin Smith papyrus related to spinal injuries [2], it was Hippocrates (460-370 BC) who was first to correlate injury to vertebra leading to limb paralysis and also the fact that it is always on the side of injured vertebrae. The detailed study of spinal anatomy, disorders and management techniques is phenomenal. Hence most medical historians credit him as the "father of spine surgery" [3].

Aulus Cornelius Celsus noted in first century AD that death may follow spinal cord injury due to trauma over cervical regions. Galen (129-210AD) observed damages of varied nature, ranging from loss of power to sensations and sparing of certain components by making incisions over the spinal cord from first cervical segment onwards. Later Paulus of Aegineta (625-690) created spine surgery instruments and wrote seven books on spinal surgery. Avicenna (980-1037) described with illustrations the cervical spine and wrote about the management of its disorders. Vesalius first described an intervertebral disc in 1543 in his work known as "De humani Corporis Fabrica" with a plate depicting the spinal column and intervertebral discs [4, 5].

Initially cervical lesions were managed by posterior approaches. Elsberg in 1925, Stookey in 1928, Semmes and Murphy in 1943, Spurling and Segerberg in 1953 described the posterior approach trying to fix various cervical pathologies [5, 6].

It was Robinson and Smith in 1955 that popularised the anterior approach with anterior disc removal and fusion using the autologous grafts [7]. The risks involved in posterior approaches along with the technical advances in form of micro instruments, microscopes, etc. helped in this evolution. Cloward soon thereafter modified the technique and introduced instrumentation for interbody fusion using autologous grafts [8]. Hirsch in 1960 introduced anterior cervical discectomy without fusion [9].

Epidemiology

An important study by Okada et al. carried out from 1995-2007 revealed progression of degeneration with aging being the only consistent factor responsible. Sex, smoking, weight, sports, alcohol and body mass index were not found to be of much significance. Also 34.1% people developed symptoms during this period [10].

Teraguchi et al. in 2014, carried out an epidemiological study on intervertebral disc degeneration in Japan in population over 40 years using MRI of spine as a measurement technique and found that the prevalence to be 51.5% at C5/6, 43.5% at C6/7and 38.6% at C4/5 in men. In women it was 46%, 33.3% and 35.8% respectively [11].

Another study by Matsumoto et al. of 497 asymptomatic patients revealed that almost 90% people over 60 years, irrespective of sex, with abnormal findings on MRI studies [12].

Another study by Saifi et al. quoting the national inpatient database from USA for the period of 2006-2013, sites a figure of 1,27,00 cases of anterior cervical discectomy with fusion (ACDF) and 1,565 cases of complete disc arthroplasty for the year 2013, being carried out every year making it as one of the commonest of the spinal surgeries [13].

Anatomical Aspects

The human spine has 33 vertebrae. Of these, cervical spine is made of the upper 07 vertebrae. The cervical spine has typical (C3-C6) and atypical vertebrae (C1, C2, and C7). The cervical discs start at C2-C3 up to C7-D1 level. Cervical discs along with vertebral body and arch form the cervical canal that encloses the spinal cord. The typical intervertebral disc includes an inner nucleus pulposus and an outer annulus fibrosus. The outermost end plates anchor these discs to the adjacent vertebrae. These are considered to be important as they help in aid of cervical spine mobility as well as stabilisation.

Cervical disc disease includes a group of conditions ranging from herniated nucleus pulposus (HNP) to internal disc disruption (IDD) to degenerative disc disease (DDD), DDD primarily include degenerative annulus tears and nuclear degradations. IDD leads to annulus fissures but no external disc deformations. HNP or disc herniations indicate external movement of the disc material usually causing compromise of the cervical canal, cord or roots [14]. While the former two are primarily responsible for the pain and stiffness in the axial skeleton the herniated discs most commonly present with radiculopathy or myelopathy which in turn are responsible for radicular pains, paraesthesias and motor or even sphincter deficits.

Indications for Anterior Approach

Although traditionally the posterior approaches were more commonly used but with passage of time and better understanding of the anatomy as well as the disease process, the anterior approaches have gained wider acceptance across the scientific community.

The important indications for using the anterior approaches are primarily when there is anterior compression from prolapsed intervertebral discs (PIVDs) leading to compressive myelopathy or myelo-radiculopathy without any significant posterior disease, when the disease is associated with ossified posterior longitudinal ligament (OPLL) and if the disease process is primarily anterior such as subluxation or kyphosis of degenerative nature or infections with epidural abscesses. Relative indications that may be considered include failure of posterior surgeries such as inadequate decompression, development of kyphosis and instability. The contraindications would include anatomical considerations, active local infections and posterior pathologies such as malignancies, pott's spine, facetal dislocation, etc. [15, 16, 17].

The success of anterior approach comes from the fact that the surgical procedure is simpler, with lesser complication rates, better decompression, fusion and stabilisation at the same time with all these leading to a better clinical and radiological outcome in the long run.

Technical Aspects of Anterior Approach

Some important anatomical aspects need to be understood, whether it is the standard technical aspects or it involves the newer advances. First thing to note is existence of fascial layers anteriorly, namely superficial layer or the investing layers of deep fascia, pretracheal layer and the prevertebral layers. The fascias delineate the various planes for the surgical procedures. The next important aspect is to remember certain important anatomical marks such as the thyroid and cricoid cartilage, hyoid bone, carotid tubercles, sympathetic ganglions, recurrent laryngeal nerve, sternocleidomastoid, omohyoids, inferior thyroid artery and carotid artery. These structures are helpful during the surgery and also to avoid complications leading to a safer surgery.

The salient steps of anterior cervical discectomy with fusion (ACDF) include the following. Patient is positioned supine and neck kept in extension. We prefer a transverse incision, usually on the right side, at the level of the planned discectomy. Next fine dissection is done going along deep fascia, platysma to pretracheal fascia. Next sternocleidomastoid and carotids are laterally retracted whereas trachea, oesophagus and thyroid are medially retracted and proceed so as to reach prevertebral fascia. This is divided in midline and the anterior aspect of the spine is thus exposed. Next we elevate the longus colli and bilaterally apply the Casper retractors after site confirmation.

Next we make an incision on the disc and then gradually carry out the discectomy. It is gradually done until the posterior longitudinal ligaments as well as sequestered disc are removed. Next we expose the iliac bone and harvest a bone graft which is snugly placed in disc space after adequate distraction. It is prudent to place a titanium plate anteriorly and screwed a level above and below to ensure that the graft piece is not displaced. All procedures should preferably be done under radiological guidance. After a good haemostasis, closure should be done in multiple layers.

The role of plating has its own controversies. It provides a rigid fixation, promotes a better rate of fusion, prevents extrusion of the graft and prevents development of segmental kyphosis. However, the increased cost factors and implant related issues are rare but possible.

Complications

Cunha et al. in 2014 analysed their series and noted 18% of patients having had complications, the commonest ones being dysphonia followed by dysphagia [18].

Tasiou et al. in 2017 published their study of complications in 114 patients over a period of five years. Their overall complication rate was 13.2%.

Commonest ones in descending order being adjacent intervertebral disc degeneration, dysphagia, post operative hematomas, dural injuries, oesophageal perforation and operative site superficial infections [19].

Epstein et al. in 2019 published their study based on multiple studies where they concluded that the overall complications rates of ACDF ranging from 13.2 to 19.3%. The important ones included dysphagia, post-operative hematomas, exacerbation of myelopathy, adjacent disc degeneration, recurrent laryngeal nerve palsy, cerebrospinal fluid (CSF) leaks, local wound infections, increased radiculopathy, Horner's syndrome, respiratory insufficiency, oesophageal perforation and lastly instrument failure. Rare complications included aseptic spondylodiscitis, meningitis, epidural abscess and new nerve root lesions. Pseudoarthrosis was seen to depend upon the total number of fusion levels (up to 4.3% in I level, 24% in 2 levels, 42% in 3 levels and up to 56% in IV levels fusion). Re-do surgeries were required in up to 11.1% of cases, especially those with pseudoarthrosis. Mortality was noted to be at 0.1% [20].

Newer Advances in Anterior Approaches

Anterior cervical discectomy and fusion (ACDF) is presently considered as the "gold standard" in the management of cervical disc diseases [21]. However, in the recent years, as the time progressed, advances have crept into this field. These in turn have been mostly propelled due to either certain complications such as the widely noted adjacent level disease next to the fused cervical segments leading to newer motion preserving techniques (complete disc replacements or arthroplasty) or avoidance of another site surgery for harvesting of grafts (titanium or other material cervical cages with or without prefilled bone particles). There has also been a gradual progress towards minimal invasive techniques in form of endoscopic discectomy and fusion in recent times as has been a trend in all medical fields worldwide.

The following important trends or advances in anterior approaches can be considered:

1. Use of allograft and bone morphogenic proteins
2. Interbody cages and spacers for cervical fusion
3. Total disc replacement (Cervical disc arthroplasty)
4. Percutaneous cervical endoscopic discectomy
5. Imaging & 3-D navigation system development

Allograft or Allogenic Bone Grafts

Allografts are the bone grafts obtained from living or cadaveric donors. They are commonly harvested from femoral, ilium, tibia, fibula, etc. These are then processed for sterility and storage by various processes such as freeze drying. Xenografts are a variant in which case the bone grafts are obtained from another species.

Although the autologous bone grafts have been the gold standard till now, allograft and the synthetic material grafts are slowly replacing them as their fusion rates are comparable to the autologous [22, 23]. They are available in various forms ranging from to morselised chips to struts or even large blocks. They can be available as bicortical, cortico-cancellous or only cancellous as per the requirements. They are preferred due to avoidance of additional morbidity, easy availability and capability to facilitate bone formation. Addition of bone stimulating factors for them to give desired results and fear of transmission of infections are certain limitations.

Demineralized bone matrix (DBM) is another allograft derived product which has collagen, proteins, calcium phosphates and growth stimulating factors. They have good osteoconductive and osteoinductive properties and available as powder, gel, granules, etc. However, since they do not a posses a good structural property, they are mostly used as graft extenders in combination with autologous or allogenic grafts [22, 24].

Cellular bone matrices (CBM) or viable cellular allograft are a new emerging variant that overcome many of the issues related to allogenic grafts. Fridenstein in 1966 had first identified the mesenchymal cells from the bone marrow, which are a type of stem cells that differentiate into chondroblasts and osteoblasts [26]. These materials has osteoconductive, osteoinductive and osteogenetic properties as they retain the mesenchymal cells during their preparation process. They have a good osteogenetic potential, are derived from the cadaveric donors and available as sponge or granules. However, they are yet to get clearance for human trials and regulatory authorities before they reach surgical practice. However, they do hold a lot of promise [22, 25].

Interbody Cages and Spacers

Interbody cages and spacers can owe their origin to Bagby, who in 1988 proposed a bagby bone basket, initially designed for horse spines and subsequently adapted to human lumbar spines that would allow the growth of bone inside a spacer made of stainless steel [28]. By next decade, the interbody cages and spacers were introduced in the cervical spine surgeries.

The common design in them all was a hollow implant, of various materials, in various shapes and sizes. They could be filled with autologous bone pieces on the table or came prefilled with allograft bone or newer osteoinductive materials. Further these were threaded or non-threaded. Over the years, standalone designs have become the mainstay method for single level ACDF with excellent long-term results.

Role of anterior plating: It has been noted that the rates of fusion are excellent in cases of single level ACDF using standalone designs or spacers. However, the rates of fusion are very poor with high rates of arthrodesis when multiple level of ACDF with non-union rates, going up to as high as 40%. However, addition of anterior plating leads to a solid stabilisation and therefore an excellent fusion along with lower subsidence rates and maintained disc height in multilevel discectomy. Its limitations include dysphagia and rare screw migrations [27, 30].

Cage design evolution: Here the basic concept is a hollow implant which were threaded (screws) or non-threaded (box or vertical ring shapes) with option of anterior plating. The earliest one to be introduced were made of titanium alloy, cylinder shaped cages that were filled on table with autologous bone. The issues noted soon thereafter were related to the cage subsidence, decreased maximum distractive height and inadequate stability in neck movements.

These were soon followed by box shaped designs with contact surfaces roughened for better stability as well as fusion. These were soon modified into wedge or trapezoid shapes for improved stability during the neck movements [29, 31]. Another variant, popularly known as the wing cages had a cylindrical centre with lateral flat wings on both. It showed a good contact but due to poor stability slowly went out of favor.

Biomechanics related to sizes: The intervertebral discs in the cervical spine are about one third the size of the vertebral bodies. Also, posterior disc height is least and maximal in the midline. This in turn is responsible for maintenance of the cervical lordosis. Also, the disc height as well as the lateral width increases as we go inferiorly from C2/C3 to C6/C7. The cages work by relieving neural compression as they restore the disc height and the canal diameter. However excessive distraction can lead to poor clinical outcomes in form of persistent neck pain, paraesthesias and poor union or fusion in future. So, most modern cages or implants are designed in such a way that they go to a maximum of 2-3 mm beyond the baseline heights or width. So, most of them are 5-8 mm in disc heights, 12-16 mm in depth and 12-20 mm. So, an ideal cage should be stable, restore adequate height and alignment with minimal complications and provide good fusion [31, 32, 33].

Cage material evolution: Three materials have found a role primarily in making of the cervical cage and implants. They include carbon fiber reinforced polymers (CF-P), titanium (Ti) with its alloys and polyetheretherketone (PEEK). Titanium was initially used with enough of experience from the orthopedic implants as they are non-corrosive, low density and allows good osteointegration. However, the mid-1990s saw emergence of the alternative CF-P initially and PEEK cages or implants subsequently. They were noted to be radiolucent with elasticity similar to the bone and therefore led to lower stress as well as less subsistence as compared to titanium [34, 35]. However, as of today, there are supporters of both and ideal cage material remains a matter of controversy.

In recent times, there is has been advances in terms of the cage materials and combinations. Recent advances include composite Ti/PEEK cages where the PEEK spacer with ridged titanium endplates. The titanium has better bioactivity whereas PEEK scores in terms of translucency and elasticity. Another advance is streamlining of anterior plate with standalone cages with a zero-profile cage and integrated low-profile plate to reduce the local complications. Variations includes PEEK spacer with anterior plates and internal screws treads or PEEK spacer with self-locking guided plate system. Further, newer advance soon to become common in clinical practice includes absorbable designs that utilizes polylactic acid, polyflycolic acid copolymers which have initial rigidity and gradually degrade to form a good arthrodesis with complete absorption in post-operative period radiologically [36]. So, cage design optimization is expected to lead to an ideal design.

Total Disc Replacement (Cervical Disc Arthroplasty)

It was Fernstom who first tried to implant a ball bearing made of stainless steel. He, from 1966 onwards, went on to implant a total of 191 lumbar and 13 cervical such implants before finally abandoning it due to unacceptable complications [37].

However, the initial enthusiasm soon died down and remained so over the next few decades as ACDF gained popularity, being well described and with results noted to be more favorable and predictable. It was only towards 1990s, that the idea of motion preserving implants re-surfaced in late 90s since the cases with adjacent segmental degeneration (ASD) [38, 39] were noted with increasing frequency and considered as among the commonest of complications of ACDF. As we know, the adjacent segment degeneration is almost seen in 20-30% of cases. Zhu et al. did a meta-analysis on comparing ACDF with CDR and noted a very significant reduction of this common complication [40]. The second important benefit is reduced heterotrophic calcification and preservation of complete range of motions. However, it being a newer technology, its long term effects in term of safety, indications and complications needs to be further assessed.

Biomechanics of ADR: As the name implies, the hallmark of this method of treatment is its ability to preserve motion and provide stability, without associated complications of ACDF. These prostheses are commonly divided as unconstrained and semi-constrained based on their degree of allowed motions. The designs and the materials include metal on metal, metal on polymer, ceramic on ceramic, ceramic on polymer and polymer composite designs. The designs need to be as close as possible to the normal intervertebral discs. While creating these artificial discs, the kinematics, material properties, stiffness, durability and finally compatibility to the imaging modalities need to be considered. The kinematics are very important as our aim is to be closest to the natural intervertebral disc alongwith adequate range of motions (ROM). The important biomechanical parameters that need to be measured must include the operative site ROM, adjacent segment ROM, intra-discal pressures, loading over the facets, postural changes to the spine and the patterns of coupling to achieve a situation where the spinal segment which has undergone instrumentation is behaving like a normal natural segment [41, 42].

Artificial disc replacement (ADR) started to gain popularity soon thereafter and today it is one of the important treatment modalities in cases of cervical disc diseases. The damaged badly degenerated disc is replaced by an artificial disc implant and is an effective alternative to ACDF. Over the years, a number of RCTs and other studies have shown an advantage with ADR as compared to ACDF.

The Cummins-Bristol device, a stainless steel, metal on metal, ball n socket joint was introduced in 1991 [43]. It was used in almost 18 cases with few of them having hardware related complications and almost all of them had dysphagia. It was then taken over by Medtronic who revised it based on biomechanics to create a titanium disc with 5-degree freedom, ball in trough configuration and renamed it as Prestige disc which continues to have a following till this day. The next to follow and which actually revolutionized this field was Bryan's disc created by Vince Bryan. This disc made of biconvex polyurethane core and titanium endplate shells. It had a complex system of implantation and had adequate ROM [44].

There are a number of devices presently in the market, with all major companies making their own devices, most of the newer ones having inferior ball in superior socket devices.

Currently some of the popular artificial discs available are Prestige and Bryan's disc by Medtronic, Prodisc-C by Synthes, Mobi-C by Zimmer, CerviCore by Stryker and Secure-C by Globus. Almost all of them have similar safety, durability and complications [42, 45]. Most newer devices have inner articular surfaces made of polymers such as ultrahigh molecular weight polyethylene (UHMWPE) along with outer sockets made of stainless steel, titanium (Ti) and cobalt-chromium-molybdenum (CCM) sockets that are sprayed with titanium plasma coating (Table 1).

The common indications being single and occasionally double level cervical disc disease. The main contraindications are significant facetal degeneration. Commonest complications noted being hardware failure and artificial disc retropulsion into the spinal canal. The aim in future is to have discs which are closest to the natural ones in terms of biomechanics, able to and maintain alignment, easy to implant and facilitate imaging for follow up cases. The aim is to provide equivalence to ACDF or maybe go beyond so as to become the gold standard in future.

Table 1. Popular cervical arthroplasty devices available

Device Name	Type/ Classification	Material Used	Manufacturer
Bryans Disc	Unconstrained	Titanium shell with Polyurethane nucleus	Medtronic Inc
Prestige LP disc	Unconstrained	Titanium-ceramic composite	Medtronic Inc
ProDisc-C	Semi constrained	CCM endplate with UHMWPE inlay	Depuy-Synthes
CerviCore	Semi constrained	CCM metal on metal	Stryker Spine
Secure-C	Semi constrained	CCM endplate with UHMWPE inlay	Globus Medical
PCM	Semi constrained	CCM endplate with UHMWPE inlay	NuVasive Inc

Technical aspects of CDR: Before deciding for the CDR, it is advisable to discuss the technique as well as cost factors and possible complications with the patient and his family. A CT scan or good quality digital radiographs pre-operatively are helpful. The patient is kept supine with neck in extension. Anterior cervical discectomy is next carried out as per the standard techniques. The posterior longitudinal ligament is cut so as to achieve a good cervical decompression. The end plates are now roughened up. The artificial discs are next placed snugly in the prepared disc space under C-arm guidance, the technical aspects of each variant being different. The neck should be brought to the neutral position while placing the artificial disc. Haemostasis and closure are finally carried out as per the standard protocol once again. Post-operative antibiotics, analgesics and Philadelphia collar usage are all hospital or surgeon specific.

Cervical Endoscopic Discectomy

Endoscopy has revolutionized the modern surgical approaches. Now, it is gaining ground in the field of neurosurgery with the latest entrant being spinal endoscopies. Cervical disc disease can be approached via the anterior discal or the posterior interlaminar access. The anterior approach has been found to be safer and shown better long-term results. The technology being new, has limited data yet on various surgical outcomes, but found to be comparable in terms of results with reduced complications, lesser hospitalization, lesser tissue trauma, lesser blood loss, early functional recovery and overall patient comfort factors.

While Hijikata and Kambin described lumber percutaneous nucleotomy, it was Tajima in 1989, who first described the anterior percutaneous endoscopic cervical discectomy (PECD) [46]. This could be carried out via an anterior approach or a posterior approach depending upon the pathology. The aim is decompression of the neural elements under visualization through a percutaneous endoscopic approach. We can now treat various cervical disc diseases such as central, paracentral or even foraminal disc herniations, using endoscopic drill or lasers. It can thus provide treatment which can be said to be comparable presently to ACDF and CDR, with advantages of lesser time, minimal tissue damage and faster recovery.

Indications for endoscopic discectomy: The common indications being prolapsed intervertebral discs (PIVD) at C3-4 to C7-D1 levels, lateral to central soft discs, radiculopathy being the chief complaint, preserved disc space of more than 4mm, no significant bony spurs and failure of conservative therapy of more than six months [47].

Contraindications

The chief contraindications for the endoscopic discectomy being spinal instability, myelopathy or severe deficits, migrated discs, calcified or sequestered discs, severely collapsed disc spaces, ossified posterior longitudinal ligaments (OPLL), past history of anterior spinal surgery, associated co morbidities such as fractures, malignancies, etc.

Technological Concepts

Patient is kept supine with neck in extension and right cervical access as the preferred route. Use of the C-arm with anteroposterior and lateral views is a must. Instruments include an endoscope with 0-25-degree view, light source, working channels for grasping forceps, dissectors, radiofrequency coagulator and side firing laser. Another channel ensures a continuous saline irrigation for better visibility, neural protection and hemostasis.

The next step is to place a needle into the disc planned to be removed. This is done by ensuring the carotid complex to be kept laterally whereas the tracheoesophageal complex is pushed medially fort the operator's finger to reach the anterior part of the vertebral body. Next, a spinal needle is pushed into 5 mm of disc space and then level is confirmed by fluoroscopy. Next intra-operative discography is done to delineate the herniations of nucleus pulposus and a guide wire is next introduced via the cannulated needle. A 2-3 mm skin incision is made around this which is then followed by sequential dilatations so as to create a space and place a working cannula. Through this annulus is cut and followed by discectomy using micro forceps and lasers. The end stage is to see the dural sac. This is followed by closure after ensuring a good hemostasis [48, 49].

Complication

The complication rate is fairly low but can be serious ones, especially those related to the access. Vascular injury, oesophageal injury, dysphagia, nerve injury, local hematoma, cord compression and local wound infection are the complications reported. Tzaan et al. reported a 2% complication in 107 patients [50]. Ruetten et al. found dysphagia in 5 cases in ACDF versus 2 cases in PECD. Also, they noted revision rates to be 6.1% in ACDF versus 7.4% with PECD [51]. Recurrence has been found to be commonest cause of revision in endoscopic surgeries as noted by Lee et al. too [54].

Overall, PECD has been reported to have a good success rate as noted by Ahn et al. (88.3%), Oh et al. (87%) and Tzaan et al. (91%) [52, 53, 50]. However, there is a steep learning curve. Hence, a generous usage of fluoroscope during the guide wire and dilators placement helps in achieving good results. Also, for safety, the working cannula is ideally placed in midline and should not go beyond posterior vertebral line.

Other important variants which are gradually generating interest is the anterior trans-corporeal approach, which involves endoscopic approach to a disc which has migrated significantly superiorly or inferiorly [55]. Another method gaining interest is the anterior cervical foraminotomy being less invasive and non-fusion technique as it provides a foraminal decompression for unilateral radiculopathy. And then, there is combination approach as advocated by Fujimoto et al. in where they have combined microsurgical discectomy with laminoplasty with good results [56]. However, all these newer variants need more studies and the data has to be compared with the gold standard techniques, so as to be accepted widely.

Conclusion

Cervical disc disease is a fairly common disorder affecting a majority of the middle aged and elderly population worldwide. However, most of them are asymptomatic. It's only those who have significant disc prolapse causing herniations or severe tension over the ligaments need some intervention. Clinical evaluation followed by radiology, preferably MRI that helps in the diagnosis. The commonest sites involved are C5/6, C6/7 and C4/5 respectively

Management for majority of the cervical disc disorders is conservative but a small yet significant number with clinical features of myelo-radiculopathy will need surgery. Anterior route is preferred approach as compared to the posterior approach. The anterior approach started in 1950s with management protocols by Robinson and Smith to be later modified by Cloward in form of ACDF that has gradually gained worldwide acceptance.

As the technology advanced, newer form of management of these came, initially with allograft and other materials, to be soon followed by artificial spacers that would take away the need for bone graft harvesting causing additional morbidity. Artificial cervical discs have brought a revolution and now minimal invasive form with endoscopic discectomy have all led to better fusions, reduced morbidity and an improved quality of life.

References

A Dweik, E Van den Brande, T Kossmann and AIR Maas. History of cervical spine surgery: from nihilism to advanced reconstructive surgery. *Spinal Cord*, (2013). 51, 809–814; 2013.107;

Ahn Y, Lee SH, Chung SE, et al. Percutaneous endoscopic cervical discectomy for discogenic cervical headache due to soft disc herniation. *Neuroradiology*, 2005; 47:924-30.

Ahn Y. Percutaneous endoscopic cervical discectomy using working channel endoscopes. *Expert Rev Med Devices*, 2016; 13: 601-10. 10.1080/17434440.2016.1180245 [PubMed].

Ali A. Baaj, M.D., Juan S. Uribe, M.D., Fernando L. Vale, M.D., Mark C. Preul, M.D., and Neil R. Crawford, Ph.D. History of cervical disc arthroplasty. *Neurosurg Focus*, 27 (3): E10, 2009.

An HS, Evanich CJ, Nowicki BH, Haughton VM. Ideal thickness of Smith-Robinson graft for anterior cervical fusion: a cadaveric study with computed tomographic correlation. *Spine*, 1993; 18(14): 2043–7.

Anastasia Tasiou, Theofanis Giannis, Alexandros G. Brotis, Ioannis Siasios, Iordanis Georgiadis, Haralampos Gatos, Eleni Tsianaka, Konstantinos Vagkopoulos, Konstantinos Paterakis, Kostas N. Fountas. Anterior cervical spine surgery-associated complications in a retrospective case-control study. *J Spine Surg*, 2017 Sep; 3(3): 444–459.

Bagby GW. Arthrodesis by the distractioncompression method using a stainless steel implant. *Orthopedics*., 1988; 11(6): 931–4.

Brenke C, Kindling S, Scharf J, Schmieder K, Barth M. Short-term experience with a new absorbable composite cage (beta-tricalcium phosphate-polylactic acid) in patients after stand-alone anterior cervical discectomy and fusion. *Spine* (Phila Pa 1976). 2013; 38(11): E635–40.

Cabraja M, Oezdemir S, Koeppen D, Kroppenstedt S. Anterior cervical discectomy and fusion: comparison of titanium and polyetheretherketone cages. *BMC Musculoskelet Disord*., 2012; 13: 172.

Caspar W, Barbier DD, Klara PM. Anterior cervical fusion and Caspar plate stabilization for cervical trauma. *Neurosurgery*., 1989; 25(4): 491– 502.

Chang UK, Kim DH, Lee MC, Willenberg R, Kim SH, Lim J: Changes in adjacent-level disc pressure and facet joint force after cervical arthroplasty compared with cervical discectomy and fusion. *J Neurosurg Spine*, 7: 33–39, 2007.

Chou Y-C, Chen D-C, Hsieh WA, Chen W-F, Yen P-S, Harnod T, et al. Efficacy of anterior cervical fusion: Comparison of titanium cages, polyetheretherketone (PEEK) cages and autogenous bone grafts. *J Clin Neurosci*., 2008; 15(11): 1240–5.

Cloward RB. The anterior approach for removal of ruptured cervical disks. *J Neurosurg*, 1985; 15: 602–617

Comron Saifi, Arielle W Fein, Alejandro Cazzulino, Ronald A Lehman, Frank M Phillips, Howard S An, K Daniel Riew Trends in resource utilization and rate of cervical disc arthroplasty and anterior cervical discectomy and fusion throughout the United States from 2006-2013. *Spine J.*, 2018 Jun; 18(6): 1022-1029.

Deng ZL, Chu L, Chen L, Yang JS. Anterior transcorporeal approach of percutaneous endoscopic cervical discectomy for disc herniation at the C4-C5 levels: a technical note. *Spine J.*, 2016 May; 16(5): 659-66. doi: 10.1016/j.spinee.2016.01.187. Epub 2016 Feb 2. PMID: 26850173.

Elizabeth Chong, Matthew H Pelletier, Ralph J Mobbs & William R Walsh. The design evolution of interbody cages in anterior cervical discectomy and fusion: a systematic review. *BMC Musculoskeletal Disorders*, 16, Article number: 99 (2015).

Elsberg CA. Tumors of the spinal cord and the symptoms of irritation and compression of the spinal cord and nerve roots: pathology, symptom a t o l o g y, diagnosis and treatment. New York: Paul B Hoeber, 1925: 195-198.

Fernstrom U: Arthroplasty with intercorporal endoprothesis in herniated disc and in painful disc. *Acta Chir Scand Suppl*, 357: 154–159, 1966.

Friedenstein AJ, Chailakhjan RK, Lalykina KS. The development of fibroblast colonies in monolayer cultures of guinea-pig bone marrow and spleen cells. *Cell Tissue Kinet.*, 1970; 3(4): 393–403.

Fujimoto Y, Baba I, Sumida T, Tanaka N, Oka S, Kawagoe H. Microsurgical transdural discectomy with laminoplasty: new treatment for paracentral and paracentroforaminal cervical disc herniation associated with spinal canal stenosis. *Spine* (Phila Pa 1976), 2002; 27: 715–721.

Goffin J, Casey A, Kehr P, Liebig K, Lind B, Logroscino C, et al.: Preliminary clinical experience with the Bryan cervical disc prosthesis. Neurosurgery 51:840–847, 2002.

Goffin J, Geusens E, Vantomme N: Long-term follow-up after interbody fusion of the cervical spine. *J Spinal Disord Tech*, 17: 79–85, 2004.

Hilibrand AS, Carlson GD, Palumbo MA, Jones PK, Bohlman HH: Radiculopathy and myelopathy at segments adjacent to the site of a previous anterior cervical arthrodesis. *J Bone Joint Surg Am*, 81: 519–528, 1999.

Hirsch C. Cervical disc rupture: diagnosis and therapy. Acta Orthop Scand 1960; 30:172-186.

Irvine DH, Foster JB, Newell DJ, Klukvin BN. Prevalence of cervical spondylosis in general practice. *Lancet.*, 1965; 285(7395): 1089–92.

Javier Quillo-Olvera, Guang-Xun Lin, Jin-Sung Kim. Percutaneous endoscopic cervical discectomy: a technical review. *Ann Transl Med.*, 2018 Mar; 6(6): 100.

Justin D. Cohen MD, Linda E. Kanim MA, Andrew J. Tronits MD, Hyun W. Bae MD. Allografts and Spinal Fusion. *Int J Spine Surg.*, 2021 Apr; 15(Suppl 1): 68–93.

Knoeller SM, Seifried C. Historical perspective: history of spinal surgery. *Spine*, 2000; 25:2838- 2843.

Korinth MC. Treatment of cervical degenerative disc disease - current status and trends. *Zentralbl Neurochir.*, 2008 Aug; 69(3): 113-24.

Le H, Thongtrangan I, Kim DH: Historical review of cervical arthroplasty. *Neurosurg Focus*, 17(3) :E1, 2004.

Lee JH, Lee SH. Clinical and radiographic changes after percutaneous endoscopic cervical discectomy: a long-term follow-up. *Photomed Laser Surg*, 2014; 32:663-8.

M. Teraguchi, N. Yoshimura, H. Hashizume, S. Muraki, H. Yamada, A. Minamide, H. Oka, Y. Ishimoto, K. Nagata, R. Kagotani, N. Takiguchi, T. Akune, H. Kawaguchi, K. Nakamura, M. Yoshida. Prevalence and distribution of intervertebral disc degenerationover the entire spine in a population-based cohort: theWakayama Spine Study. *Osteoarthritis and Cartilage*. Volume 22, Issue 1, January 2014, Pages 104-110

Marcelo Lemos Vieira da Cunha, Francisco Alves de Araújo Júnior, Cássio Czottis Grapiglia, Denildo César Amaral Veríssimo, Roberta Rehder, Samir Ale Bark, Luis Alencar Biurrum Borba. Complications of the anterior approach to the cervical spine. *Coluna/Columna*, 13 (3) • Jul-Sep 2014.

Marketos SG, Skiadas P. Hippocrates: the father of the spine surgery. *Spine*, 1999; 24: 1381-1387.

Martin H. Pham, Vivek A. Mehta, Alexander Tuchman, Patrick C. Hsieh, "Material Science in Cervical Total Disc Replacement", *BioMed Research International*, vol. 2015, Article ID 719123, 9 pages, 2015.

Matgé G. Cervical cage fusion with 5 different implants: 250 cases. *Acta Neurochir.*, 2002; 144(6): 539–50.

Matsumoto M, Fujimura Y, Suzuki N, Nishi Y, Nakamura M, Yabe Y, Shiga H. MRI of cervical intervertebral discs in asymptomatic subjects. *J Bone Joint Surg Br.*, 1998 Jan; 80(1): 19-24. [PubMed: 9460946].

Michael B Furman, MD, MS; Chief Editor: Dean H Hommer, MD. *Cervical Disc Disease.*, Updated 16 Apr 2020. Medscape, Accessed in 01-08-2021.

N Muthukumar. Surgical management of cervical spondylotic myelopathy. *Neurology India*, Year: 2012 | Volume: 60 | Issue : 2 | Page : 201-209.

Nancy E. Epstein. A Review of Complication Rates for Anterior Cervical Diskectomy and Fusion (ACDF). *Surg Neurol Int*. 2019; 10: 100.

Oh HS, Hwang BW, Park SJ, et al. Percutaneous endoscopic cervical discectomy (PECD): An analysis of outcome, causes of reoperation. *World Neurosurg*, 2017; 102: 583-92.

Okada E, Matsumoto M, Ichihara D, Chiba K, Toyama Y, Fujiwara H, Momoshima S, Nishiwaki Y, Hashimoto T, Ogawa J, Watanabe M, Takahata T. Aging of the cervical spine in healthy volunteers: a 10-year longitudinal magnetic resonance imaging study. *Spine* (Phila Pa 1976). 2009 Apr 01; 34(7): 706-12. [PubMed: 19333104].

Ramesh Chandra. Anterior Surgical Approach to Cervical Spine with Fusion: An Appraisal of 55 Cases. *NIMHANS Journal.*, Volume: 06 Issue: 2S December 1988 Page: 141-148.

Ruetten S, Komp M, Merk H, et al. Full-endoscopic anterior decompression versus conventional anterior decompression and fusion in cervical disc herniations. *Int Orthop*, 2009; 33: 1677-82.

Scholz M, Schnake K, Pingel A, Hoffmann R, Kandziora F. A new zero-profile implant for stand-alone anterior cervical interbody fusion. *Clin Orthop Relat Res*., 2011; 469(3): 666–73.

Sharma SB, Luke Kim JS, Siddappa ND, Jabri HE. Current status of full-endoscopic spine surgery in cervical spine: Anterior and posterior approach. *Indian Spine J*, 2020; 3: 41-53.

Skovrlj B, Guzman JZ, Al Maaieh M, Cho SK, Iatridis JC, Qureshi SA. Cellular bone matrices: viable stem cell-containing bone graft substitutes. *Spine J.*, 2014; 14(11): 2763–2772.

Smith GW, Robinson RA. The treatment of certain cervical-spine disorders by anterior removal of the intervertebral disc and interbody fusion. *J Bone Joint Surg.*, 1958; 40(3): 607–24.

Suchomel P, Barsa P, Buchvald P, Svobodnik A, Vanickova E. Autologous versus allogenic bone grafts in instrumented anterior cervical discectomy and fusion: a prospective study with respect to bone union pattern. *Eur Spine J.*, 2004; 13(6):510–515.

Tajima T, Sakamoto H, Yamakawa H. Diskectomy cervicale percutanee. *Rev Med Orthop*, 1989; 17: 7-10.

Taku SUGAWARA, Anterior Cervical Spine Surgery for Degenerative Disease: A Review. *Neurol Med Chir* (Tokyo). 2015 Jul; 55(7): 540–546.

The history of spinal surgery for disc disease, An illustrated timeline. Igor de Castro, Daniel Paes dos Santos, Daniel de Holanda Christoph, José Alberto Landeiro. *Arq Neuropsiquiatr*, 2005; 63(3-A): 701-706.

Tzaan WC. Anterior percutaneous endoscopic cervical discectomy for cervical intervertebral disc herniation: outcome, complications, and technique. *J Spinal Disord Tech*, 2011; 24: 421-31.

Urist MR. Bone: formation by autoinduction. *Science.*, 1965; 150(3698): 893–899.

Wilke HJ, Kettler A, Claes L. Primary stabilizing effect of interbody fusion devices for the cervical spine: an *in vitro* comparison between three different cage types and bone cement. *Eur Spine J.*, 2000; 9(5): 410–6.

Zhu Y, Zhang B, Liu H, Wu Y, Zhu Q. Cervical Disc Arthroplasty Versus Anterior Cervical Discectomy and Fusion for Incidence of Symptomatic Adjacent Segment Disease: A Meta-Analysis of Prospective Randomized Controlled Trials. *Spine* (Phila Pa 1976), 2016 Oct 1; 41(19): 1493-1502.

Chapter 9

Spinal Dysraphism and Congenital Non-Dysraphic Malformations

Priyadarshi Dikshit[1,*], Pragya Gupta[2], Rudrashish Haldar[2], Ved Prakash Maurya[1], Arun Kumar Srivastava[1] and Rajkumar[1]

[1]Department of Neurosurgery, Sanjay Gandhi Post-Graduate Institute of Medical Sciences, Lucknow, India

[2]Department of Anaesthesiology, Sanjay Gandhi Post-Graduate Institute of Medical Sciences, Lucknow, India

Abstract

'Spinal dysraphism' is a blanket denomination referring to a spectrum of disparate disorders stemming from errors in spinal cord development or that of the surrounding mesenchymal structures, including the vertebral column. The usage of the term spina bifida interchangeably with spinal dysraphism would be imprecise. The conventional practice of grouping a wide range of pathology under one term is an oversimplification of the subject and often seems unjust to the disease pathogenesis. Although each disorder included in this spectrum has developmental roots, the extent of embryological pathophysiology is peculiar in each, thus mandating a tailored treatment strategy. Unsurprisingly, the outcomes can be quite contrasting. It cannot be overemphasized that a limpid understanding of the basic embryology, pathological anatomy, and the pathophysiology related to each anomaly is paramount in every disorder for planning an optimal treatment strategy. The care provider should focus on the dysraphism part and include a complete evaluation for any

* Corresponding Author's Email: vpmsurgery@gmail.com

In: Neurosurgery Research
Editors: Amit Agrawal, Pradeep Chouksey, Adesh Shrivastava et al.
ISBN: 978-1-68507-837-9

associated systemic anomaly, focusing on cardiovascular, musculoskeletal, respiratory, and genitourinary systems. This anomaly allows for plenary management with apt anaesthesiologic and surgical management planning.

Most of the afflicted individuals require long term follow-up and rehabilitation measures owing to the extent of dysraphism related deficits as well as due to associated syndromic manifestations. Proper counselling of parents is crucial in alleviating the apprehension regarding the developmental anomaly that is not infrequently associated with disfigurement and a mediocre outcome despite best management. In the present chapter, we try to convey the essence of embryological basis in spinal dysraphism, treatment planning, anaesthetic considerations, follow-up strategy, and measures to stave off delayed complications.

Introduction

Conventional teaching described categorization of spinal dysraphism states into two major groups: the Spina bifida Aperta and the Spina bifida Occulta (Table 1) (French 1983). With the advent of better ante-natal diagnostic modalities, earlier ante-natal detection rates of spina bifida aperta has become significantly high leading to early terminations of pregnancy thus decreasing incidence of such cases. In similar lines with increasing availability and quality of magnetic resonance imaging (MRI), the incidence of spina bifida occulta has been witnessed to be increasing. The clear understanding of the pathophysiology of the spinal dysraphism states has made significant change in the management of these disorders with a tailored approach for each disorder subtype. Moreover, the earlier detection of the disorder using effective screening programs with the help of clinical assessment and radiological diagnostic modalities has helped limit the neurological disability and thus somewhat liberating these disorders from associated despondency.

Embryological Basis of Spinal Dysraphism

The embryonic period lasts for the first eight weeks of gestation, during which organogenesis occurs and is followed by the fetal life, wherein precise and orchestrated development of each organ-related tissue along with enlargement of the fetus to the point of optimal maturity face the extra-uterine life. Embryogenesis of the human central nervous system stems from the neural plate, a specialized mid-line region on the dorsal surface of the embryonic plate, by the third week period of gestation (POG). The margins of the neural plate fold to form the neural tube, the broad cranial end of which forms the cerebral vesicles, and the extended narrow caudal portion extends to form the spinal cord till the region of the S2 spinal cord segment. The segments below the level of S2 develop by a process known as secondary neurulation (Sadler 2012).

Table 1. Conventional classification of spinal dysraphism

Spina Bifida Aperta
• Myeloschisis
• Myelomeningocele
• Hemi-meningomyelocele
• Meningocele
• Type 2 Chiari Malformation
Occult spinal dysraphism
• Dermal sinus
• Tethered cord
• Lipomyelomeningocele
• Lumbo-sacral lipoma
• Diastematomyelia
• Neuro-enteric cyst
• Anterior (sacral) meningocele
• Occult posterior spina bifida

Based on the POG, spinal cord development can be broadly subdivided into three phases:

i. Development during gastrulation (second to third week POG).
ii. Development during primary neurulation (third to fourth week POG).
iii. Development during the phase of secondary neurulation (fifth to sixth week POG) (Sadler 2005; Tortori-Donati, Rossi, and Cama 2000).

Phase of Gastrulation

After the formation of the embryonic disc with the epiblast cells lining the side of the amniotic sac and the hypoblast cells towards the yolk sac, there is the formation of an area of proliferating epiblast cells towards the caudal end of the embryonic disc in the midline. The proliferating cells of the primitive node gradually replace the hypoblast cells, thus forming the endoderm. After this, start insinuating between the epiblasts (future ectoderm) and the hypoblasts, giving rise to the mesoderm. The mesoderm builds up in the space between the ectoderm and endoderm except for the region of the pro-chordal plate where the epiblasts and hypoblasts are adherents (this region corresponds to the future buccopharyngeal membrane). The mesoderm further differentiates into the axial mesoderm, the paraxial mesoderm, and the lateral plate mesoderm.

Of importance in the purview is the formation of pre-notochordal cells (axial mesoderm), which invaginate directly cranial from the primitive knot and end at the region of the pro-chordal plate. A depression soon appears in the primitive knot. It invaginates along the pre-notochordal cells forming a tube-like structure known as the neuro-enteric canal. It then assimilates with the endoderm to communicate the yolk sac with the amniotic sac. After this transient communication, the neuro-enteric canal involutes and detaches off the ectoderm and the endoderm to form a cellular cord-like structure known as the notochord.

The notochord influences the overlying ectoderm to transform into the future neural plate, which marks the genesis of the cerebral vesicles and spinal cord. Regulation of the dorsal mesoderm in the middle and caudal regions of the embryo is made by the BRACHYURY (T) gene expressed in the pre-notochordal cells and the notochord. In the absence of the BRACHYURY gene product, there occurs shortening of the embryonic axis with caudal agenesis/ dysgenesis with the grade of the malformation depending on the time of loss of the gene product during embryonic development.

Phase of Primary Neurulation

By the third week of POG, a slipper-shaped area of thickened ectoderm appears rostral to the region of the primitive node. The lateral margins of this thickened plate (the neural plate) begin elevating, and soon the neural plate furrows inward with its lateral edges approximating each other, creating the neural tube. The neural plate margin fusion process is believed to start in the cervical spinal cord region, which then proceeds in both cranial and caudal directions in a "zipper-like" fashion. The neuropores communicate with the overlying amniotic cavity until the primary neurulation process is complete.

Upon neurulation, the neural tube pinches off and separates from the adjacent neuroepithelium by a process known as disjunction. The closure of the cranial neuropore occurs by the 25th day POG (somite stage 18- 20), while the caudal neuropore closes within the next three days (Sadler 2012; 2005). Non-closure of the caudal neuropore leads to an open myelocele and reflects a severe form of spinal cord dysraphism. In contrast, non-closure of the cranial neuropore leads to anencephaly, often incompatible with life.

The lumen of the neural tube, which represents the future spinal canal, remains continuous with that of the rostral cerebral vesicles. In the developing spinal cord, the neuroectodermal cells form a pseudostratified epithelium with the cells connected by junctional complexes at the luminal side of the tube. The neuroepithelial cells start proliferating and give rise to specialized cells, neuroblasts, which start palisading around the lumen of the developing neural tube and segregate into an inner layer known as the mantle zone and an outer layer known as the marginal zone. Later during further development, the mantle zone forms the gray matter of the spinal cord. In contrast, the marginal zone gets populated by the nerve fibers emerging from the neuroblasts that eventually get myelinated and form the white matter.

With further growth of the neuroblasts in a more centrifugal fashion around the central canal, there appears two ventral thickening of the central gray matter (mantle zone) known as the basal plates and two dorsal thickenings known as the alar plates, and both separated on each side by a sulcus known as the sulcus limitans. The basal plates harbour the future anterior horn cells and function as the motor centres of the spinal cord, while the alar plates serve as the sensory centres of the spinal cord. The spinal cord's midline ventral and dorsal portions are devoid of the proliferating neuroblasts and harbour pathways for the crossover of nerve fibers across the midline to the contralateral side. In addition to the basal and alar plates, another intermedio-lateral horn is formed in the region of the thoracic spinal cord segments (T1 – T12) and the upper lumbar segments (L1, L2). These represent the future sympathetic outflow of the autonomic nervous system. The central neuroepithelial cells differentiate into ependymal cells, which line the central canal.

Phase of Secondary Neurulation

Totipotent axial mesodermal cells near the caudal end of the neural tube formation, also known as the caudal cell mass, develop in the BRACHYURY gene product under the influence of the adjacent notochord. These cells gradually coalesce and form a cord-like structure that cavitates and transforms into a tube-like structure. This caudal tube-like structure then becomes continuous with the neural tube. The caudal part of this secondary neurulation structure undergoes regression (retrogressive differentiation). It forms a thin band known as the filum terminale that spans from the tip of conus medullaris to the coccyx region (coccygeal medullary vestige) (Melvin et al. 2000;

Schoenwolf 1979; Sadler 2012). POG after the secondary neurulation process as described above is complete by the third month, and the spinal cord extends the entire spinal column length.

Development and Derivatives of the Neural Crest

During the neural plate development, along the elevating lateral edges of the former, another longitudinal elevation in proximity is known as the neural crest. The neural crest is formed by the proliferating neuroectodermal cells, and the crest extends throughout the length of the neural tube. The crest cells migrate laterally and differentiate mainly into neuroblasts forming the sensory ganglia (dorsal root ganglia) and other cell types, including the Schwann cells and melanocytes. These cells develop central and peripheral processes. The central process penetrates the neural tube and may either end in the dorsal horn (alar plate) or may ascend to higher centres traversing through the marginal zone of the developing neural tube. The peripheral processes join to form the rami and trunks of the spinal nerves and migrate to the periphery to reach the sensory end organs. As mentioned before, in addition to forming the sensory ganglion cells, the neural crest cells give rise to the Schwann cells, meninges, melanocytes, odontoblasts, and mesenchyme of the pharyngeal arches.

Further Development of the Spinal Cord

By the third month of POG, the spinal cord stretches across the entire length of the spinal canal, with the spinal nerve roots passing through the neural foramina at the same level of the respective spinal segments. With the increase in gestational age, the crown-rump length increases rapidly, and the growth of the vertebrae and dura mater far exceeds that of the neural tube leading to cranial pulling of the spinal cord. This process results in an oblique course of the dorsal and ventral roots emerging towards their respective neural foramina from the spinal cord. The spinal cord termination gradually ascends to the L2-L3 vertebral level while the dural sac extends caudally till the S2 vertebral level. Below the termination of the spinal cord, the ventral and dorsal roots below the level of L2 aggregate and reminisce a horse's tail (cauda equina).

Peri-Neural Tube Sclerotome Formation

After the third week of POG, the paraxial mesoderm gets sorted into segments known as the somitomeres, the precursor tissues of the future somites. This segmentation process of the paraxial mesoderm progresses in a cephalon-caudal fashion, and within each somitomeres unit thus formed, there is a concentric arrangement of cells around a central mass of cells. By the end of the fifth week POG, 44 pairs (one on each side of the neural tube) of somites are formed: four occipital, eight cervical, 12 thoracic, five lumbar, five sacral, and ten coccygeal somite pairs. The NOTCH and WNT gene products influence the formation of the somitomeres and somites.

After the formation of somites from their precursors, the somitomeres; undergo a process known as epithelization, forming a doughnut-shaped mass with a small central lumen. The cells from the ventral and medial portions of this doughnut-shaped somite re-differentiate into mesenchymal fibroblast-like cells under the influence of FGF8 and WNT3a proteins and start surrounding the notochord and the neural tube. Then under the influence of the NOGGIN and Sonic Hedgehog (SHH) produced by the notochord, the ventromedial cells give rise to sclerotome cells (Melvin et al. 2000; Pang and Thompson 2011; Sadler 2012). These cells later differentiate into the vertebrae and ribs. Cells in the ventrolateral and dorsomedial portions of the somites develop into myotomes and contribute to the lateral musculature (along with lateral plate mesoderm contributing to the lateral and limb muscles) and paraxial musculature, respectively. The cells in between the ventrolateral and dorsomedial cell groups give rise to the dermatomal derivatives.

During the fourth week of POG, the sclerotomal cells migrate and surround the notochord and spinal cord to join with similar cells from the contralateral side to form a pre-neural tube sclerotomal mass in each somite segment level. This sclerotomal mass then undergoes re-segmentation in which the sclerotomal mass sub-divides into cranial and caudal halves. Each caudal half of a sclerotome joins the cranial half of the subjacent sclerotome to form the future vertebral body. Thus, each vertebral body develops from the caudal half of a somite and the cranial half of the subjacent somite. Thus, explaining the fissure of Von Ebner, the vascularity of a typical vertebral body and the passage of spinal nerves in the intervertebral level (Pang and Thompson 2011; Aoyama and Asamoto 2000).

Embryonic Pathophysiology Based Classification of Spinal Dysraphism

Understanding the intricate development of the spinal cord and the surrounding vertebral column is complex. A broad spectrum of spinal anomalies (grouped as spinal dysraphism) can result from any form of derangement in the infinitude steps involved, and each step and degree of derangement can lead to a unique morphology. However, to simplify this into a more comprehensible and pragmatic classification, the following classification can guide us to a bird's eye view of the diverse spectrum of spinal dysraphism (Table 2) (Acharya et al. 2017; S. Rufener, Ibrahim, and Parmar 2011).

Table 2. Embryological classification of spinal dysraphism

A. Disorders related to notochord
- a. Neuro-enteric cysts
- b. Dorsal Enteric fistula
- c. Split cord malformations (diastematomyelia)

B. Disorders related to caudal cell mass
- a. Caudal regression syndrome
- b. Segmental spinal dysgenesis

C. Disorders of Primary Neurulation
- a. Premature disjunction
    - i. Lipomeningomyelocele
    - ii. Lipomyelocele
    - iii. Intra-dural lipoma.
- b. Non-disjunction
    - i. Myelocele
    - ii. Meningomyelocele
    - iii. Dorsal dermal sinus
- c. Combined anomalies of primary neurulation and gastrulation
    - i. Hemimyelocele
    - ii. Hemimyelomeningocele

D. Disorders due to derangement of the secondary neurulation process
- a. Low lying tethered cord
- b. Persistent terminal ventricle
- c. Thickened filum terminale/Tight filum terminale
- d. Intra-sacral/ anterior sacral meningocele
- e. Terminal myelocystocele

Clinical Features

As myriad is the spectrum of the spinal dysraphism disorder, so multitudinous are the clinical manifestations of this group of disorders. The manifestations may be inconspicuous with only an overlying pigmented patch or a tuft of hair in cases of spina bifida occulta or can be devastating with paraplegia and bladder and bowel incontinence. The diagnosis and presentation can be early in the intrauterine period with ante-natal imaging, as in the case of occult cases of spinal dysraphism to delayed onset in late childhood in cases of low-lying tethered cord. Many of the cases of spinal dysraphism may be accompanied by cranial anomalies such as Chiari malformation and associated syringomyelia with/ without hydrocephalus. As emphasized earlier, each spinal dysraphism subtype deserves a volume for separate and elaborate descriptions of clinical features and management protocols; however, the same is beyond the scope of this chapter. The cutaneous manifestations of occult spinal dysraphism can be grouped into those with a high index of suspicion and those with a low index of suspicion (Table 3).

Table 3. Cutaneous markers of spinal Dysraphism

Cutaneous markers with high index of suspicion:
1. Hypertrichosis
2. Atypical Dimples (> 1 inch above the anal verge)
3. Acrochordons/ pseudo nails
4. Sub-cutaneous Lipomas
5. Cutaneous cavernous hemangiomas
6. Aplasia cutis/ dysplastic skin (scar)
7. Midline Dermal sinus/ Dermoid cyst
Cutaneous markers with low index of suspicion:
1. Cutaneous telangiectasia
2. Port-wine stain (capillary hemangiomas)
3. Hyperpigmented patches
4. Melanotic nevi
5. Teratoma

Spinal dysraphism has been traditionally classified into closed and open types based on the integrity of the overlying skin. The closed types are further subclassified into those with and those without a subcutaneous swelling/mass. The open spinal dysraphism types present with a mass over the back, often diagnosed at birth with or without CSF leak from the mass. The overlying skin myelomeningocele is often dysplastic and thin, it tends to rupture during labor, and a planned caesarian section can avoid this. This highlights the importance of a prenatal diagnosis not just for the decision of early termination of pregnancy but for avoiding a dreaded complication associated with these disorders, as any rupture can lead to life-threatening meningitis. The defects can be anywhere in the vertebral column, including the thoracolumbar region, the lumbar region, lumbosacral region, pure-thoracic region, sacral, and cervical regions in decreasing order of incidence (Figure 1).

Disorders of primary neurulation tend to involve the thoracic or thoracolumbar region, lumbar region, or even higher levels. In contrast, sacral region studies are usually associated with secondary neurulation defects. High cervical defects have been reported to be up to 4% cases. (Steinbok 1995; Venkataramana 2011a).

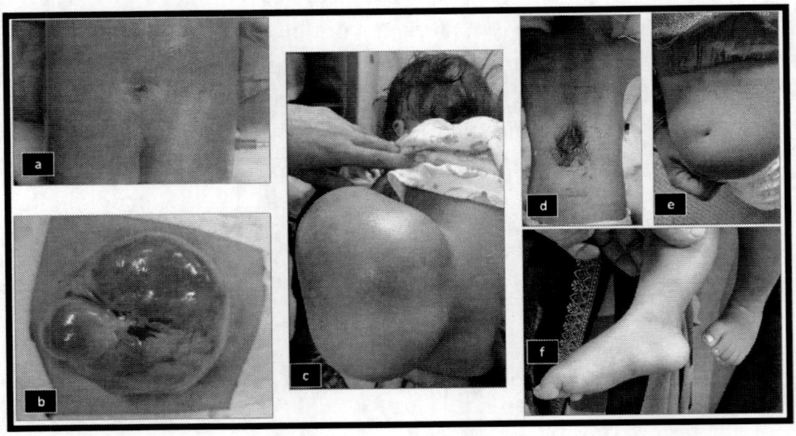

Figure 1. a) Clinical photograph of a two-year-old child with an isolated dimple over lower lumbar segment. On close observation, the dimple measured about 8 mm with history of serous discharge from the dermal sinus. b) The intraoperative image of an eight-month-old child with lobulated swelling over the lumbar region. The trans-illumination test suggests few traversing nerve roots without active cerebrospinal fluid leak from the swelling. c) Clinical photograph of a one-year-old child with a huge lumbosacral lobulated swelling. Transillumination test was negative with paraplegia and the size of swelling exceeds the size of child's head. d) The operation room photograph of a seven-year-old girl shows an isolated tuft of hair over thoracolumbar region. The intraoperative impression revealed type- I split cord malformation. e) The clinical photograph of a ten-month-old girl revealed a diffuse lumbar swelling crossing the midline. An isolated non-discharging sinus is present over the right lateral aspect of the swelling. f) The clinical photograph of the paraplegic feet of a child with lipomyelomeningocele revealed the typical varus deformity in both the feet.

Depending on the level of the defect, the motor, sensory and autonomic (bladder and bowel) deficits vary and in severe cases at each level, there is complete motor loss with areflexia, hypoesthesia/anaesthesia below the level of the lesion associated with bladder and bowel sphincter weakness or even atonic sphincter, sometimes causing rectal prolapse. Not infrequently, there is an associated small posterior fossa with tonsillar herniation leading to syringomyelia with/without syringobulbia leading to the brainstem and lower cranial nerve dysfunction in addition to manifestations of central cord syndrome with or without respiratory distress. In subjects having a less dramatic presentation, the long-standing syringomyelia leads to paraxial muscle weakness and kyphoscoliosis in addition to the myelopathy and manifestations of central cord syndrome. In addition to neurogenic kyphoscoliosis, there are frequent associations of vertebral segmental anomalies, hemivertebrae, Klippel Feil anomaly, and deformities of the rib-cage and distal limb anomalies (club foot, CTEV). The presence of a large head indicated associated hydrocephalus in such cases.

Prenatal Diagnosis

Testing of maternal serum alpha-fetoprotein (AFP) alone performed three times at the 12th week POG, 22nd week POG, and 32nd week POG has detection rates of up to 80% for spina bifida and up to 90% for anencephaly. In addition to AFP, antenatal ultrasonography can also identify up to 90% of spinal meningomyelocele cases. Together these two modalities can yield a high detection rate of over 90% and grossly lethal anomalies are almost always detected, leading to termination of pregnancy (Candenas et al. 1995; Boyd et al. 2000). Contemporary practice is witnessing a growing usage of fetal MRI leading to more accurate detection of dysraphism disorders, including midline or posterior fossa anomalies. However, the accurate prediction of post-natal outcomes is still not feasible despite these advancements. Only in a few selected cases is the need for amniocentesis justified for detecting spinal dysraphism (Anderson et al. 1994).

Post-Natal Radiological Assessment

Early imaging is the rule in each case of spinal dysraphism for time management and planning appropriate intervention and prediction of outcome.

MRI of the affected spinal region with whole spine screening remains the investigation of choice for assessing the severity of dysraphism. Additional cranial screening is done to rule out hydrocephalus, small posterior fossa, and Chiari malformation. X-ray of the spinal column in a standing position in cases associated with kyphoscoliosis is used to assess the degree of scoliosis. CT of the involved spinal segment helps determine the vertebral anomaly's extent, such as hemivertebra/ block vertebrae/ Klippel Feil anomaly. It is also valuable for morphological assessment of bony spur in cases of (diastematomyelia) type 1 split cord malformation (Figure 2). In the following sections, we will outline, in short, the various spinal dysraphism disorders.

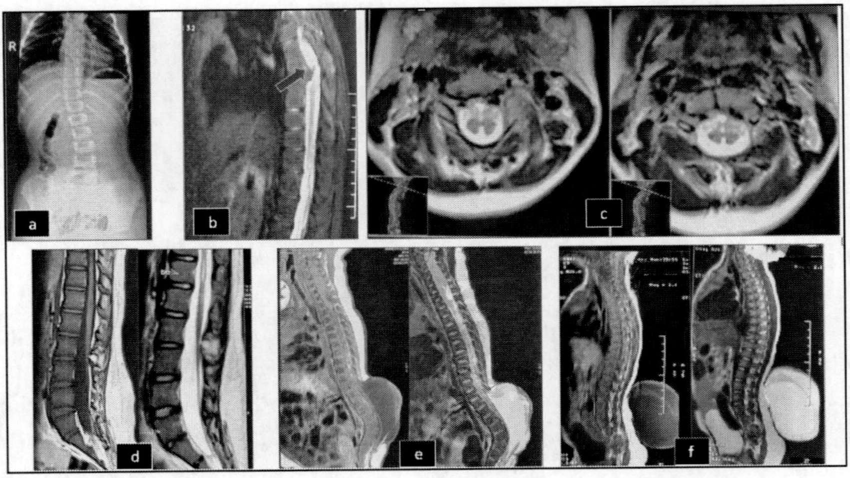

Figure 2. a) The x- ray spine of a seven-year-old girl with recurrent tethering who was operated for meningomyelocele at the age of 15 days of life. The presence of thoracolumbar scoliosis indicates a long-standing pathology. b and c) The sagittal section of MRI spine indicates a dorsal bony spur noted at D5-D6 level [a purple arrow]. The axial section of same patient revealed type-I split cord malformation. d) The sagittal section of MRI spine suggests a low-lying cord with thickened filum terminale. The subcutaneous fat is hyperintense on T1WI and T2WI. A ventrolateral arachnoid cyst is noted at the lumbosacral region, T1 hypo and T2 hyperintense. e) The sagittal section of MRI spine revealed a lesion which is hypointense on T1WI and hyperintense on T2WI with significant lumbar kyphotic deformity. f) The sagittal section of MRI spine revealed a lesion at lumbar region with narrow pedicle which is hypointense on T1WI and hyperintense on T2WI with terminal portion of cord entering into the swelling. The presence of septations is well appreciated.

Anomalies of Notochord Development

Neuro-Enteric Cyst

This rare disorder results from abnormal persistence of the neuro-enteric canal, which is present in the early phase of notochordal development prior to its involution. The typical result is a mucous-lined cystic mass in the spinal canal over the cervical and thoracic regions. The neuro-enteric cysts may be associated with a fistula/ sinus tract through the primitive osseous canal of Kovalevsky and vertebral segmental anomalies in more severe variants.

Split Cord Malformation

Split cord malformation (SCM) refers to a bifid state of the spinal cord. It can be of two types: Type 1 (Diastematomyelia) SCM. A thick Osseo-cartilaginous septum separates two separate thecal sacs and often a bony spur emanating from them the posterior vertebral surface, and each thecal sac harbors a hemi-cord.

Type 2 (Diplomyelia) SCM has a single thecal sac encasing both Hemi-cords, occasionally separated by a thin fibrous septum.

Anomalies of Gastrulation and Caudal Cell Mass

Caudal Regression Syndrome (CRS)

This disorder results from the combined anomaly of gastrulation and primary neurulation and represents a complex dysraphism state. An inherited defect in the HLX-B gene is often incriminated in this condition, and the CRS has a preponderance for children born to diabetic mothers. This condition is often associated with VACTERL and Currarino triad syndromes. There are two types of CRS:

1. *Type 1 CRS:* is characterized by a miniaturized maldeveloped terminal vertebral column, with a high lying conus and severe visceral and orthopaedic anomalies reflecting the gastrulation anomaly. The orthopaedic anomalies include small hip bones and reduced range of motion at the hip joint, underdeveloped femurs often associated with severe genu-valgum with feet tucked under the hips leading to "frog-leg" appearance. Not infrequently, there is an associated congenital talipes equinovarus anomaly. The common visceral anomalies include renal anomalies, including agenesis/ horseshoe kidney and

ureteral duplication. There may be hypospadias, cryptorchidism, recto-vaginal fistula, and bladder exstrophy. The higher termination of the spinal cord reflects the non-contribution by the caudal cell mass to spinal cord genesis, and a higher cord termination is associated with a more severe form of the disorder. The most severe reported type of CRS is the mermaid syndrome/configuration in which there is severe sacral dysgenesis/ agenesis and fused lower limbs.

2. *Type 2 CRS:* is the less severe variant of CRS and is associated with a low-lying tethered cord with a thick filum terminale (Boulas 2009).

Segmental Spinal Dysgenesis

This rare condition features segmental thoracic/thoracolumbar/lumbar vertebral or spinal cord dysgenesis/agenesis. Segmental spinal dysgenesis is associated with severe focal kyphoscoliosis, and the caudal spinal segments are dystrophic, bulky, low lying and tethered; however, the cranial spinal segments are morphologically regular.

Anomalies of Primary Neurulation: Premature Disjunction

Premature disjunction of the neural tube leads to the interposition of an abnormal amount of surrounding mesenchymal cells into the space between surface ectoderm and the neural tube, dragging the ectopic mesenchyme into the neural canal and often between the margins of the neural plate. This leads to incomplete closure of the neural tube (caudal neuropore), and the intervening mesenchyme often differentiates into lipomatous formation.

Lipo-Myelocele (LMC) & Lipo-Meningomyelocele (LMMC)

LMC and LMMC together comprise about 1/5th of all cases of closed spinal dysraphism and up to 50% of cases of occult spinal dysraphism. The main differentiating feature between the LMC and LMMC is the location of the region of the placode-lipoma interface. In an LMC, the interface is located within the spinal canal, whereas the interface lies outside the spinal canal in the case of an LMMC due to expansion of the subarachnoid space (S. L. Rufener et al. 2010; Rossi et al. 2004).

Spinal Lipoma

Spinal lipoma is a relatively simple manifestation of premature disjunction spectrum with a lipoma within the confines of the neural canal. It is of two types: terminal (filum) lipoma and intra-dural lipoma. An intra-dural lipoma is located dorsally in the midline but within the thecal sac. These lipomas are often located in the lumbar and lumbosacral regions. Terminal lipoma refers to fibro-lipomatous thickening of the filum terminale and are often asymptomatic and considered a standard variant unless associated with features of tethered cord.

Anomalies of Primary Neurulation: Non-Disjunction

Non-disjunction refers to the failure of the neural plate to separate from the surrounding surface ectoderm, leading to the formation of a neuro-ectodermal connection/ tract preventing neural and mesenchymal migration. This type leads to open neural tube defects, myelocele, meningocele, meningomyelocele, and dermal sinus tracts (Giuffre 1966).

Spinal Dermal Sinus

In this least severe type of non-disjunction disorder, there is a dermal sinus underneath an atypical surface skin dimple connecting to the conus medullaris via the subcutaneous tissues and dura mater. A similar anomaly is also found in the occipital region. This anomaly is often associated with a subtle form of focal underlying spina bifida, such as a bifid lumbar spinous process. When patent, the tract may predispose the patient to meningitis and be associated with spinal dermoid/ epidermoid in up to 50% of such cases (Wilson et al. 2016).

Meningomyelocele & Myelocele

These represent a more severe form of non-disjunction leading to non-closure of the neural tube with exposure of the neural placode leading to an open neural tube defect. Meningomyelocele accounts for 98% of open neural tube defects, and myelocele account for the remaining 2% and thus are rare. The neural placode is flush with skin in cases of myelocele with an open central canal, while the placode projects beyond the skin in cases of meningomyelocele. These conditions are associated with a neural placode and malformed and often non-developed caudal neural tissue elements.

Hemi-Myelocele & Hemi-Myelomeningocele

These represent combined anomalies of gastrulation and primary neurulation and are extremely rare. In these cases, there is diastematomyelia, and one cord fails to complete the process of neurulation due to non-disjunction.

Anomalies of Secondary Neurulation

Abnormalities in the process of secondary neurulation are mostly those associated with regression of the caudal cell mass, while non-development of the secondary neurulation process as seen with CRS is a more severe form and is often associated with gastrulation anomalies and has been described before.

Low Lying Spinal Cord and Thickened Filum with Tethered Cord

Low lying spinal cord refers to cord termination of the spinal cord below the level of L2 after the first month of infancy or the presence of a thickened filum terminale. It leads to manifestations of tethered cord syndrome following a growth spurt. T1 weighted sequences on axial images accurately detect this. A filum thickness of more than 1.5 mm (hyperintense on T1 weighted images compared to cauda equina roots) fetches the diagnosis of a thickened filum.

Anterior Sacral and Intra-Sacral Meningocele

Intra-sacral meningocele refers to an arachnoid lined cystic space-occupying lesion within an enlarged sacral spinal canal; it is often accompanied by sacral anomalies, diastematomyelia, and tethered cord syndrome. An anterior sacral meningocele is a sizeable cerebrospinal fluid (CSF) filled anterior meningeal outpouching of the sacral end of the thecal sac, often through an enlarged neural foramen. This often presents with a CSF-filled presacral mass.

Terminal Myelo-Cystocele

A large terminal spinal cord syrinx characterizes this condition associated with a low-lying spinal cord. The enlarged terminal portion of the spinal cord (harboring the syrinx) is herniating through a posterior spinal defect. The terminal syrinx is essentially a type of hydromyelia that communicates with the central canal of the cranial spinal cord. The meningocele portion of the herniated mass communicates with the rest of the spinal subarachnoid space but not with the terminal syrinx.

Epidemiology and Burden of Disease

There are many theories for developing neural tube disorders that clinically manifest as spinal dysraphism. A single etiology fails to explain the occurrence of this pathology with a myriad of presentations. Amongst the proposed reason for the development of such disorders is; decreased maternal folic acid levels, younger maternal age (teenage pregnancy) as well as pregnancy in advanced maternal age, lower socioeconomic status, increased intake of caffeine by mother during pregnancy, ethnicity (higher incidence in non- Hispanic whites and Hispanics) and maternal intake of medications (Valproate, Methotrexate, Isotretinoin, Antiretroviral drugs), maternal obesity and diabetes, as well as genetic factors. Many unknown environmental factors remain concealed and have a role in developing spinal dysraphism (Phillips, Burton, and Evans 2017; Alexander, Matthews, and Murphy 2015; Au, Ashley-Koch, and Northrup 2010).

About two decades ago, neural tube defects worldwide incidence was 4-10 per 1,000 live births. Following mandatory fortification of cereals and grains by the U.S. Food and Drug Administration (FDA), there was a significant fall in the prevalence of neural tube defects, i.e., 1-2 per 1,000 live births since 1998 (Williams et al. 2015). Certain geographical regions and social customs (consanguineous marriages) contributed to the increased incidence of spinal dysraphism in Southeast Asian countries, including the Indian sub-continent. The most recent data from hospital-based studies conducted in different cities of India suggested a prevalence of 0.5 to 11 per 1,000 live births (Greene and Copp 2009; Verma and Mathews 1983). Males are affected more than females (ratio- 1.5:1), and the incidence of hydrocephalus was less than that in the western populations (Kumar and Singh 2003). A systematic review conducted in 2020 suggested the prevalence of 2.8% to have Occult Spinal Dysraphism (OSD) with midline cutaneous stigmata amongst the pediatric population. Amongst these patients who underwent spinal ultrasonography screening, less than 1% of patients required neurosurgical intervention (Choi et al. 2020).

Anaesthetic Considerations in the Surgery for Spinal Dysraphism

Preoperative Evaluations

Because of general anaesthesia, its systemic effects, and the physiologic stress due to surgery, coexisting diseases must be identified, and potential physiological derangements are anticipated. Preoperative laboratory tests should be ordered specific to the proposed procedure. Vertebral defects may be related to other congenital anomalies in the neonate. The VACTERL syndrome- vertebral defects, anorectal malformations, cardiovascular anomalies, tracheoesophageal fistula, renal (genitourinary), and limb malformations, is seen in 13% of children with tracheoesophageal fistula.

(Milstein, Lau, and Bickers 1985). In addition to the anatomic and physiological complexities associated with paediatric patients. Significant medical history, details of previous surgical procedures, previous anaesthetic history, and details of ongoing treatments must be reviewed, emphasizing the respiratory, cardiovascular, and central nervous systems. Impairment of functional capacity of these systems can be related to or a result of the condition requiring spinal dysraphism surgery.

Airway examination is mandatory since some craniofacial anomalies usually require specialized methods to secure the airway. Congenital heart diseases may mandate echocardiography in assessing the heart function, and a paediatric cardiologist's evaluation may be necessary.

Preoperative sedatives like oral midazolam can allay separation anxiety (McCann and Kain 2001). Preoperative fasting regimens should be adequate to reduce the risk of pulmonary aspiration as well as preventing hemodynamic and metabolic instability during anaesthesia.

All gloves and equipment used should be latex-free in these children to prevent allergy (Vanderhaegen et al. 2010). Drug history should be detailed for concomitant antiepileptic therapy as it can affect the hepatic function and drug metabolism.

Induction and Maintenance of Anaesthesia

General anaesthesia involving intubation and mechanical ventilation is the usual modality. Induction may be inhalation or intravenous. The usual agent of inhalation induction is sevoflurane. If intravenous patent access is present, agents like Thiopentone or Propofol can be used (Vanderhaegen et al. 2010).

Airway Management

After induction airway should be secured using reinforced (armoured) tubes of appropriate sizes. Muscle relaxation is usually done with nondepolarizing neuromuscular blockers to facilitate intubation. To repair meningoceles and myelomeningoceles, tracheal intubation may need to be performed with the child positioned in the lateral decubitus position or supine using a padded doughnut ring to protect the neuroplaque from rupture (Conran and Kahana 1998). Cuffed tubes can be used if regular pressure monitoring is done and the nasotracheal approach can reduce kinking. Patients are then placed prone, ensuring that the endotracheal tube and intravenous lines are well connected. Eyes and pressure points should be well padded.

Vascular Access

A large-bore cannula is required in more than one limb. Inadequate venous access, failure of attempts or anticipated blood loss justifies central venous cannulation. Fluid management includes maintenance fluid, replacement of third space loss and blood loss.

Fluid and Electrolyte Management

For hemodynamic stability, the careful maintenance of intravascular volume and electrolytes during surgery is required. Acute blood loss or venous air embolism can suddenly lead to cardiovascular collapse. Normovolemia should be kept throughout the surgery. Maximum allowable blood loss should be calculated beforehand. Hematocrit values 21-25% indicate blood transfusion. Initial blood loss should be replaced with 3ml of normal saline for every 1 ml of blood loss or a colloid solution, such as 55% albumin, equal blood loss. Subject to the extent and length of vascular beds, subsequent fluid administration at 3-10 ml/kg/hr may be required.

Pediatric patients are at significant risk of hypoglycemia. Premature infants who have restricted reserves of glycogen and less gluconeogenesis require continuous infusions of glucose at 5-6mg/kg/min to maintain serum levels.

Maintenance of Anaesthesia

Any standard technique, either inhalation or intravenous, can maintain anaesthesia (Davidson et al. 2005). Muscle relaxants should be stopped or their effects allowed to diminish when monitoring of motor function during neurosurgery is carried out. Monitoring during spinal surgery in routine includes ECG, pulse oximetry, capnography and blood gases monitoring, temperature (core and peripheral), BP (usually invasive in long surgical cases) and neuromuscular block.

Central venous pressure monitoring should be carried out in patients with associated cardiac pathology and expected massive blood loss. A urinary catheter should be placed in such patients. Repeated monitoring of hemoglobin, hematocrit, acid-base status and coagulation profile may be required in some patients. Monitoring for air embolus should also be done. Spinal cord electrical monitoring should be included as part of the routine perioperative care of these patients and should be carried out throughout the surgery. Intraoperative hypothermia should be minimized by warming mattresses, hot air warming blankets and warmed intravenous fluids (Lee and Wheeler 1997).

Preservation of body heat is crucial for infants with myelomeningocele, as autonomic control below the defect level is abnormal in them. Operating ambient theatre temperature should be a minimum 27degree centigrade, and a radiant heat warmer should be used during positioning and skin draping. Placement of neonate should be done on a warm air mattress to conserve heat.

Intraoperative management aims to minimize spinal cord ischemia and compression on the spinal cord. These are attained by maintaining spinal cord perfusion pressure by monitoring blood pressure and reducing venous congestion by correctly positioning the patient to prevent abdominal compression. Both propofol and remifentanil can be used for total intravenous anaesthesia in older children.

Intraoperative Spinal Cord Monitoring

In spinal dysraphism surgery, intraoperative monitoring of spinal cord function has been viewed as a standard of care (Sala, Kržan, and Deletis 2002). Methods of monitoring the integrity of the spinal cord function intraoperatively include somatosensory evoked potential (SSEP) and motor evoked potential (MEP) (Costa et al. 2007; MacDonald 2006). Volatile anaesthetics and opioids influence SSEP and MEP values (Boisseau et al. 2002).

Any intraoperative neurophysiologic changes in monitoring (increased latency, decreased amplitude, or complete loss of waveform) should be immediately reported to the anaesthesiologist and surgeon. The team (anaesthesiologist, surgeon, neurophysiologist) should then decide how to address and deal with the changes.

Postoperative Anaesthetic Management

Conclusion of where the child should be shifted after operation depends on the pre-existing cardiac and respiratory function, intraoperative events, duration of the surgery, amount of blood loss, hypothermia, and analgesic needs. Some children require postoperative mechanical ventilation and nursing in intensive care. Opioid-based analgesia is usually used for pain after surgery (Nemergut, Yaster, and Colby 2013). This is done using a morphine infusion or a nurse-controlled analgesia infusion in young children less than seven years of age. Children, more than seven years of age may self-operate patient-controlled analgesia. Infiltration of the stitch site with local anaesthetic at the end of surgery will improve pain in the immediate postoperative period. Opioids can be supplemented with paracetamol. Non-steroidal anti-inflammatory drugs can be added if there are no contraindications to their use.

Surgical Management

The surgical intervention is the mainstay of treatment to relieve the symptoms of tethering and prevent further progression of the musculoskeletal deformity. The guiding principle for surgical management of Spinal dysraphism include:

- Total detethering of the adhered cord structure
- Reconstruction of the dural tube with adequate CSF column around the spinal cord to eliminate the chances of tethering (Figure 3).

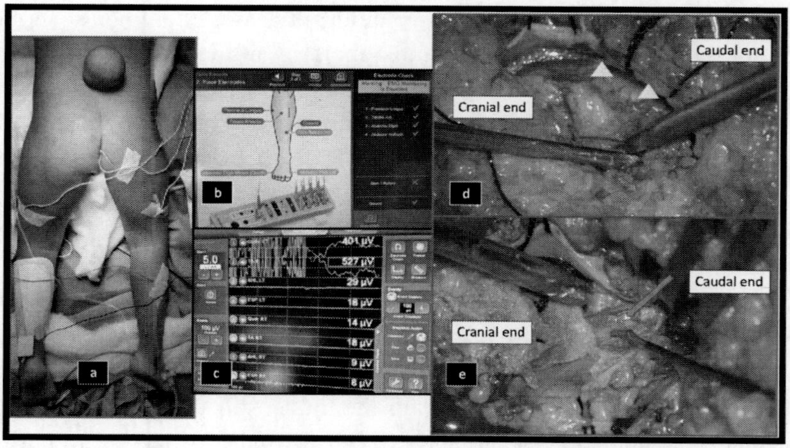

Figure 3. a) The intraoperative images of a child in prone position. The electrodes for intraoperative neuromonitoring (IONM) are placed and secured with micropores. b and c) The IONM monitor showing the arrangement of electrodes and the intraoperative electrophysiological recording during the decompression of the intradural spinal lipoma. d) The intraoperative photograph of spinal lipoma decompression with red curvilinear line showing the plane of lipoma excision. The two yellow triangles point towards the tuft of nerve fibers arising from the conus. e) This image reveals the status after adequate lipoma decompression and separating the filum terminale from rest of the nerve fibers. The filum is being stimulated with IONM probe and blue arrow point towards the filum which is separated with a cottonoids piece underneath the filum.

Post-Operative Follow-up and Rehabilitation

Following adequate surgical management, there still exists a theoretical possibility of retethering. This retethering may manifest in the form of the reappearance of clinical symptoms such as sensory-motor deficits, bladder bowel complaints or dull aching localised pain over the lower back. Even in the best hands, the incidence of retethering has been estimated to be about 20-35%. These patients require regular follow-up, and the reappearance of clinical symptoms raises the red flag. Thorough clinical examination in the form of electrophysiological and urodynamic evaluation is mandatory to quantify the amount of impairment compared to the preoperative status. The involvement of orthopaedics, cardiothoracic and vascular surgeons, and urologists help manage associated anomalies in most of these children (Venkataramana 2011b).

The associated vertebral column deformity, most commonly scoliosis, does not require surgical correction in a majority of the cases. The deformity in the foot, most common club foot, talipes equinovarus, requires close follow up with orthopaedics and physical medicine and rehabilitation to bring these children into the mainstream of society.

Conclusion

The developmental anomaly of spinal dysraphism requires teamwork to deal with the deformity and the components that require early attention to prevent further damage. A national registry for the Indian subcontinent; is mandatory to detect the actual prevalence and effects of food fortification to curb this pathology, which significantly impacts the quality of life of the individual and the family. The tertiary centre health care facilities have an essential responsibility to disseminate public awareness regarding prompt medical attention for children with dysraphic spectrum and commitment to eliminate this disabling anomaly.

Authors Declaration

The corresponding authors guarantee on behalf of all the co-authors regarding copyright issues and patients' permission to use clinical and radiological photographs.

The authors have no potential conflict of interest to declare.

References

Acharya, Ullas V, Hima Pendharkar, Dandu R Varma, Nupur Pruthi, and Shriram Varadarajan. 2017. 'Spinal Dysraphism Illustrated; Embroyology Revisited'. *The Indian Journal of Radiology & Imaging* 27 (4): 417.

Alexander, Michael A, Dennis J Matthews, and Kevin P Murphy. 2015. *Pediatric Rehabilitation: Principles and Practice*. Demos Medical Publishing.

Anderson, NG, S Jordan, MR MacFarlane, and M Lovell-Smith. 1994. 'Diastematomyelia: Diagnosis by Prenatal Sonography.' *AJR. American Journal of Roentgenology* 163 (4): 911–14.

Aoyama, Hirohiko, and Ken Asamoto. 2000. 'The Developmental Fate of the Rostral/Caudal Half of a Somite for Vertebra and Rib Formation: Experimental Confirmation of the Resegmentation Theory Using Chick-Quail Chimeras'. *Mechanisms of Development* 99 (1–2): 71–82.

Au, Kit Sing, Allison Ashley-Koch, and Hope Northrup. 2010. 'Epidemiologic and Genetic Aspects of Spina Bifida and Other Neural Tube Defects'. *Developmental Disabilities Research Reviews* 16 (1): 6–15.

Boisseau, N, M Madany, P Staccini, G Armando, F Martin, D Grimaud, and M Raucoules-Aimé. 2002. 'Comparison of the Effects of Sevoflurane and Propofol on Cortical Somatosensory Evoked Potentials'. *British Journal of Anaesthesia* 88 (6): 785–89.

Boulas, Mari M. 2009. 'Recognition of Caudal Regression Syndrome'. *Advances in Neonatal Care* 9 (2): 61–69.

Boyd, PA, DG Wellesley, HEK De Walle, R Tenconi, S Garcia-Minaur, GRJ Zandwijken, C Stoll, and M Clementi. 2000. 'Evaluation of the Prenatal Diagnosis of Neural Tube Defects by Fetal Ultrasonographic Examination in Different Centres across Europe'. *Journal of Medical Screening* 7 (4): 169–74.

Candenas, M, R Villa, R Fernandez Collar, MJ Moina, S Pintado, F Garcia Saez, and FV Alvarez. 1995. 'Maternal Serum Alpha-Fetoprotein Screening for Neural Tube Defects: Report of a Program with More than 30000 Screened Pregnancies'. *Acta Obstetricia et Gynecologica Scandinavica* 74 (4): 266–69.

Choi, Se Jin, Hee Mang Yoon, Ji Sun Hwang, Chong Hyun Suh, Ah Young Jung, Young Ah Cho, and Jin Seong Lee. 2020. 'Incidence of Occult Spinal Dysraphism among Infants with Cutaneous Stigmata and Proportion Managed with Neurosurgery: A Systematic Review and Meta-Analysis'. *JAMA Network Open* 3 (7): e207221–e207221.

Conran, Aisling M, and Madelyn Kahana. 1998. 'Anesthetic Considerations in Neonatal Neurosurgical Patients'. *Neurosurgery Clinics of North America* 9 (1): 181–85.

Costa, P, A Bruno, M Bonzanino, F Massaro, L Caruso, I Vincenzo, P Ciaramitaro, and E Montalenti. 2007. 'Somatosensory-and Motor-Evoked Potential Monitoring during Spine and Spinal Cord Surgery'. *Spinal Cord* 45 (1): 86–91.

Davidson, Andrew J, Grace H Huang, Caroline Czarnecki, Margaret A Gibson, Stephanie A Stewart, Kris Jamsen, and Robyn Stargatt. 2005. 'Awareness during Anesthesia in Children: A Prospective Cohort Study'. *Anesthesia & Analgesia* 100 (3): 653–61.

French, Barry N. 1983. 'The Embryology of Spinal Dysraphism.' *Clinical Neurosurgery* 30: 295–340.

Giuffre, R. 1966. 'Intradural Spinal Lipomas'. *Acta Neurochirurgica* 14 (1): 69–95.

Greene, Nicholas DE, and Andrew J Copp. 2009. 'Development of the Vertebrate Central Nervous System: Formation of the Neural Tube'. *Prenatal Diagnosis: Published in Affiliation with the International Society for Prenatal Diagnosis* 29 (4): 303–11.

Kumar, Raj, and SN Singh. 2003. 'Spinal Dysraphism: Trends in Northern India'. *Pediatric Neurosurgery* 38 (3): 133–45.

Lee, Benjamin, and Tamara Wheeler. 1997. 'Emergence and Recovery from Anesthesia for Pediatric Patients in the Post-Anesthesia Care Unit'. *Pediatric Annals* 26 (8): 461–69.

MacDonald, David B. 2006. 'Intraoperative Motor Evoked Potential Monitoring: Overview and Update'. *Journal of Clinical Monitoring and Computing* 20 (5): 347–77.

McCann, Mary Ellen, and Zeev N Kain. 2001. 'The Management of Preoperative Anxiety in Children: An Update'. *Anesthesia & Analgesia* 93 (1): 98–105.

Melvin, Elizabeth C, Timothy M George, Gordon Worley, Amy Franklin, Joanne Mackey, Kristi Viles, Nishu Shah, Courtney R Drake, David S Enterline, and David McLone. 2000. 'Genetic Studies in Neural Tube Defects'. *Pediatric Neurosurgery* 32 (1): 1–9.

Milstein, Jay M, Marcella Lau, and Rex G Bickers. 1985. 'Tracheal Agenesis in Infants with VATER Association'. *American Journal of Diseases of Children* 139 (1): 77–80.

Nemergut, Michael E, Myron Yaster, and Christopher E Colby. 2013. 'Sedation and Analgesia to Facilitate Mechanical Ventilation'. *Clinics in Perinatology* 40 (3): 539–58.

Pang, Dachling, and Dominic NP Thompson. 2011. 'Embryology and Bony Malformations of the Craniovertebral Junction'. *Child's Nervous System* 27 (4): 523–64.

Phillips, Leslie A, Justin M Burton, and Sarah Helen Evans. 2017. 'Spina Bifida Management'. *Current Problems in Pediatric and Adolescent Health Care* 47 (7): 173–77.

Rossi, Andrea, Roberta Biancheri, Armando Cama, Gianluca Piatelli, Marcello Ravegnani, and Paolo Tortori-Donati. 2004. 'Imaging in Spine and Spinal Cord Malformations'. *European Journal of Radiology* 50 (2): 177–200.

Rufener, Stephanie, Mohannad Ibrahim, and Hemant A Parmar. 2011. 'Imaging of Congenital Spine and Spinal Cord Malformations'. *Neuroimaging Clinics* 21 (3): 659–76.

Rufener, Stephanie L, Mohannad Ibrahim, Charles A Raybaud, and Hemant A Parmar. 2010. 'Congenital Spine and Spinal Cord Malformations—Pictorial Review'. *American Journal of Roentgenology* 194 (3_supplement): S26–37.

Sadler, TW. 2005. 'Embryology of Neural Tube Development'. In: 135:2–8. Wiley Online Library. 2012. 'Chapter 18: Central Nervous System. U Sadler TW, Langman's Medical Embriology, (Pp 287–320)'.

Sala, Francesco, Matevž J Kržan, and Vedran Deletis. 2002. 'Intraoperative Neurophysiological Monitoring in Pediatric Neurosurgery: Why, When, How?' *Child's Nervous System* 18 (6): 264–87.

Schoenwolf, Gary C. 1979. 'Histological and Ultrastructural Observations of Tail Bud Formation in the Chick Embryo'. *The Anatomical Record* 193 (1): 131–47.

Steinbok, Paul. 1995. 'Dysraphic Lesions of the Cervical Spinal Cord'. *Neurosurgery Clinics of North America* 6 (2): 367–76.

Tortori-Donati, P, A Rossi, and A Cama. 2000. 'Spinal Dysraphism: A Review of Neuroradiological Features with Embryological Correlations and Proposal for a New Classification'. *Neuroradiology* 42 (7): 471–91.

Vanderhaegen, Joke, Gunnar Naulaers, Sabine Van Huffel, Christine Vanhole, and Karel Allegaert. 2010. 'Cerebral and Systemic Hemodynamic Effects of Intravenous Bolus Administration of Propofol in Neonates'. *Neonatology* 98 (1): 57–63.

Venkataramana, NK. 2011a. 'Spinal Dysraphism'. *Journal of Pediatric Neurosciences* 6 (Suppl1): S31.2011b. 'Spinal Dysraphism'. *Journal of Pediatric Neurosciences* 6 (Suppl1): S31–40.

Verma, IC, and AR Mathews. 1983. 'Congenital Malformations in India'. *Peoples of India: Some Genetic Aspects. New Delhi: Indian Council of Medical Research*, 70.

Williams, Jennifer, Cara T Mai, Joe Mulinare, Jennifer Isenburg, Timothy J Flood, Mary Ethen, Barbara Frohnert, and Russell S Kirby. 2015. 'Updated Estimates of Neural Tube Defects Prevented by Mandatory Folic Acid Fortification—United States, 1995–2011'. *MMWR. Morbidity and Mortality Weekly Report* 64 (1): 1.

Wilson, Peyton, Erin Hayes, Andrew Barber, and Jacob Lohr. 2016. 'Screening for Spinal Dysraphisms in Newborns with Sacral Dimples'. *Clinical Pediatrics* 55 (11): 1064–70.

Chapter 10

Dynamic Lumbar Stabilization Procedure: Recent Advancements in Spinal Fusion Surgery

S. Shashivadhanan*

Military Hospital Bathinda, India

Abstract

Lumbar spine fusion surgery is an accepted modality for treating degenerative disc disease, since past four decades. Rigid lumbar spinal fixation has been considered as one of the factors in accelerating degeneration in adjacent vertebral body motion segments. It is also associated with flat back syndrome, pseudoarthrosis, osteopenia and worsening of biomechanics of spinal ligaments. The procedure lacks predictable outcome. These inconsistencies stem from a lack of understanding regarding the exact mechanism of back pain. Dynamic lumbar stabilization was developed to mitigate these problems by mimicking natural pattern of weight bearing and spine movement. Dynamic fusion works on the principle of transference of weight from the degenerated disc / facet to stabilization construct which is dynamic. This is accomplished without compromising the normal segmental motion. In spite of offering several advantages dynamic fusion lacks universal acceptance. This research paper attempts to critically evaluate dynamic fusion procedure and compare it with the conventional rigid fusion. This was a single institutional prospective study carried out from Sept 2016 to 2018. 10 patients underwent Posterior Dynamic Stabilization. The clinical outcomes of the dynamic stabilization group were compared with 10 historical controls (n = 10) who had undergone rigid lumbar fusion and shared a same clinical profile. Thrust was on

*Corresponing Author's E-mail: drshashivadhanan@gmail.com.

In: Neurosurgery Research
Editors: Amit Agrawal, Pradeep Chouksey, Adesh Shrivastava et al.
ISBN: 978-1-68507-837-9

evaluating posture related pain and improvement in functional status between the two groups. The dynamic stabilization group reported better pain relief in flexion /extension related movement while the rigid fixation group reported better pain relief in axial rotation. The group undergoing dynamic fixation showed marked improvement in functional status in comparison to rigid fixation group. Complication rates were similar in both groups. Our study showed Posterior Lumbar Dynamic stabilization to be better than rigid lumbar fixation in those patients having flexion extension posture related pain. However further confirmation requires stronger randomized trials with evaluation of long-term outcomes before conclusively proving its superiority over rigid fusion. Minimally invasive approaches for dynamic fusion must be directed towards maintaining the integrity of soft tissue structures while restoring dynamic stability and even load transmission. Disc regeneration seems a future possibility which might change the way we treat the culprit disc.

Introduction

A lumbar pedicular dynamic stabilization system (LPDSS) is an alternative to fusion for treatment of degenerative disc disease (DDD). In this study, clinical and radiological results of one LPDSS (Saphinaz, Medikon AS, Turkey) were compared with results of rigid fixation after two-year follow-up.

Methods

All patients had anteroposterior and lateral standing x-rays of the lumbar spine preoperatively and at 3 months, 12 months and 24 months after surgery. Lordosis of the lumbar spine, segmental lordosis and ratio of the height of the intervertebral disc spaces (IVS) measured preoperatively and at 3 months, 12 months and 24 months after surgery.

All patients underwent MRI and/or CT preoperatively, 3months, 12 months and 24 months postoperatively. The ratio of intervertebral disc space to vertebral body height (IVS) and segmental and lumbar lordosis were evaluated preoperatively and postoperatively. Pain scores were evaluated via Visual Analog Scale (VAS) and Oswestry Disability Index (ODI) preoperatively and postoperatively.

Results

In both groups, the VAS and ODI scores decreased significantly from preoperatively to postoperatively. There was no difference in the scores between groups except that a lower VAS and ODI scores were observed after 3 months in the LPDSS group. In both groups, the IVS ratio remained unchanged between preoperative and postoperative conditions. The lumbar and segmental lordotic angles decreased insignificantly to preoperative levels in the months following surgery.

Conclusion

Patients with LPDSS had equivalent relief of pain and maintenance of sagittal balance to patients with standard rigid screw-rod fixation. LPDSS appears to be a good alternative to rigid fixation.

Keywords: degenerative disc disease, dynamic stabilization, lumbar spine, rigid stabilization, posterior pedicle based dynamic stabilization, rigid stabilization, posterior pedicle based dynamic stabilization, rigid stabilization

Introduction

Albee first described fusion as the treatment for Potts Spine whereas Hibbs is credited for performing the first ever spinal fusion surgery for spinal deformity correction (Albee F H, 1911, Hibbs R A 1911). Since past four decades lumbar fusion has become the standard of care for treatment of degenerative diseases of lumbar spine with instability. Long term studies show that outcomes of fusion surgery are unpredictable. Moreover there are associated complications including adjacent segment disease and pseudoarthrosis. (Cheng B C et al., 2007, Kumar A 2008). 5 to 100% patients undergoing spinal fusion surgery land up with adjacent segment disease due to degeneration. (Harrop JS 2008). Dynamic stabilization of the spine was developed to solve the problem arising from rigid fusion Dynamic stabilization attempts to mimic natural spine movements. Dynamic construct is known to take away load from degenerated disc or facet without compromising on segmental motion. This is the philosophy governing dynamic stabilization devices. This also translates to reduced stress on the adjacent segments (Gardner A & Pande K C 2002, Lee C K 1988, Hilibrand AS and Robbins M 2004).

It has been hypothesized that Posterior Dynamic stabilization controls abnormal motion, promoting normal load transmission thereby preserving global spine movement. This will prevent progression of adjacent segment degeneration. It might also help in reversal of early disc degenerative changes. (Sengupta DK 2005). Posterior dynamic fixation devices aim at reducing burden on the posterior facets and annulus of intervertebral disc. They also limit motion in certain defined planes. Rigid stabilization, has so far failed, to completely address the problem of, mechanical back pain arising from spinal instability. Pedicle screw-based posterior dynamic stabilization evolved in order to mitigate this problem. Studies of these devices have shown promising results in the short term.

From the anatomical stand point, low back pain may arise from pain sensitive structures which include vertebral endplates, periosteum, annulus, facet joints, and soft tissues. Studies have proven, that clinical outcome following fusion, are worse as compared to radiological outcomes (Fritzell P et al. 2002). Many patients fail to improve in spite of successful radiological spinal fusion (Boos N 1997). Rigid lumbar spinal fixation has been considered as one of the factors in accelerating degeneration in adjacent vertebral body motion segments. These issues made patients and care givers search for alternative treatment modalities (Cunningham BW 1997).

Kirkaldy-Willis and Farfan in 1982 theorized the three stage concept of lumbar spine degeneration. The starting point seems to be disc degeneration leading to abnormal load distribution across the disc space (Mulholland RC 2002 15). Proponents of fixed fusion reasoned that pain occurred due to instability which happened due to abnormal movement and believed abnormal mobility to be the main cause for pain. Therefore curtailing mobility seemed the logical treatment for pain relief. In the short term they were proven right but over a period of time their unpredictable outcomes have raised many questions. Failure to address the problem of abnormal weight transmission across the disc space seems to be an important factor resulting in failure of rigid fusion procedures. In recent past, many posterior dynamic stabilization systems have been developed as a viable alternative to rigid fusion of lumbar spine.

In 2002, Stoll and colleagues developed the dynamic neutralization system (Dynesys). The system has titanium alloy pedicle screw, cord of polyester material, and spacer made of polycarbonate urethane. The cord resists undue spine flexion and the spacer resists undue spinal extension. They work in tandem so as to maintain spinal motion within physiological limits. The spacer also avoids discal compression during extension, thereby preventing foraminal compromise. This also reduces load on the posterior part of annulus of disc. (Stoll TM 2002, Delamate RB 2006, Schnake KJ 2006).

Materials and Methods

It this pilot study, 10 patients were subjected to dynamic fusion and their outcomes were compared with 10 historical controls who shared a similar clinical profile. It was carried out in a single service hospital from Sep 2017 to Sep 2018.Patients operated using the Dynesys dynamic neutralization system, were allotted to the dynamic fusion Group (total 10) and those undergoing conventional lumbar fusion were allotted to the Fixed Fusion Group (total 10). All underwent single level fusion. All procedures were performed under general anesthesia. Patients were placed prone so as to maintain lumbar lordosis. Fusion was carried out using mid line approach, separating lamina from the muscular attachments. For foraminal stenosis, fecetectectomy, Flavectomy and discectomy was performed on case to case basis.

Patient Population

Of the 10 patients in each group, 07 were men and 03 were women. At the time of surgery, mean age of patients was 61.0 ± 12.9 years. The duration of mean clinical and radiological follow-up was 6 months. 69.5 Kg was the mean weight of patients with their weights ranging between 56 to 88 kg.

Inclusion criteria: All patients with painful degenerated lumbar disc disease following failed conservative management were included in the study. Patients with painful spondylolysis or mobile sagittal instability (up to Grade One spondylolisthesis from 1st to 5th Lumbar vertebra) were included. Only cases requiring single level fusion were considered.

Exclusion criteria: Patients less than 18 years and more than 70 years of age, those having tumors, primary infections or inflammatory etiologies, congenital neural tube defects, visceral diseases, history of previous spinal trauma or previous lumbar surgeries were excluded from the study.

Pain relief outcomes was analyzed using Visual analogue scale (VAS) pertaining to low back pain and Oswestry disability index (ODI).

Complication were grouped as those occurring within the first 24 hours and those within 7 days during post-operative period. Patients were reevaluated after 6 months and pain scores were analyzed.

Observation

7th post-operative day pain scores showed that there was 75% improvement in the posture related (flexion/extension) radicular pain in the Dynamic Lumbar fusion group. In comparison, the rigid fusion group showed no improvement in posture related (flexion/extension) radicular pain. At the same time the Dynamic Lumbar fusion group showed no improvement in pain arising due to axial rotation. The patients under fixed fusion group reported significant improvement in pain arising due to axial rotation.

Table 1. Comparison of posture related vertebral and radicular pain in the Rigid Fusion and Dynamic Fusion Group

	Preoperative pain status			Post operative pain status		
	Posture related (flexion/extension) vertebral pain	Posture related (flexion/extension) radicular pain	posture related (axial rotation)	posture related (flexion/extension) vertebral pain	posture related (flexion/extension) radicular pain	posture related (axial rotation) pain
Rigid fusion (total 10)	90%	60%	70%	70%	40%	50%
Dynamic fusion (toal 10)	100%	80%	70%	80%	10%	70%

Table 2. Comparison of functional capacity (movement related) score (maximum of 10) before and after surgery

	Functional capacity score (Before Surgery)	Functional Capacity score (6 months after surgery)
Rigid Fusion	3/10	5/10
Dynamic Fusion	3/10	7/10

Functional Capacity measured as a subjective score measured in a scale of 0 to10 where 0/10 meant absolutely disability and 10/10 meant no functional disability during movement. Dynamic fusion group reported better improvement in their movement related functional capability.

Table 3. Complication in two groups

	Intra operative period	First 7 post-operative day	6 Months following surgery
Rigid Fusion	Nil	Nil	Nil
Dynamic Fusion	Nil	Nil	Nil

Result

Our study showed that during short term, dynamic fusion group provided significant reduction in posture related pain during flexion and extension. However, it did not improve pain during to axial rotation. The Fixed fusion group reported more significant pain relief on axial rotation. At the end of 6 months following surgery, the dynamic fusion group had significantly more improvement in their functional status. As the technique of surgical exposure was same in both procedures there were no difficulties or complications encountered in both groups. There was marginal increase in duration of radiation exposure in the dynamic fusion group.

Discussion

Intervertebral Disc is the largest avascular structure in adults having two principle biomechanical roles. One is to transmit load in an isotropic manner thereby preventing abnormal load transmission. The second role is to allow a controlled range of motion there by preventing neural compression on the adjacent structures. The spinal muscles also seem to play a significant role in maintaining global spine movement. Studies have shown that relative loading patterns rather than absolute patterns of loading were implicated in pain generation during the degenerative cascade. (McNally D S & Adams M A 1992). A common observation validating this fact is that, as the spine ages, the aged disc redistributes the weight evenly thereby resulting in spontaneous pain relief (McNally D S et al. 1996, Modic M T 1990). At the bone implant interface, owing to controlled motion, there is increased surface stress leading to fracture at this site. (Goel V K 1991). Doing rigid fixation without analysis of painful movement renders the motion segment totally immobile. This approach of “sledge hammer to crack a nut” is not only overkill but might prove detrimental in the long term. This approach may interfere with maintenance of sagittal balance during various postures as spine is a dynamic entity. Fusion has been implicated in accelerating disease of adjacent motion segments. Posterior distracting procedures have resulted in spinal deformities like flat back syndrome (Okuda S et al. 2004). Pseudoarthrosis (15-96%) (Etminan M et al. 2002), osteopenia due to fusion device (McAfee et al. 1997) and destruction in biomechanical properties of the spinal ligaments (Kotani Y et al., 1998). Dynamic stabilization proposes to replicate the success of large volume Interbody fusions, without the loss of movement by creating a near normal loading pattern. Dynamic systems, therefore, may work by altering the load transmission across the degenerated disc while maintaining movement within normal physiological limits. Altering load transmission across the degenerated disc may prove beneficial for regeneration of the disc.

Dynamic stabilization of the spine was developed to solve the problem arising from rigid fusion. Dynamic stabilization attempts to mimic natural spine movements. Dynamic construct is known to take away load from degenerated disc or facet without compromising on segmental motion. This is the philosophy governing dynamic stabilization devices.

This study evaluated the clinical and radiological results for a relatively new posterior dynamic screw stabilization system used to treat chronic low back pain in degenerative disc disease (DDD) patients. Six month follow up has shown that dynamic screw stabilization had better short term clinical outcomes as compared to rigid posterior lumbar stabilization systems.

Dynamic stabilization devices have come into the lumbar fusion arena since past two decades. It is hypothesized that Dynamic stabilization devices, help in maintaining neutral posture of the affected spinal segment and controls sagittal plane bending at same level. They modify the load distribution within the segment, particularly within the intervertebral disc (McNally DS et al. 2006). The Dynesys Dynamic Stabilization System (DSS) (Zimmer Spine, Inc., Warsaw, IN, USA), has shown to partly achieve some of the goals of dynamic stabilization. (Beastall J et al. 2008) In degenerative disc disease there is an increased load transmission across the anterior column of spine. With Dynamic fusion the axis of rotation is shifted posteriorly leading to posterior redistribution of load. It is probable that that reduced anterior load transmission might provide better chances of regeneration to the degenerated disc (Bozku H et al. 2010).

Reversal of the degenerative process can offer true cure to the problem of degenerated lumbar disc. So far all existing modalities of treatment attempt to treat the secondary effects of degeneration. Only gene therapy holds promise in reversing the disc degeneration, so as to restore its normal load bearing and transmission function (Nishida K at al 1998, Goupille P et al. 1998). Studies carried out by Cienciala et al. have shown that during three year follow up of patients with Dynesys, there was disappearance of disc bulge with near total reversal of canal stenosis with restoration of posterior longitudinal ligament (Cienciala J 2010).

Our experience shows that Dynamic Fusion does not require fusion of healthy adjacent transition segment. This may not be the case in rigid fusion. (For example, for an unstable segment localized at L4 /L5, single level dynamic fusion would suffice addressing the L4/5 segment and leave the healthy LS /S1 level which may not be the case in rigid fusion). Secondly in case of unsuccessful outcomes the dynamic system can be converted to rigid system without much tissue disruption. Proponents of rigid fusion might argue that the purpose of implant is to provide temporary stabilization till permanent fusion takes place. The existing dynamic fusion implants may not be able to provide dynamic stabilization throughout life. Even if that be the case, going by Wolfe's law, eventually increased compressive loads during flexion will lead to bony fusion across the Interbody space. This might transform the dynamic fusion into a rigid fusion. We also feel that the dynamic fusion can be used in those cases of painful degenerative disc disease with no demonstrable sagittal instability where in, the decompressive procedure per say would render the segment unstable (e.g., foraminal stenosis due to sagittalized facet requiring bilateral medial facetectomy).

So far, existing literature on this subject appears inconclusive and does not establish clear superiority of fusion over rigid fusion in the long term. There are very few randomized trials comparing merits and demerits of both of these systems. Their methodology of quality comparison, independent randomization, binding and follow up leaves a lot to be desired.

Conclusion

The Dynamic fusion is a newer method which attempts to address problems associated with rigid fusion. Current available data does not establish its superiority in the long term. Dynamic fusion addresses some of the short falls of rigid fusion. However, it lacks universal validation. Current understanding of all the pain mechanism in degenerative disc disease still remains shrouded in mystery. As the exact cause of pain remains elusive so also is the cure. What also need cognizance are the osseoligamentous construct and para spinal muscle which play a definite role in maintaining delicate spinal stability during adoption of various postures. Minimally invasive approaches must be directed towards maintaining the integrity of these soft tissue structures while restoring dynamic stability and even load transmission. Disc regeneration seems a future possibility which might change the way we treat the culprit disc.

There is some evidence to show that dynamic stabilization slows the disc degenerative process. It might help in rehydration once compressive load is taken off. Further prospective and randomized clinical trials are needed to prove the superiority of dynamic stabilization system over the conventional rigid fixation systems. Furthermore defining that subset of patients, timing of intervention and duration of follow up is the main challenge. All these aspects need to be clearly defined before drawing conclusions.

To summarize, our experience and existing body of literature shows that Dynamic lumbar stabilization appears to be a better alternative to rigid lumbar fixation in patients having flexion extension posture related pain and canal stenosis. We recommend its use in addressing cases where instability results following surgical neural decompression. However it requires stronger randomized trials with evaluation of long term outcomes before conclusively proving its superiority over rigid fusion.

Conflict of Interest

None

References

Albee F H, "Transplantation of a portion of the tibia into the spine for Pott's disease," *Journal of the American Medical Association*, vol. 57, p. 11, article 885, 1911.

Beastall J, Karadimas E, Siddiqui M, et al. The Dynesys lumbar spinal stabilization system; a preliminary report on positional magnetic resonance imaging findings. *Spine.* 2007;32(6):685–90.

Boos N, Webb JK. Pedicle screw fixation in spinal disorders: A European view. *Eur. Spine J.* 1997; 6:2–18.

Bozku H, Senoğlu M, Baek S, et al. Dynamic lumber pedicle screw-rod stabilization in vitro biomechanical comparison with standard rigid pedicle screw-rod stabilization. *J. Neurosurg. Spine.* 2010; 12:183–9.

Cheng B C, Gordon J, Cheng J, and Welch W C, "Immediate biomechanical effects of lumbar posterior dynamic stabilization above a circumferential fusion," *Spine*, vol. 32, no. 23, pp. 2551–2557, 2007.

Cienciala J, Chaloupka R, Repko M, and Krbec M, "Dynamic neutralization using the dynesys system for treatment of degenerative disc disease of the lumbar spine," *Acta Chirurgiae Orthopaedicae et Traumatologiae Cechoslovaca*, vol. 77, no. 3, pp. 203–208, 2010.

Cunningham B W, Kotani Y, McNulty P S, et al. The effect of spinal destabilization and instrumentation on lumbar intradiscal pressure: An in vitro biomechanical analysis. *Spine.* 1997;22:2655–63.

Delamater R B, Maxwell J, Davis R, Sherman J, and Welch W, "Nonfusion application of the Dynesys system in the lumbar spine: early results from IDE multicenter trial," *Spine Journal*, vol. 6, supplement 1, article S77, no. 5, 2006. View at Google Scholar.

Etminan M, Girardi F, Khan S, et al. Revision strategies for lumbar pseudarthrosis. *Orthoped. Clin. North Am.* 2002;33(2):381–92.

Fritzell P, Hägg O, Wessberg P, et al. Swedish Lumbar Spine Study Group. Chronic low back pain and fusion; a comparison of three surgical techniques: A prospective multicenter randomized study from the Swedish lumbar spine study group. *Spine.* 2002; 27: 1131–41.

Gardner A and Pande K C, "Graf ligamentoplasty: a 7-year follow-up," *European Spine Journal,* vol. 11, supplement 2, pp. S157–S163, 2002.

Goel V K, Lim T H, Gwon J, et al. Effects of rigidity of an internal fixation device. A comprehensive biomechanical investigation. *Spine.* 1991; 16: 155–61.

Goupille P, Jayson MI, Valat J P, Freemont A J (1998) Matrix metalloproteinases: the clue to intervertebral disc degeneration? *Spine* 23: 1612- 1626).

Harrop J S, Youssef J A, Maltenfort M et al. "Lumbar adjacent segment degeneration and disease after arthrodesis and total disc arthroplasty," *Spine*, vol. 33, no. 15, pp. 1701–1707, 2008.

Hibbs R A, "An operation for progressive spinal deformities," *New York Medical Journal*, vol. 93, pp. 1013–1016, 1911.

Hilibrand A S and M. Robbins M, "Adjacent segment degeneration and adjacent segment disease: the consequences of spinal fusion?" *Spine Journal*, vol. 4, supplement 6, pp. S190–S194, 2004.

Kotani Y, Cunningham B W, Cappuccino A, et al. The effects of spinal fixation and destabilization on the biomechanical and histologic properties of spinal ligaments. An in vivo study. *Spine.* 1998;23:672–82

Kumar A, Beastall J, J. Hughes J et al. "Disc changes in the bridged and adjacent segments after Dynesys dynamic stabilization system after two years," *Spine*, vol. 33, no. 26, pp. 2909–2914, 2008

Lee C K, "Accelerated degeneration of the segment adjacent to a lumbar fusion," *Spine*, vol. 13, no. 3, pp. 375–377, 1988.

McAfee P C, Farey I D, Sutterlin C E, et al. The effect of spinal implant rigidity on vertebral bone density. A canine model. *Spine.* 1991;16:190–97.

McNally D S, Adams M A (1992) internal intervertebral disc mechanics as revealed by stress profilometry. *Spine* 17:66-73.

McNally D S. Rationale for dynamic stabilization. In: Kim D H, Cammisa F P, Fessler R G, editors. *Dynamic Reconstruction of the Spine*. 1st. Thieme: New York; 2006. pp. 237–43.

McNally D S, Shackleford I M, Goodship A E, et al. In vivo stress measurement can predict pain on discography. *Spine* 1996; 21:2580–7.

Modic M T. Degenerative disc disease and back pain. *Magnetic Resonance Imaging Clin. North Am*. 1999;7:481–91, viii.

Mulholland RC, Sengupta DK. Rationale, principles and experimental evaluation of the concept of soft stabilization. *Eur. Spine J.* 2002;11(2):198–205.

Nishida K, Kang J D, Suh J K, Robbins P D, Evans C H, Gilbertson L G (1998) Adenovirus-mediated gene transfer to nucleus pulposus cells. Implications for the treatment of intervertebral disc degeneration. *Spine* 23:2437-2442; [discussion 2443].

Okuda S, Iwasaki M, Miyauchi A, et al. Risk factors for adjacent segment degeneration after PLIF. *Spine* 2004; 29:1535–40.

Schnake K J, Schaeren S, and Jeanneret B, "Dynamic stabilization in addition to decompression for lumbar spinal stenosis with degenerative spondylolisthesis," *Spine*, vol. 31, no. 4, pp. 442–449, 2006.

Sengupta D K, "Dynamic stabilization devices in the treatment of low back pain," *Neurology India*, vol. 53, no. 4, pp. 466–474, 2005.

Stoll T M, Dubois G, and Schwarzenbach O, "The dynamic neutralization system for the spine: a multi-center study of a novel non-fusion system," *European Spine Journal*, vol. 11, supplement 2, pp. S170–S178, 2002.

Chapter 11

Ankylosing Spondylitis and Rheumatoid Arthritis

Orlin Pavlov[1], MD and Kalina Koleva[2], MD
[1]Department of Neurosurgery, Klinikum Fulda, University Medicine Marburg, Marburg, Germany
[2]Department of Pharmacology and Toxicology, Medical University of Sofia, Sofia, Bulgaria

Abstract

Ankylosing spondylitis (AS) and rheumatoid arthritis (RA) represent one of the most common entities, encountered by the spine surgeons. Several important pathways in the process of chronic inflammation have been identified. These pathways play an important role in sustaining AS and RA. Several new drug classes have been developed, including tumour necrosis factor inhibitors (TNFis) and biological disease-modifying antirheumatic drugs (bDMARDs), which are blocking IL-17. These novel approaches are currently applied in the treatment of AS und RA. Two Anti-TNF and one Anti-IL-17A pharmacological agents have been currently approved in USA. Interestingly, DMARD and the other biologic agents have shown to decrease the incidence of cervical spine involvement in the cases of RA. However, once the process of chronic inflammation in the cervical spine has begun, it is not possible to stop the progression only with DMARD.

There is a shifting paradigm to a more aggressive treatment of patients with fractures and AS. The patients with history of trauma and AS need extensive diagnostic procedures to rule out a fracture. Aggressive treatment *via* stabilization techniques is aimed due to the high rate of hardware failure. On the other hand, RA affects the cervical spine

In: Neurosurgery Research
Editors: Amit Agrawal, Pradeep Chouksey, Adesh Shrivastava et al.
ISBN: 978-1-68507-837-9

in numerous ways, all leading to instability and neurologic deficit. Those patients remain surgical candidates.

Ankylosing Spondylitis

Ankylosing spondylitis (AS) is a chronic immune-mediated inflammatory arthritis, which belongs to the group of chronic spondyloarthritis. AS occurs mainly in male patients in their thirties and affects the sacroiliac joints and the axial skeleton. The HLA-B27 allele is known to have a strong association with the disease (Chen et al. 2017). It is already estimated that a wide spectrum of the HLA-B alleles plays a crucial role in the development and the sustainment of the chronic immune response. Several important pathways in the process of chronic inflammation have been identified. These pathways play an important role in sustaining AS. Several new drug classes have been developed, including tumour necrosis factor inhibitors (TNFis) and biological disease-modifying antirheumatic drugs (bDMARDs), which are blocking IL-17.

Advances in Conservative Treatment

From a surgical point of view, AS represents a bone altering disease, where bone formation and bone resorption coexist. This leads to the formation of bone erosions and syndesmophytes. This process is mediated by IL-17, which promotes osteoclastogenesis directly and through the activation of receptor activator of nuclear factor kappa B (RANK) (Chabaud and Miossec 2001, Lubberts et al. 2001). TNF-α triggers bone destruction through the RANK-RANK ligand (RANK-RANKL) system and inhibits bone formation *via* the overexpression of Dickkopf-related protein 1 (DKK1) (Sato et al. 2006), which then suppresses the WNT bone pathway (Sato et al. 2006, Baron and Rawadi 2007). The effects of IL-17 lead not only to bone destruction but also to a bone formation, especially on the sites with mechanical stress. The biological therapies are based on the above-mentioned cascade. Two Anti-TNF and one Anti-IL-17A pharmacological agents have been currently approved in USA for the treatment of AS. Infliximab, firstly mentioned in 2016 in PLANETAS study and Etanercept, firstly mentioned in 2017, which belong to the group of Anti-TNF, are among the most promising pharmacological agents (Park et al. 2016, Emery et al. 2017). The results of the treatment with Secukinumab, which belongs to the group of anti-IL-17, were published in 2017 in MEASURE 1 study. There are several anti-IL-17 pharmacological agents, which are currently under investigation: Ixekizumab, Brodaluma, Ustekinumab and ABT-122 (Garcia-Montoya, Gul, and Emery 2018). In USA, the Brodalumab and Ustekinumab are stopped from further investigation due to safety issues or lack of effectiveness. ABT-122 is a combined anti-IL-17A/TNF-α, which just passed Phase II clinical trials and Phase III clinical trial is scheduled to begin in 2022.

Advances in Diagnostic Management

"Less Is More"

Reinhold et al. conducted a literature review regarding the spine fractures in the patients with AS. Based on this literature review, the recommendations of the Spine Section of the German Society for Orthopaedics and Trauma (DGOU) were developed (Reinhold et al. 2018). The continuous spinal bone remodelling, with simultaneous ectopic bone formation and osteopenia, is the main reason for increased fracture risk in the patients with AS. According to these recommendations, any patient with AS, after a minor or major trauma with new pain, needs to undergo a further evaluation with X-Ray, CT or MRI, despite his/her neurological status. Patients with AS after trauma and pain without any neurological symptoms must undergo X-Ray plus CT. X-Ray misses common hyperextension fracture, which is why an additional CT (3 levels above and below the level of injury) is recommended. If no fracture is detected in these modalities, then an MRI is mandatory to rule out a fracture. However, if a fracture is already diagnosed with X-Ray and CT, then a CT-scan/MRI of the whole spine needs to be performed. The reason behind this recommendation is that multisegment or multilevel injuries occur in 6% to 8% in these patients (Zdichavsky et al. 2005). After completing the diagnostic phase, the therapeutic strategy needs to be developed.

If a patient with AS after trauma develops a new neurologic deficit, then the diagnostic protocol is straightforward. The risk to sustain a spinal cord injury, nerve root lesions, intramedullary edema or spinal epidural hematoma is 11.4 times higher with AS, compared to the general spine trauma population (Alaranta, Luoto, and Konttinen 2002). The patient needs to undergo X-Ray, CT-scan and MRI of the spine. After the assessment of the fracture, an emergency surgical intervention is required. It is recommended to use the AO Spine classification for the assessment of the fractures. The M2 case-specific modifier (TL system) is designated for patients with ASD (SA, DISH), rheumatologic conditions, or osteopenia/osteoporosis (Vaccaro et al. 2013, Reinhold et al. 2018). If no fracture is present, then an extensive neurologic diagnostic needs to be performed.

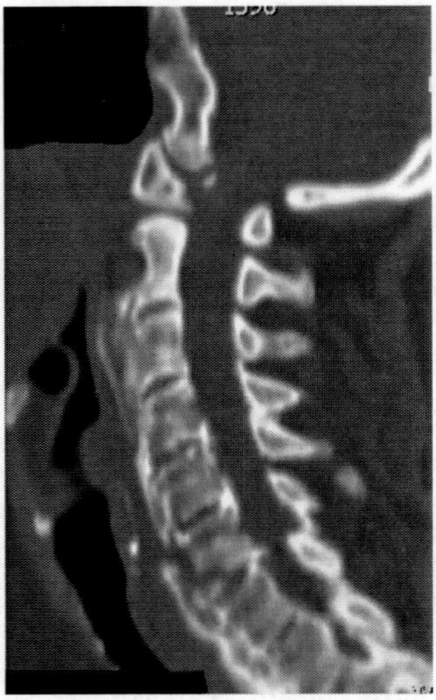

Figure 1. depicts a CT of a 81-years patient, who presents herself after a fall with neckpain and without any neurologic deficit. CT shows a dislocation fracture of C6 (Type B fracture).

Advances in Surgical Management

The advances in the surgical management are based on the experience with imaging modalities and follow-ups of the patients with AS after trauma. The patients with cervical fractures remain the most difficult group, regarding the development of treatment strategy. DGOU recommends for unstable B- and C-Type fractures a combined anterior-posterior instrumentation. When a ventral stabilization is not possible, then a longer construct (3 levels above and 3levels below the level of the fracture) is recommended for internal fixation. The recommendations do not specify whether masa lateralis or pedicle screws should be used.

The treatment of fractures in thoracolumber (TL) segment begins with reduction-closed or open. A good closed reduction could be achieved on the operating table with appropriate pads, correcting the deformity up to a point.

Large gaps could be closed by changing the position of the operating table. In some extreme cases, as in B3 type fractures, an inclined upright sitting position might be necessary (Reinhold et al. 2018). After the reduction of the fracture, a transpedicular screw fixation follows (at least 2 levels above and below the level of the fracture). A careful planning of the surgical strategy is mandatory, in order to avoid implant-related problems, such as screw loosening, implant failure, etc. From a biomechnaical point of view, usually monoaxial pedicle screw systems are recommended, in order to achieve a better fracture reduction and obtain higher intrinsic construct stability (Reinhold et al. 2018). Despite the good surgical planning and execution, the surgeon has to be prepared for at least 15% screw loosening rates (Balling and Weckbach 2015). The recent studies have shown that AS coexists with osteoporosis in 25% of the cases (Klingberg et al. 2014). In the cases of poor bone quality, it is recommended to extend the internal fixation on 3 levels below and above the level of the fracture, in order to achieve a good destribution of the forces on more vertebrae. Augmentation techniques are also avaible to aid the spinal stabilization.

Achieving a good reduction of the fracture is not always possible. In those cases, *in situ* internal fixation has to be performed. In order to avoid early implant failure or pseudarthrosis, a ventral stabilization has to be carried out. From biomechanical point of view, the expandable cages with anterior angular stable plating system are recommended to achieve the best possible biomechanical stability. One should avoid wedge osteotomy in correcting a preexisting deformity, because this technique could further jeopardize the biomechanical stability.

Rheumatoid Arthritis

Rheumatoid arthritis (RA) is a chronic systemic inflammatory disease, which primarily affects bones, ligaments and joints. The extraskeletal manifestation of the disease affects the cardio-vascular, pulmonary, hematologic and gastrointestinal system. RA affects most commonly the small joints, but the second most commonly affected region is the cervical spine (Wasserman, Moskovich, and Razi 2011, Joaquim and Appenzeller 2014). The most recent studies suggest that around 80% of the patients will have some kind of cervical spine involvement within the first two years of the diagnosis of RA (Joaquim and Appenzeller 2014). The chronic inflammation in the cervical spine leads to the formation of pannus, which results in bony erosions and ligament laxity.

The upper cervical spine could be affected in one of the three ways: atlantoaxial instability, cranial settling and subaxial subluxation or a combination of three. All these pathological findings represent a cervical instability (Joaquim and Appenzeller 2014). C2 vertebrae could be additionally affected by RA, causing atraumatic erosions or fractures in dens axis (Mallory, Halasz, and Clarke 2014). These findings further contribute to the development of atlantoaxial instability. When left untreated, the cervical spine involvement is the main reason for worsening of quality of life. Complications as hydrocephalus, cardiac arrest and neurological deterioration are the drug treatment limiting factors. Interestingly, DMARD and the other biologic agents have shown to decrease the incidence of cervical spine involvement. However, once the process of chronic inflammation in the cervical spine has begun, it can't be stopped with any biological agents (Mallory, Halasz, and Clarke 2014). In those cases, surgery is required, in order to achieve atlantoaxial and craniocervical stabilization.

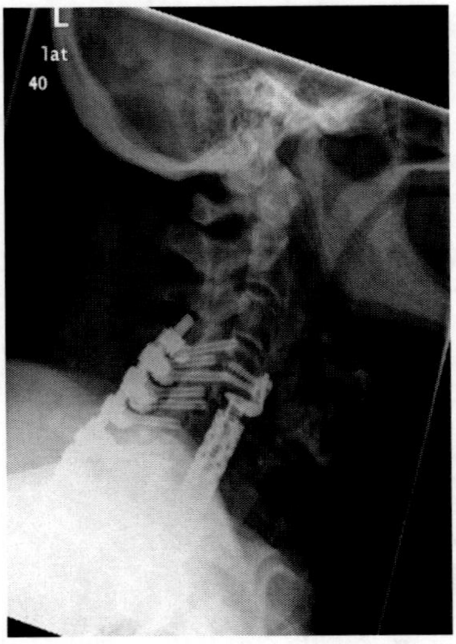

Figure 2. depicts a postoperative X-Ray after a circumferential reconstruction of C5 and C6 Author's Archive.

Advances in Surgical Treatment

Sunahara et al. reported a series of 21 patients with untreated atlantoaxial instability (AAI), who refused to undergo a surgical treatment. None of these patients showed any improvement over the course of observation. 16 patients showed further neurological deterioration with myelopathy (Sunahara et al. 1997). This is one of the many case series, which demonstrate the importance of surgical treatment in the cases of cervical spine involvement.

In patients with AAI, C1-C2 fixation remains a golden standard. Several techniques to achieve C1-C2 fusion are already famous: Gallie's technique (Wiring and grafting), with its modifications, Magerl's technique (transarticular screw fixation C1/C2), Goel and Laheri's technique (plate and screw fixation) and Harms and Melcher's technique (C1 lateral mass screws and C2 pedicle or pars screws). The different techniques have been widely discussed in biomechanical and clinical studies. A salvage method for fixation in C2 has been developed (translaminar screw fixation) in the cases where no pedicle or pars screws are possible. The first screw is inserted by placing a pilot hole at the junction of the spinous process and lamina along the cranial margin of the lamina, for the second screw on the contralateral side, a caudal margin of the lamina is chosen (Gillick, Wainwright, and Das 2015). In the cases of cranial settling and vertical migration of the dens, a occipitocervical fixation is required (Lipson 1985). *Grob* first described this technique in 1991, which involves occipital plating and cervical screws (Grob et al. 1991, Gillick, Wainwright, and Das 2015). In those cases, it is of utter importance that the head is fixed in neutral position. A hyperextension results in *in situ* fixation of the head with extension- "Stargazer position" and hyperflexion results in aberrant position of the kin to the sternum. Decompression of the spinal canal could be achieved simultaneously throughout a laminectomy of C1. Schmitt-Sody, M et al. published one of the largest Series of dorsal stabilizations in RA, where 12 occipitocervical stabilizations procedures were performed. In these series, most of the patients received short-segment occipitocervical stabilization (C0 up to C3/C4) and only 3 patients received a long stabilization, extending from C0 to thoracic region (Schmitt-Sody et al. 2008). Interestingly, in these series, only two of patients developed subaxial subluxation (SAS), which is a much lower percentage than reported in literature. RA alters the biomechanical properties of the other segments as well, which requires a larger construct, in order to achieve fusion and to reduce the risk for further complications. Hirano et al. suggested that stopping too short to the thoracic spine would result in significant subaxial disease progression (Hirano et al. 2010).

Cranial settling (CS) is the next step of the atlantoaxial instability, which causes a ventral compression of the cervicomedullary junction. An odontoidectomy is required in those cases, in order to achieve adequate decompression. There are two main ways to achieve a ventral decompression in CS-transoral-transpharyngeal approach (TTA) or endoscopic approach with resection of the dens. The TTA provides surgical access to the anterior clivus, C1 and C2. Transoral approaches provide the fundamental anatomy and technique upon which the more complex jaw-splitting approaches are based (Hsu et al. 2010). The use of a transnasal approach to access the anterior structures of the upper neck was first reported in an anatomical study by Alfieri et al. in 2002 (Alfieri, Jho, and Tschabitscher 2002). The first use of this technique for a decompression of the anterior cervical structures was used 3 years later by Kassam et al. (Kassam et al. 2005). For the endoscopic approaches a good assessment of the preoperative images is necessary. The use of navigation techniques provides accurate intraoperative localization of pathology, thereby increasing the chance of a complete odontoidectomy (Harminder et al. 2018). The data in literature is limited to case series and case reports. Up to this point, there are no prospective clinical trials utilizing this technique. One of the main advantages of the endoscopic-endonasal approach is the fact that all of the complications, related to the transoral approach, are avoided. At our institution, we developed a new approach to achieve a ventral decompression and stabilization. A new combined transoral-transcervical approach was developed to maximize exposure and surgical corridor, allowing not only decompression but also stabilization *via* cage and plate. This case report is planned for publication by the end of 2022. This approach offers significant advantages over the extended transoral approach with jaw-splitting techniques and offers a wide working angle.

The SAS is another complication of RA. It could begin *de novo* or after a monosegmental dorsal fusion (C1/C2). Clarke et al. and Ito et al. have reported a very high level of SAS after a monosegmental dorsal instrumentation-39% and 57, 6% respectively (Clarke et al. 2006, Ito et al. 2009). In the case series of Ito et al., a transarticular screw fixation was used, whereas *Clarke* et al. used C1-C2 fusion. The incidence of subaxial instability in patients with RA, who underwent cervical arthrodesis, may be higher than previously reported, indicating the need for a continuous follow-up (Clarke et al. 2006). After the subaxial subluxation has occurred, the surgeon needs to address two entities-cervical deformity and spinal canal compression. The optimal treatment of

SAS remains multilevel laminectomy plus dorsal fusion. *Roy-Camille, Magerl, An,* and *Anderson* have each described variations of screw placement that differ by their entry point into the lateral mass and their trajectory (Roy-Camille 1991, Magerl and Seemann 1987, Gillick, Wainwright, and Das 2015).

The initial treatment of patients with RA remains conservative (Mallory, Halasz, and Clarke 2014). This is due to the advances made in the pharmacological therapy. Since rheumatologist are the ones referring the patient to the spine surgeons, early identification of SAS is mandatory. The surgical treatment is indicated in the cases of craniocervical instability. The mortality of rheumatoid patients undergoing cervical spine surgery has significantly improved over the last 30 years. Between 1980 and 1990 the 10-year survival rate was 35%, compared to 55% in the decade of 2000-2010 (P = 0.001, LogRank) (Bhatia et al. 2014). With the advances in neuroanesthesia and postoperative care, the rate of perioperative complications is diminishing.

Conclusion

Identifying the surgical candidates among patients with trauma begins with careful anamnesis. Patients with AS require a more aggressive diagnostic work-up to rule out an unstable fracture. Aggressive treatment *via* stabilization is aimed due to the high rate of hardware failure. On the other hand, RA affects the cervical spine in numerous ways, leading to cervical instability and neurologic deficit. Despite the higher mortality and morbidity rate, these patients remain surgical candidates.

References

Alaranta, H., S. Luoto, and Y. T. Konttinen. 2002. "Traumatic spinal cord injury as a complication to ankylosing spondylitis. An extended report." *Clin. Exp. Rheumatol.* 20 (1):66-8.

Alfieri, A., H. D. Jho, and M. Tschabitscher. 2002. "Endoscopic endonasal approach to the ventral cranio-cervical junction: anatomical study." *Acta Neurochi.r (Wien)* 144 (3):219-25; discussion 225. doi: 10.1007/s007010200029.

Balling, H., and A. Weckbach. 2015. "Hyperextension injuries of the thoracolumbar spine in diffuse idiopathic skeletal hyperostosis." *Spine (Phila Pa 1976)* 40 (2):E61-7. doi: 10.1097/brs.0000000000000676.

Baron, R., and G. Rawadi. 2007. "Targeting the Wnt/beta-catenin pathway to regulate bone formation in the adult skeleton." *Endocrinology* 148 (6):2635-43. doi: 10.1210/en. 2007-0270.

Bhatia, Robin, Nikolas Haliasos, Pierluigi Vergara, Caroline Anderson, and Adrian Casey. 2014. "The surgical management of the rheumatoid spine: Has the evolution of surgical intervention changed outcomes?" *Journal of Craniovertebral Junction & Spine* 5 (1):38-43. doi: 10.4103/0974-8237.135221.

Chabaud, M., and P. Miossec. 2001. "The combination of tumor necrosis factor alpha blockade with interleukin-1 and interleukin-17 blockade is more effective for controlling synovial inflammation and bone resorption in an ex vivo model." *Arthritis Rheum.* 44 (6):1293-303. doi: 10.1002/1529-0131(200106)44:6<1293::aid-art221> 3.0.co;2-t.

Chen, B., J. Li, C. He, D. Li, W. Tong, Y. Zou, and W. Xu. 2017. "Role of HLA-B27 in the pathogenesis of ankylosing spondylitis (Review)." *Mol. Med. Rep.* 15 (4):1943-1951. doi: 10.3892/mmr.2017.6248.

Clarke, M. J., A. A. Cohen-Gadol, M. J. Ebersold, and M. E. Cabanela. 2006. "Long-term incidence of subaxial cervical spine instability following cervical arthrodesis surgery in patients with rheumatoid arthritis." *Surg. Neurol.* 66 (2):136-40; discussion 140. doi: 10.1016/j.surneu.2005.12.037.

Emery, Paul, Jirí Vencovský, Anna Sylwestrzak, Piotr Leszczynski, Wieslawa Porawska, Asta Baranauskaite, Vira Tseluyko, Vyacheslav M. Zhdan, Barbara Stasiuk, Roma Milasiene, Aaron Alejandro Barrera Rodriguez, Soo Yeon Cheong, and Jeehoon Ghil. 2017. "52-week results of the phase 3 randomized study comparing SB4 with reference etanercept in patients with active rheumatoid arthritis." *Rheumatology (Oxford, England)* 56 (12):2093-2101. doi: 10.1093/rheumatology/kex269.

Garcia-Montoya, Leticia, Hanna Gul, and Paul Emery. 2018. "Recent advances in ankylosing spondylitis: understanding the disease and management." *F1000Research* 7:F1000 Faculty Rev-1512. doi: 10.12688/f1000research.14956.1.

Gillick, John L., John Wainwright, and Kaushik Das. 2015. "Rheumatoid Arthritis and the Cervical Spine: A Review on the Role of Surgery." *International Journal of Rheumatology* 2015:252456-252456. doi: 10.1155/2015/252456.

Grob, D., J. Dvorak, M. Panjabi, M. Froehlich, and J. Hayek. 1991. "Posterior occipitocervical fusion. A preliminary report of a new technique." *Spine (Phila Pa 1976)* 16 (3 Suppl):S17-24.

Harminder, Singh, Rote Sarang, Jada Ajit, D. Bander Evan, J. Almodovar-Mercado Gustavo, I. Essayed Walid, Härtl Roger, K. Anand Vijay, H. Schwartz Theodore, and P. Greenfield Jeffrey. 2018. "Endoscopic endonasal odontoid resection with real-time intraoperative image-guided computed tomography: report of 4 cases." *Journal of Neurosurgery JNS* 128 (5):1486-1491. doi: 10.3171/2017.1.JNS162601.

Hirano, K., Y. Matsuyama, Y. Sakai, Y. Katayama, S. Imagama, Z. Ito, N. Wakao, H. Yoshihara, Y. Miura, M. Kamiya, K. Sato, H. Nakamura, and N. Ishiguro. 2010. "Surgical complications and management of occipitothoracic fusion for cervical destructive lesions in RA patients." *J. Spinal Disord. Tech.* 23 (2):121-6. doi: 10.1097/BSD.0b013e3181993315.

Hsu, W., J. P. Wolinsky, Z. L. Gokaslan, and D. M. Sciubba. 2010. "Transoral approaches to the cervical spine." *Neurosurgery* 66 (3 Suppl):119-25. doi: 10.1227/01.neu.0000365748.00721.0b.

Ito, H., M. Neo, T. Sakamoto, S. Fujibayashi, H. Yoshitomi, and T. Nakamura. 2009. "Subaxial subluxation after atlantoaxial transarticular screw fixation in rheumatoid patients." *Eur. Spine J.* 18 (6):869-76. doi: 10.1007/s00586-009-0945-5.

Joaquim, A. F., and S. Appenzeller. 2014. "Cervical spine involvement in rheumatoid arthritis - a systematic review." *Autoimmun. Rev.* 13 (12):1195-202. doi: 10.1016/j.autrev.2014.08.014.

Kassam, A. B., C. Snyderman, P. Gardner, R. Carrau, and R. Spiro. 2005. "The expanded endonasal approach: a fully endoscopic transnasal approach and resection of the odontoid process: technical case report." *Neurosurgery* 57 (1 Suppl):E213; discussion E213. doi: 10.1227/01.neu.0000163687.64774.e4.

Klingberg, E., M. Nurkkala, H. Carlsten, and H. Forsblad-d'Elia. 2014. "Biomarkers of bone metabolism in ankylosing spondylitis in relation to osteoproliferation and osteoporosis." *J. Rheumatol.* 41 (7):1349-56. doi: 10.3899/jrheum.131199.

Lipson, S. J. 1985. "Cervical myelopathy and posterior atlanto-axial subluxation in patients with rheumatoid arthritis." *J. Bone Joint Surg. Am.* 67 (4):593-7.

Lubberts, E., L. A. Joosten, B. Oppers, L. van den Bersselaar, C. J. Coenen-de Roo, J. K. Kolls, P. Schwarzenberger, F. A. van de Loo, and W. B. van den Berg. 2001. "IL-1-independent role of IL-17 in synovial inflammation and joint destruction during collagen-induced arthritis." *J. Immunol.* 167 (2):1004-13. doi: 10.4049/jimmunol.167.2.1004.

Magerl, F, and PS Seemann. 1987. "Cervical spine I, Strasbourg 1985."

Mallory, G. W., S. R. Halasz, and M. J. Clarke. 2014. "Advances in the treatment of cervical rheumatoid: Less surgery and less morbidity." *World J. Orthop.* 5 (3):292-303. doi: 10.5312/wjo.v5.i3.292.

Park, W., D. H. Yoo, J. Jaworski, J. Brzezicki, A. Gnylorybov, V. Kadinov, I. G. Sariego, C. Abud-Mendoza, W. J. Escalante, S. W. Kang, D. Andersone, F. Blanco, S. S. Hong, S. H. Lee, and J. Braun. 2016. "Comparable long-term efficacy, as assessed by patient-reported outcomes, safety and pharmacokinetics, of CT-P13 and reference infliximab in patients with ankylosing spondylitis: 54-week results from the randomized, parallel-group PLANETAS study." *Arthritis Res. Ther.* 18:25. doi: 10.1186/s13075-016-0930-4.

Reinhold, Maximilian, Christian Knop, Christian Kneitz, and Alexander Disch. 2018. "Spine Fractures in Ankylosing Diseases: Recommendations of the Spine Section of the German Society for Orthopaedics and Trauma (DGOU)." *Global Spine Journal* 8 (2 Suppl):56S-68S. doi: 10.1177/2192568217736268.

Roy-Camille, R. 1991. "Rationale and technique of Internal Fixation in Trauma of the Cervical Spine." *Spinal trauma.*

Sato, K., A. Suematsu, K. Okamoto, A. Yamaguchi, Y. Morishita, Y. Kadono, S. Tanaka, T. Kodama, S. Akira, Y. Iwakura, D. J. Cua, and H. Takayanagi. 2006. "Th17 functions as an osteoclastogenic helper T cell subset that links T cell activation and bone destruction." *J. Exp. Med.* 203 (12):2673-82. doi: 10.1084/jem.20061775.

Schmitt-Sody, M., C. Kirchhoff, S. Buhmann, P. Metz, C. Birkenmaier, H. Troullier, V. Jansson, and A. Veihelmann. 2008. "Timing of cervical spine stabilisation and outcome in patients with rheumatoid arthritis." *International Orthopaedics* 32 (4):511-516. doi: 10.1007/s00264-007-0349-2.

Sunahara, N., S. Matsunaga, T. Mori, K. Ijiri, and T. Sakou. 1997. "Clinical course of conservatively managed rheumatoid arthritis patients with myelopathy." *Spine (Phila Pa 1976)* 22 (22):2603-7; discussion 2608. doi: 10.1097/00007632-199711150-00004.

Vaccaro, A. R., C. Oner, C. K. Kepler, M. Dvorak, K. Schnake, C. Bellabarba, M. Reinhold, B. Aarabi, F. Kandziora, J. Chapman, R. Shanmuganathan, M. Fehlings, and L. Vialle. 2013. "AOSpine thoracolumbar spine injury classification system: fracture description, neurological status, and key modifiers." *Spine (Phila Pa 1976)* 38 (23):2028-37. doi: 10.1097/BRS.0b013e3182a8a381.

Wasserman, B. R., R. Moskovich, and A. E. Razi. 2011. "Rheumatoid arthritis of the cervical spine-clinical considerations." *Bull. NYU Hosp. Jt. Dis.* 69 (2):136-48.

Zdichavsky, M., M. Blauth, C. Knop, U. Lange, C. Krettek, and L. Bastian. 2005. "[Ankylosing spondylitis. Therapy and complications of 34 spine fractures]." *Chirurg* 76 (10):967-75. doi: 10.1007/s00104-005-1023-0.

Chapter 12

Hirayama Disease

M. Manoranjitha Kumari[1,*], R. Gopikrishnan[1] and A. S. Ramesh[2]

[1]Assistant Professor Neurosurgery, Jawaharlal Institute of Postgraduate Medical Education and Research, Puducherry, India

[2]Additional Professor and Head of the Department of Neurosurgery, Jawaharlal Institute of Postgraduate Medical Education and Research, Puducherry, India

Abstract

Hirayama disease (HD) is a self-limiting neurological illness of young males causing wasting of the unilateral upper limb muscles, predominantly the hand and forearm. It is also known as "Monomelic amyotrophy." Even though an uncommon clinical condition, it is increasingly recognized nowadays. HD presents with an insidious onset and has a slowly progressive natural history. The greater degree of flexion movement of the neck, resulting in compression of the spinal cord due to anterior shifting of the dura, is thought to be the underlying pathophysiology causing neural damage. Clinical findings of segmental spinal muscular atrophy and Flexion Extension views of Magnetic Resonance Imaging (MRI) cervical spine showing anterior displacement of posterior cervical dura along with increased flow voids due to venous congestion in the posterior epidural space confirm the diagnosis. Since flexion of the neck is the reason for the neurological disruption, it is imperative to prevent neck flexion either by surgery or by applying a cervical collar to arrest the neural damage. There are controversies regarding the role of surgery in this self-limiting disease; however,

*Corresponding Author's Email: manoranjithakumaridr@gmail.com.

In: Neurosurgery Research
Editors: Amit Agrawal, Pradeep Chouksey, Adesh Shrivastava et al.
ISBN: 978-1-68507-837-9

studies have proven the role of early surgery to halt the disease progression. Because it is rare and has a better prognosis than its close mimics motor neuron disease, good clinical knowledge is mandatory to diagnose early and halt the progression.

Introduction

Hirayama disease (HD) is an uncommon neurological condition. It was initially described by Hirayama et al. as "Juvenile muscular atrophy of unilateral upper extremity" in 1959 based on their early experience with 12 patients (K. Hirayama et al. 1963). Subsequently, numerous HD cases were reported from Asian countries, predominantly Japan (Keizo Hirayama 2008; Huang et al. 2008). It is a self-limiting condition with a benign course that closely resembles motor neuron disease, often affecting male patients in their teens. The classical presentation is progressive asymmetrical weakness and atrophy of the upper limb, mainly in the distal group of muscles. Radiological studies with MRI imaging done in neck flexion position revealed anterior displacement of the posterior dural sleeve of the cervical spinal canal, resulting in compression of the lower cervical segment of the spinal cord; Contrast-enhanced MRI revealed venous dilation and congestion in the posterior epidural space (Zhou et al. 2010; S. Pradhan and Gupta 1997). There is no clinical consensus regarding the best management of Hirayama disease yet.

Epidemiology and Demographics

HD is primarily a disease of the Asian population and is mainly reported from Japan, China, Malaysia, Taiwan, Sri Lanka, and India. Few cases and series have been reported from North America and Europe in the last two decades due to the increased migration of people (Ghosh et al., 2011; K. Hirayama 2000). HD predominantly affects young males (M: F 20:1), mostly in their teenage or early twenties (Tashiro et al. 2006). The weakness and wasting of the upper limb muscles, especially the hand and forearm, start insidiously during adolescence and progress slowly over several years to become evident in early adulthood (Tashiro et al. 2006; Kieser, Cox, and Kieser 2018). Hirayama noticed that the peak period of disease onset is roughly two years later than the peak of the longitudinal growth curve of adolescents in Japan. He presumed that there is a disparity between the length of the vertebral column and the spinal dura during the growth spurt (K. Hirayama 2000). Tashiro and colleagues proposed that male preponderance of this condition can be due to a sudden increase in males' longitudinal growth during adolescence compared with female counterparts (Tashiro et al. 2006). Though HD is non-familial in most instances, nine familial cases have been reported in English literature (Atchayaram, Vasudev, and Goel 2009).

Clinical Features and Differential Diagnosis

HD is a self-limiting disease with a progressive course that becomes static within a period of six or lesser years. It is seen predominantly in males aged between 15 and 25 years (Keizo Hirayama 2008; Tashiro et al. 2006). Clinically, patients will present with unilateral upper limb weakness and atrophy of muscles innervated by C7 to T1, but in some cases, the involvement can be bilateral and asymmetrical. The involved hand shows polyminimyoclonus on the attempted extension of the fingers and minimal transient deterioration of weakness during cold exposure (cold paresis). The patients may show normal cranial nerve, cerebellar, lower limb, sensory functions, superficial and deep tendon reflexes with preserved bladder. Electromyographic (EMG) studies show chronic denervation patterns of affected muscle groups (K. Hirayama 2000; Keizo Hirayama 2008).

In 1984, Gowrie Devi and colleagues from South India, in the initial series, reported 13 patients of Monomelic Amyotrophy with classical findings of HD. On long-term follow-up, none of these patients had disease progression in other limbs even after 15 years (Gourie-Devi, Suresh, and Shankar 1984). In 2003, the same author reported 44 patients who had disease progression up to 5 years in 79.5%, up to 8 years in 4.6% and subtle involvement of the opposite hand in 15.9% with a mean follow-up period of 9.7 years (2.5-23 years). None of the patients experienced new symptoms or deficits after attaining a static course (Gourie-Devi and Nalini 2003). None of the patients had lower limb involvement as well. Pradhan et al. and Raval et al. observed unilateral features in 90% of cases, whereas Sonwalkar et al. and Hassan et al. noticed bilateral features in most cases (75% and 55%, resp.) (Sunil Pradhan 2009; Raval et al. 2010; Sonwalkar et al. 2008; K. M. Hassan, Sahni, and Jha 2012). Hasan and colleagues observed sparing of brachioradialis (oblique amyotrophy) in all their cases, whereas other authors have reported 37.5% to 67.5% in their study. Cold paresis was an important finding noted in 35% in one study and 55% in another (Raval et al. 2010; Kaukab Maqbool Hassan and Sahni 2013). Very few patients had sensory symptoms such as dysesthesia of hands 9-12% (K. M. Hassan, Sahni, and Jha 2012).

HD should be differentiated from HD mimics such as Amyotrophic lateral sclerosis (ALS), spinal muscular atrophy (SMA), X-linked spinobulbar atrophy, and O'Sullivan-McLeod syndrome. The absence of lower motor neuron features and the lack of relentless progression differentiate it from ALS (Shneider and Hirano 2019). Historically, HD was thought to be a form of SMA. However, SMA occurs in children under 18 months of age except for SMA 3, which manifests after 18 months. Moreover, survivor motor neuron 1 (SMN 1) mutations seen in SMA were not found in patients with HD. Unlike HD, which affects C7-T1 myotomes, SMA affects tongue muscles, axial, respiratory, and limb muscles. Kennedy disease or X-linked spinobulbar atrophy affects predominantly males in their third or fourth decade of life. It usually involves the bulbar and proximal limb muscles (Shneider and Hirano 2019). O'Sullivan-McLeod syndrome involves the small muscles of the hand and evolves over a more extended period (25-40 years). (O'Sullivan and McLeod 1977).

Pathophysiology

The pathophysiology of HD is different from progressive motor neuron diseases and other degenerative diseases. Because of the disease's rareness and normal life expectancy of these patients, there have been very few cases of HD that have undergone autopsy to date. Several hypotheses have been put forward to explain the pathophysiology. Hirayama and colleagues were the first ones to do the autopsy on a 38-year-old patient who succumbed due to lung carcinoma with HD diagnosed at the age of 15. The autopsy revealed macroscopic evidence of flattening of the spinal cord at the lower cervical segment. Microscopically there was evidence of reduced anteroposterior diameter of the anterior horns, decreased numbers of large and small neurons with features of astrogliosis and central necrosis with no evidence of cavity formation predominantly noted at the C7 and C8 segments. They also noticed different stages of degenerative changes in the surviving neurons. Other intramedullary structures were found to be normal. They concluded that these pathological findings were strongly suggestive of ischemic cervical myelopathy of the lower cervical cord, excluded the possibility of motor neuron disease, and gave the term "juvenile focal cervical poliopathy." (K. Hirayama et al. 1987).

Subsequently, many authors have substantiated the findings described by Hirayama in his autopsy report with their imaging findings. Several authors have hypothesized that all these pathophysiological changes occur due to increased flexion movement of the cervical spine with tight, non-elastic cervical dura. Xiaojuan Xua and colleagues from China in 2011, for the first time, reported that patients with HD had a high degree of range of movement during neck flexion in the cervical X-ray (X. Xu et al. 2011). In his cervical radiological study, done in 31 HD cases and 40 controls, he found a higher degree of segmental and overall cervical flexion movements in HD patients than controls (X. Xu et al. 2011). All the patients in his study had forward displacement of posterior dura, spinal cord atrophy, widening of epidural space with flow voids in 58% of the cases (X. Xu et al. 2011). The presence of the tight dura, separation of the posterior dura from the subjacent lamina are thought to be the reason for the anterior displacement of the dura during neck flexion (Sonwalkar et al. 2008; C. J. Chen et al. 1998; C.-J. Chen et al. 2004).

According to Chen and colleagues, flexion and extension of the neck cause some difference in the length of the spinal canal (C.-J. Chen et al. 2004). During neck flexion, there is an increase in length of the anterior wall of the spinal canal about 1.5 cm, and 5 cm at the posterior wall, measured from T1 to the upper surface of the Atlas. The dura is firmly attached to the periosteum of the foramen magnum above, dorsal aspects of coccyx below, and freely suspended in the epidural space in the rest of the spinal canal. For a normal individual during flexion movement of the neck, this length discrepancies between the vertebral canal and the dura can be compensated by the slack dura without causing any forward shifting. Since the dura is not slack but tight in patients with HD, the dura's forward movement during neck flexion leads to cord compression and other multiple subclinical ischemic events on the anterior horn cells. These explanations may explain the forward shifting dura hypothesis; however, it is insufficient to explain asymmetrical cord involvement. Shinomiya and colleagues proposed another hypothesis called "posterior epidural ligament factor." They demonstrate two types of ligaments in the spinal epidural space, one being fine elastic and another one is a large ligament. These ligaments situated in the posterior epidural space between the posterior dural sac and the ligamentum flavum, are abundantly present between C1 & C2 and start decreasing from C2 and almost become sparse at C6 and C7 (Shinomiya et al. 1995). This differential distribution of these ligaments in the epidural space could be the reason for resistance against the detachment of dura mater from subjacent yellow ligament resulting in asymmetrical cord involvement. Atul Goel and colleagues observed multilevel spinal instability, including Atlantoaxial instability, in five patients with Hirayama disease who underwent posterior spinal fixation. They claim that Atlantoaxial instability may be related to the instability of sub-axial spinal segments or may even be the primary reason behind the pathogenesis for HD (Goel, Dhar, and Shah 2017).

Some authors have conducted genetic studies on HD as this disease has male predilections, occurring in particular ethnic groups, and closely resembling motor neuron disease. Misra and colleagues in 2005 studied 15 male patients from 14 families and concluded that the survivor motor neuron (SMN) gene deletion is absent in HD. Nevertheless, the disease occurs exclusively in male patients, and the presence of HD in 2 brothers of the same family suggests a possibility of x chromosome involvement. Hence, it needs further research on this subject (Misra et al. 2005). Some studies show that the patients with HD have elevated levels of serum total immunoglobulin E, and it has been postulated that HyperIgEamia precipitates HD (T.-H. Chen et al. 2010).

Among all the proposed pathogenesis, the theory of cervical spinal cord compression by the abnormally tight dura during flexion movement of the neck is the most accepted one. Due to repeated trauma to the spinal cord because of the tight anteriorly displaced dura during every flexion movement against the body of the vertebra causes impaired perfusion and neuronal loss (Lapresle 1969).

Diagnosis

Thorough clinical knowledge of the disease is of utmost importance to arrive at a diagnosis. HD has to be differentiated from motor neuron diseases. Dynamic MRI of the cervical spine is the gold standard technique to confirm the diagnosis; however, electrophysiological studies are indispensable to differentiate HD from other motor neuron diseases.

MRI Protocol and Image Analysis

Imaging of the cervical spine should be acquired with the patient lying supine, with the neck in neutral and flexed positions. The optimal flexion required is more than 25 degrees, and some authors prefer 30-40 degrees. Placing MRI-compatible support behind the nape of the neck can achieve adequate flexion (Boruah et al. 2018; Hou et al. 2012). Imaging protocol should include Sagittal T2- and T1- weighted images, sagittal and coronal short inversion recovery images, and axial T2- and T1-weighted fast spin-echo, axial 2D T2-weighted gradient recalled-echo sequences along with post gadolinium fat-suppressed sagittal T1-weighted sequences (Boruah et al. 2018; Lai et al. 2011). Asymmetrical thinning of the spinal cord in mid-sagittal MRI without any obvious canal stenosis or disc bulge in a young individual with wasting of hands and forearm should prompt the clinician to order flexion MRI images. Anterior displacement of posterior dura is an essential finding in flexion MRI to confirm the diagnosis. In their study done in Hirayama patients, Vincent Lai and colleagues found a significantly higher degree of anterior shifting of the posterior dural sac ranging from 6.1 to 7.8mm during neck flexion, which is far higher than the control group (Lai et al. 2011). Other findings included asymmetrical cervical cord flattening (68.9%), wide and prominent epidural space (100%), posterior epidural flow voids (46.7%), all of which did not appear in neutral MRI (Goel, Dhar, and Shah 2017). During flexion, it is assumed that there is increased pressure in the anterior epidural space, collapsing the epidural veins in the anterior epidural space, thereby enlarging the posterior epidural veins, which disappears in extension or neutral position. There was no venous obstruction in the cervical epidural space of patients with HD, as confirmed by Elsheikh et al. in his two patients with spinal angiography (Elsheikh et al. 2009). In some chronic patients, there appears to be atrophy of the spinal cord and hyperintensities in T2 weighted images resulting in snake eye appearance of the anterior horns (33%) (Lai et al. 2011). These MRI features suggest a late stage of HD, which indicates a worse prognosis (H. Xu et al. 2019). Apart from the pathology within the spinal canal, there seems to be pathology in spine biomechanics as well. In their retrospective study on 44 patients with HD concerning the sagittal balance of the cervical spine, Jian Song et al. found that HD patients had less C2–C7 Cervical lordosis angle, T1 slope, and cervical tilt angle when compared to their counterparts. These measurements became normalized after surgery (Song et al. 2020).

Electrophysiological Findings

There are various neurophysiological tests that can be performed to diagnose HD, and they are indispensable. Electromyographic studies show denervation patterns of the affected muscles. Ninety percent of the patients show acute or chronic denervation patterns of the unaffected homonymous muscle groups, suggesting a bilateral disease progression. There will be an increased fiber density with jitter in the progressive stage. In non-progressive stages, the jitter reduces due to the maturation of reinnervation (K. Hirayama 2000). In the Nerve conduction study, conduction velocity may be normal in most patients; very few show abnormalities in conduction velocity, 2.8% in the ulnar nerve, 5.4% in the median nerve (Huang et al. 2008). There will be evidence of abnormality in the amplitude of compound action potentials, 67.6% for the ulnar and 27% for the median nerve (Huang et al. 2008). Sensory nerve conductions are found to be normal in HD. F waves may show a mild increase in latency. There may also be low persistence with a singular high amplitude waveform, indicating reinnervation or denervation of the muscle (K. Hirayama 2000). Patients with HD can have an abnormal Soleus H reflex. The ratio between the maximum amplitude of the H reflex and the maximum amplitude of the M reflex (Hmax/Mmax) and vibratory inhibitory index of H reflex has a positive correlation with duration of illness and degree of forward shifting of the spinal cord (Zheng et al. 2017). Motor evoked potentials might show prolonged latency and reduced amplitude after transcranial stimulation. Somatosensory evoked potentials show abnormal conduction. Most of the electrophysiological abnormalities get aggravated during neck flexion.

Illustrative Case

A 20-year-old third-year engineering college student presented with a history of difficulty in writing, buttoning, unbuttoning his shirts, and the tremulousness of fingers for two years. He felt that it is more difficult to grip objects in the right than the left hand. The symptoms started two years ago, progressed for one year, and became static for the last one year. There was no history of sensory impairment. On examination, he was thin built, tall stature, and had a long neck. There was thinning of bilateral forearm muscles, the right side more affected than the left. Thenar and hypothenar muscles on the right hand were atrophic. There was tremulousness of fingers on attempted extension (Figure 1). Elbow flexion and extension were normal bilaterally. Bilateral wrist flexion and extension were 4+. Handgrip was 60% on the right and 80% on the left side. The lower limb motor examination was normal. There were no sensory deficits. Deep tendon reflexes were normally elicited. His cervical spine X-ray and Neutral MRI cervical spine showed evidence of loss of lordosis (Figure 2- A&B). Flexion MRI of the cervical spine showed forward shifting of posterior dura with prominent epidural space, which is a pathognomonic feature of HD (Figure 2-4). Since the patient's disease has become non-progressive in the last one year, he was treated conservatively with a cervical collar. He showed improvement in handgrip and writing at a six months follow-up period.

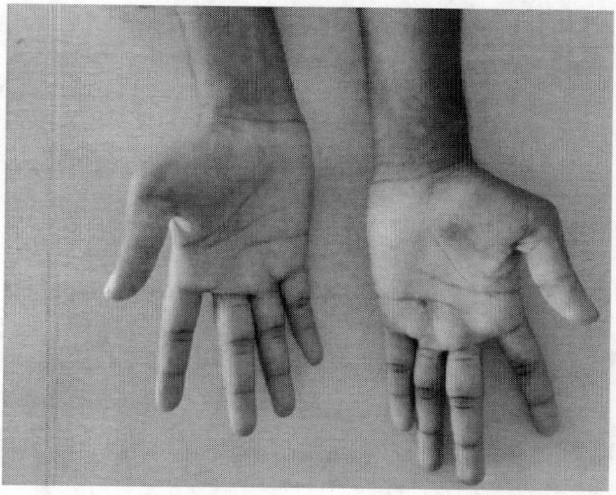

Figure 1. Wasting of the thenar and hypothenar muscles of both hands, right more than the left.

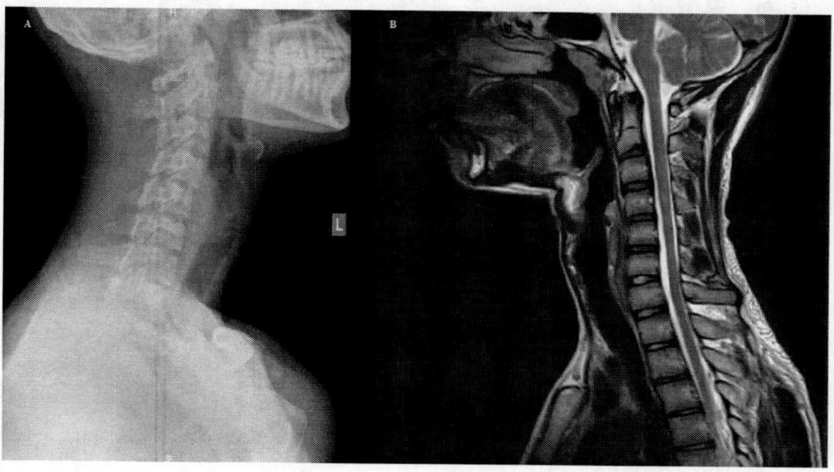

Figure 2. A&B showing X-ray and MRI of the cervical spine in neutral position showing loss of lordosis.

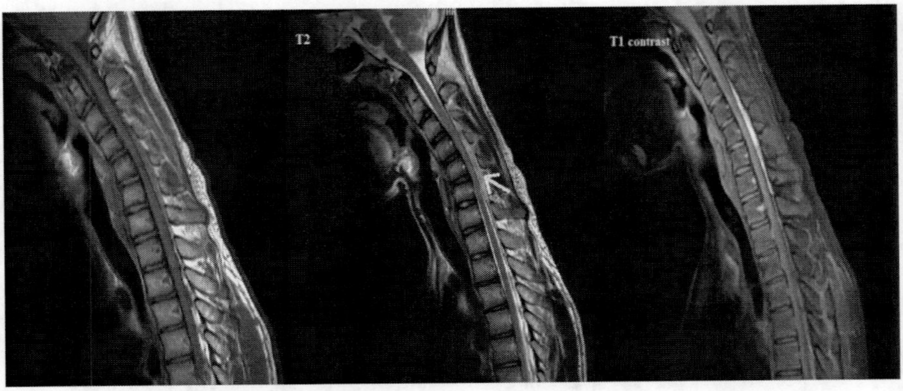

Figure 3. Flexion MRI in three sequences shows the hallmark sign of forward shifting of the posterior dura, and wide posterior epidural space (yellow arrow), which enhances with contrast.

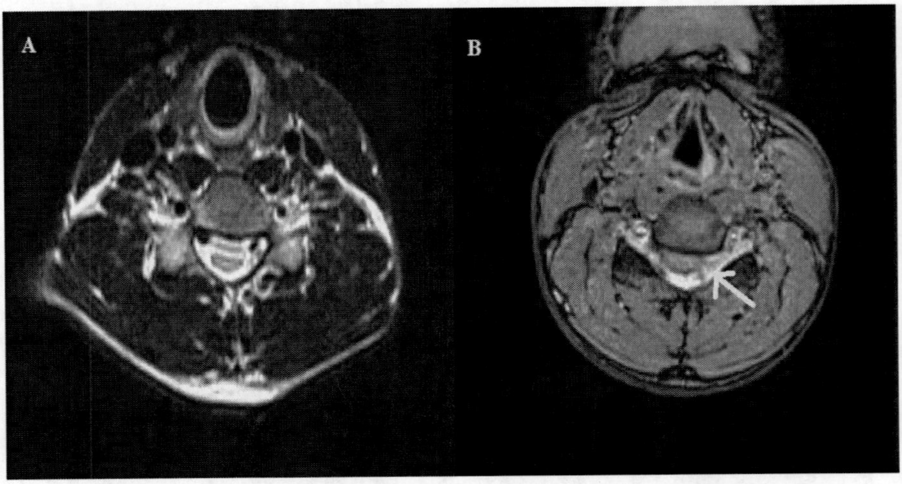

Figure 4. A- T2 Axial in neutral position shows flattened cord with intramedullary hyperintensity. B. Axial image was taken during neck flexion, showing detached epidural space, prominent flow voids (yellow arrow), and obliteration of anterior thecal space.

Table 1. Literature evidence on various treatment modalities

Author	N*	Management	Comments
(Brandicourt et al. 2018)	3	Posterior laminectomy and excision of venous plexus	Improvement in two patients, stable disease in the third patient
(Arrese et al. 2009)	1	C3-C6 Laminectomy and lax duraplasty	Stable disease
(Tokumaru and Hirayama 2001)	38	Cervical collar	No progression in all patients
(Agundez et al. 2015)	4	3 patients managed conservatively 1 patient underwent C5-C6 Anterior cervical discectomy and fusion	Spontaneous improvement in 3 conservatively managed patient Stable disease in operated patient
(Antonioni, Fonderico, and Granieri 2020)	1	Symptomatic treatment with medical therapy and cervical collar	Improvement in symptoms
(Srivastava et al. 2020)	1	Lateral mass instrumentation	Neurological improvement noted at one year follow up
(Konno et al. 1997)	5	Duraplasty with posterior spinal fusion	Improvement in all patients
(Ito, Takai, and Taniguchi 2014)	6	Laminoplasty with duraplasty	Improvement in all patients
(Goel, Dhar, and Shah 2017)	5	Multilevel posterior spinal stabilization with laminectomy	All patients showed improvement in hand grip

*N- number of patients treated

Treatment

There is no clinical consensus regarding the best management of Hirayama disease. However, numerous case series and reports on the management of Hirayama disease exist. Conservative management is recommended for most cases as the condition is self-limiting and usually doesn't progress beyond five years. Surgery may be necessary when the disease is severe or progressive. In patients with a short duration of illness and minimal cord atrophy, cervical collar application improves symptoms (Tokumaru and Hirayama 2001).

However, no randomized control study compares patients treated with cervical collar application and surgery. Regarding surgical management, both anterior and posterior approaches, with or without corpectomy, fusion, or duraplasty, have been reported to arrest or reverse the symptoms effectively. The following table (Table 1) enumerates various surgical options and their outcome described in the literature. In patients with severe progressive myelopathy, anterior cervical discectomy and fusion improved symptoms, mainly by restricting neck flexion (Agundez et al. 2015). Data comparing the effectiveness and superiority of one surgical procedure over the other is lacking. A randomized control study by Lu et al. comparing anterior cervical discectomy and fusion with anterior cervical corpectomy and fusion revealed no significant difference in outcome between these two procedures (Lu et al. 2013). Lyu et al. attempted to establish guidelines for the management of HD. They recommend that surgical treatment is preferred if the disease is progressive or progresses after a period of arrest or if the patient is not ready to wear the collar for an extended period (Lyu et al. 2020).

Conclusion

Despite being a benign nature and self-limiting course, few subsets of patients with HD would require treatment either with a cervical collar or with surgery. Hence timely identification of symptoms and diagnosis by doing flexion MRI cervical spine and categorizing patients for either surgery or conservative management based on the clinical context would prevent further ischemia of the cord due to repeated flexion induced injury.

References

Agundez, M., I. Rouco, J. Barcena, B. Mateos, J. Barredo, and J. J. Zarranz. 2015. "Hirayama Disease: Is Surgery an Option?" *Neurologia (Barcelona, Spain)*, 30 (8): 502–9. https://doi.org/10.1016/j.nrl.2013.05.005.

Antonioni, Annibale, Mattia Fonderico, and Enrico Granieri. 2020. "Hirayama Disease: A Case of an Albanian Woman Clinically Stabilized Without Surgery." *Frontiers in Neurology*, 11: 183. https://doi.org/10.3389/fneur.2020.00183.

Arrese, I., J. J. Rivas, J. Esteban, A. Ramos, and R. D. Lobato. 2009. "A Case of Hirayama Disease Treated with Laminectomy and Duraplasty without Spinal Fusion." *Neurocirugia (Asturias, Spain)*, 20 (6): 555–58; discussion 558.

Atchayaram, Nalini, M. K. Vasudev, and Gaurav Goel. 2009. "Familial Monomelic Amyotrophy (Hirayama Disease): Two Brothers with Classical Flexion Induced Dynamic Changes of the Cervical Dural Sac." *Neurology India*, 57 (6): 810–12. https://doi.org/10.4103/0028-3886.59488.

Boruah, D. K., A. Prakash, B. B. Gogoi, R. R. Yadav, D. D. Dhingani, and B. Sarma. 2018. "The Importance of Flexion MRI in Hirayama Disease with Special Reference to Laminodural Space Measurements." *AJNR. American Journal of Neuroradiology*, 39 (5): 974–80. https://doi.org/10.3174/ajnr.A5577.

Brandicourt, P., J. C. Sol, S. Aldéa, F. Bonneville, P. Cintas, and D. Brauge. 2018. "Cervical Laminectomy and Micro Resection of the Posterior Venous Plexus in Hirayama Disease." *Neuro-Chirurgie*, 64 (4): 303–9. https://doi.org/10.1016/j.neuchi.2018.04.004.

Chen, C. J., C. M. Chen, C. L. Wu, L. S. Ro, S. T. Chen, and T. H. Lee. 1998. "Hirayama Disease: MR Diagnosis." *AJNR. American Journal of Neuroradiology*, 19 (2): 365–68.

Chen, Chi-Jen, Hui-Ling Hsu, Ying-Chi Tseng, Rong-Kuo Lyu, Chiung-Mei Chen, Ying-Chih Huang, Li-Jen Wang, Yon-Cheong Wong, and Lai-Chu See. 2004. "Hirayama Flexion Myelopathy: Neutral-Position MR Imaging Findings--Importance of Loss of Attachment." *Radiology*, 231 (1): 39–44. https://doi.org/10.1148/radiol.2311030004.

Chen, Tai-Heng, Chih-Hsing Hung, Tsyh-Jyi Hsieh, Shiang-Ru Lu, San-Nan Yang, and Yuh-Jyh Jong. 2010. "Symmetric Atrophy of Bilateral Distal Upper Extremities and HyperIgEaemia in a Male Adolescent with Hirayama Disease." *Journal of Child Neurology*, 25 (3): 371–74. https://doi.org/10.1177/0883073809336876.

Elsheikh, Bakri, John T. Kissel, Gregory Christoforidis, Matthew Wicklund, Dimitri T. Kehagias, E. Antonio Chiocca, and Jerry R. Mendell. 2009. "Spinal Angiography and Epidural Venography in Juvenile Muscular Atrophy of the Distal Arm 'Hirayama Disease.'" *Muscle & Nerve*, 40 (2): 206–12. https://doi.org/10.1002/mus.21307.

Ghosh, Partha S., Manikum Moodley, Neil R. Friedman, A. David Rothner, and Debabrata Ghosh. 2011. "Hirayama Disease in Children from North America." *Journal of Child Neurology*, 26 (12): 1542–47. https://doi.org/10.1177/0883073811409226.

Goel, Atul, Arjun Dhar, and Abhidha Shah. 2017. "Multilevel Spinal Stabilization as a Treatment for Hirayama Disease: Report of an Experience with Five Cases." *World Neurosurgery*, 99 (March): 186–91. https://doi.org/10.1016/j.wneu.2016.11.143.

Gourie-Devi, M., and A. Nalini. 2003. "Long-Term Follow-up of 44 Patients with Brachial Monomelic Amyotrophy." *Acta Neurologica Scandinavica*, 107 (3): 215–20. https://doi.org/10.1034/j.1600-0404.2003.02142.x.

Gourie-Devi, M., T. G. Suresh, and S. K. Shankar. 1984. "Monomelic Amyotrophy." *Archives of Neurology*, 41 (4): 388–94. https://doi.org/10.1001/archneur.1984.04050160050015.

Hassan, K. M., Hirdesh Sahni, and Atul Jha. 2012. "Clinical and Radiological Profile of Hirayama Disease: A Flexion Myelopathy Due to Tight Cervical Dural Canal Amenable to Collar Therapy." *Annals of Indian Academy of Neurology*, 15 (2): 106–12. https://doi.org/10.4103/0972-2327.94993.

Hassan, Kaukab Maqbool, and Hirdesh Sahni. 2013. "Nosology of Juvenile Muscular Atrophy of Distal Upper Extremity: From Monomelic Amyotrophy to Hirayama Disease--Indian Perspective." *BioMed Research International*, 2013: 478516. https://doi.org/10.1155/2013/478516.

Hirayama, K. 2000. "Juvenile Muscular Atrophy of Distal Upper Extremity (Hirayama Disease)." *Internal Medicine (Tokyo, Japan)*, 39 (4): 283–90. https://doi.org/10.2169/internalmedicine.39.283.

Hirayama, K., M. Tomonaga, K. Kitano, T. Yamada, S. Kojima, and K. Arai. 1987. "Focal Cervical Poliopathy Causing Juvenile Muscular Atrophy of Distal Upper Extremity: A Pathological Study." *Journal of Neurology, Neurosurgery, and Psychiatry*, 50 (3): 285–90. https://doi.org/10.1136/jnnp.50.3.285.

Hirayama, K., T. Tsubaki, Y. Toyokura, and S. Okinaka. 1963. "Juvenile Muscular Atrophy of Unilateral Upper Extremity." *Neurology*, 13 (May): 373–80. https://doi.org/10.1212/wnl.13.5.373.

Hirayama, Keizo. 2008. "[Juvenile muscular atrophy of unilateral upper extremity (Hirayama disease)--half-century progress and establishment since its discovery]." *Brain and Nerve = Shinkei Kenkyu No Shinpo*, 60 (1): 17–29.

Hou, Chao, Hongbin Han, Xiaohong Yang, Xiaojuan Xu, Hui Gao, Dongsheng Fan, Yu Fu, Yu Sun, and Bo Liu. 2012. "How Does the Neck Flexion Affect the Cervical MRI Features of Hirayama Disease?" *Neurological Sciences: Official Journal of the Italian Neurological Society and of the Italian Society of Clinical Neurophysiology*, 33 (5): 1101–5. https://doi.org/10.1007/s10072-011-0912-x.

Huang, Ying-Chih, Long-Sun Ro, Hong-Shiu Chang, Chiung-Mei Chen, Yih-Ru Wu, Jian-Der Lee, and Rong-Kuo Lyu. 2008. "A Clinical Study of Hirayama Disease in Taiwan." *Muscle & Nerve*, 37 (5): 576–82. https://doi.org/10.1002/mus.20980.

Ito, Hirotaka, Keisuke Takai, and Makoto Taniguchi. 2014. "Cervical Duraplasty with Tenting Sutures via Laminoplasty for Cervical Flexion Myelopathy in Patients with Hirayama Disease: Successful Decompression of a 'Tight Dural Canal in Flexion' without Spinal Fusion." *Journal of Neurosurgery. Spine*, 21 (5): 743–52. https://doi.org/10.3171/2014.7.SPINE13955.

Kieser, David C., P. J. Cox, and S. C. J. Kieser. 2018. "Hirayama Disease." *European Spine Journal: Official Publication of the European Spine Society, the European Spinal Deformity Society, and the European Section of the Cervical Spine Research Society*, 27 (6): 1201–6. https://doi.org/10.1007/s00586-018-5545-9.

Konno, S., S. Goto, M. Murakami, M. Mochizuki, H. Motegi, and H. Moriya. 1997. "Juvenile Amyotrophy of the Distal Upper Extremity: Pathologic Findings of the Dura Mater and Surgical Management." *Spine*, 22 (5): 486–92. https://doi.org/10.1097/00007632-199703010-00004.

Lai, Vincent, Yiu Chung Wong, Wai Lun Poon, Ming Keung Yuen, Yat Pang Fu, and Oi Wah Wong. 2011. "Forward Shifting of Posterior Dural Sac during Flexion Cervical Magnetic Resonance Imaging in Hirayama Disease: An Initial Study on Normal Subjects Compared to Patients with Hirayama Disease." *European Journal of Radiology*, 80 (3): 724–28. https://doi.org/10.1016/j.ejrad.2010.07.021.

Lapresle, J. 1969. "[Clinical and neuropathological aspects of circulatory disorders of the spinal cord]." *Bulletin Der Schweizerischen Akademie Der Medizinischen Wissenschaften*, 24 (5): 512–28.

Lu, Feizhou, Hongli Wang, Jianyuan Jiang, Wenjun Chen, Xin Ma, Xiaosheng Ma, Xinlei Xia, and Lixun Wang. 2013. "Efficacy of Anterior Cervical Decompression and Fusion Procedures for Monomelic Amyotrophy Treatment: A Prospective Randomized Controlled Trial: Clinical Article." *Journal of Neurosurgery. Spine*, 19 (4): 412–19. https://doi.org/10.3171/2013.4.SPINE12575.

Lyu, Feizhou, Chaojun Zheng, Hongli Wang, Cong Nie, Xiaosheng Ma, Xinlei Xia, Wei Zhu, et al. 2020. "Establishment of a Clinician-Led Guideline on the Diagnosis and Treatment of Hirayama Disease Using a Modified Delphi Technique." *Clinical Neurophysiology: Official Journal of the International Federation of Clinical Neurophysiology*, 131 (6): 1311–19. https://doi.org/10.1016/j.clinph.2020.02.022.

Misra, U. K., J. Kalita, V. N. Mishra, A. Kesari, and B. Mittal. 2005. "A Clinical, Magnetic Resonance Imaging, and Survival Motor Neuron Gene Deletion Study of Hirayama Disease." *Archives of Neurology*, 62 (1): 120–23. https://doi.org/10.1001/archneur.62.1.120.

O'Sullivan, D. J., and J. G. McLeod. 1977. "Distal Chronic Spinal Muscular Atrophy Involving the Hands." *Clinical and Experimental Neurology*, 14: 256–59.

Pradhan, S., and R. K. Gupta. 1997. "Magnetic Resonance Imaging in Juvenile Asymmetric Segmental Spinal Muscular Atrophy." *Journal of the Neurological Sciences*, 146 (2): 133–38. https://doi.org/10.1016/s0022-510x(96)00296-1.

Pradhan, Sunil. 2009. "Bilaterally Symmetric Form of Hirayama Disease." *Neurology*, 72 (24): 2083–89. https://doi.org/10.1212/WNL.0b013e3181aa5364.

Raval, Monali, Rima Kumari, Aldrin Anthony Dung Dung, Bhuvnesh Guglani, Nitij Gupta, and Rohit Gupta. 2010. "MRI Findings in Hirayama Disease." *The Indian Journal of Radiology & Imaging*, 20 (4): 245–49. https://doi.org/10.4103/0971-3026.73528.

Shneider, Neil A., and Michio Hirano. 2019. "Motor Neuron Diseases." In *CURRENT Diagnosis & Treatment: Neurology*, edited by John C.M. Brust, 3rd ed. New York, NY: McGraw-Hill Education. neurology.mhmedical.com/content.aspx?aid=1159971054.

Song, Jian, Zhong-Yi Cui, Zhen-Hao Chen, and Jian-Yuan Jiang. 2020. "Analysis of the Effect of Surgical Treatment for the Patients with Hirayama Disease from the Perspective of Cervical Spine Sagittal Alignment." *World Neurosurgery*, 133 (January): e342–47. https://doi.org/10.1016/j.wneu.2019.09.025.

Sonwalkar, Hemant A., Rakesh S. Shah, Firosh K. Khan, Arun K. Gupta, Narendra K. Bodhey, Surjith Vottath, and Sukalyan Purkayastha. 2008. "Imaging Features in Hirayama Disease." *Neurology India*, 56 (1): 22–26. https://doi.org/10.4103/0028-3886.39307.

Srivastava, Sudhir Kumar, Nandan Marathe, Aditya Raj, Sunil Bhosale, and Kiran Dhole. 2020. "Surgical Management of Hirayama Disease: A Rare Entity with Unusual Clinical Features." *Asian Journal of Neurosurgery*, 15 (2): 405–8. https://doi.org/10.4103/ajns.AJNS_291_19.

Tashiro, Kunio, Seiji Kikuchi, Yasuo Itoyama, Yukio Tokumaru, Gen Sobue, Eiichiro Mukai, Ichiro Akiguchi, Kenji Nakashima, Jun-ichi Kira, and Keizo Hirayama. 2006. "Nationwide Survey of Juvenile Muscular Atrophy of Distal Upper Extremity (Hirayama Disease) in Japan." *Amyotrophic Lateral Sclerosis: Official Publication of the World Federation of Neurology Research Group on Motor Neuron Diseases*, 7 (1): 38–45. https://doi.org/10.1080/14660820500396877.

Tokumaru, Y., and K. Hirayama. 2001. "[Cervical collar therapy for juvenile muscular atrophy of distal upper extremity (Hirayama disease): results from 38 cases]." *Rinsho Shinkeigaku = Clinical Neurology*, 41 (4–5): 173–78.

Xu, Haocheng, Minghao Shao, Fan Zhang, Cong Nie, Hongli Wang, Wei Zhu, Xinlei Xia, Xiaosheng Ma, Feizhou Lu, and Jianyuan Jiang. 2019. "Snake-Eyes Appearance on MRI Occurs during the Late Stage of Hirayama Disease and Indicates Poor Prognosis." *BioMed Research International*, 2019: 9830243. https://doi.org/10.1155/2019/9830243.

Xu, Xiaojuan, Hongbin Han, Hui Gao, Chao Hou, Dongsheng Fan, Yu Fu, and Yu Sun. 2011. "The Increased Range of Cervical Flexed Motion Detected by Radiographs in Hirayama Disease." *European Journal of Radiology*, 78 (1): 82–86. https://doi.org/10.1016/j.ejrad.2010.08.012.

Zheng, Chaojun, Yu Zhu, Feizhou Lu, Dongqing Zhu, Shuo Yang, Xiaosheng Ma, Xinlei Xia, Robert Weber, and Jianyuan Jiang. 2017. "Changes in the Soleus H-Reflex Test and Correlations between Its Results and Dynamic Magnetic Resonance Imaging Abnormalities in Patients with Hirayama Disease." *Clinical Neurophysiology: Official Journal of the International Federation of Clinical Neurophysiology*, 128 (12): 2375–81. https://doi.org/10.1016/j.clinph.2017.09.103.

Zhou, Bo, Lei Chen, Dongsheng Fan, and Dong Zhou. 2010. "Clinical Features of Hirayama Disease in Mainland China." *Amyotrophic Lateral Sclerosis: Official Publication of the World Federation of Neurology Research Group on Motor Neuron Diseases*, 11 (1–2): 133–39. https://doi.org/10.3109/17482960902912407.

Chapter 13

Biologics of Spinal Fusion

Aishik Mukherjee, Rupant Kumar Das and Dibyendu Kumar Ray*

AMRI Hospitals, Salt Lake, Kolkata, India

Abstract

Spinal fusion, one of the most frequently performed procedures in spine surgery is required for various pathological conditions of the spine. Fusion aims to prevent or correct segmental instability by promoting a bony union of two or more spinal segments. Failed segmental fusion is one of the principal causes of poor outcomes in spine surgery often leading to persistent or recurrent symptoms and therefore increased disability. The biology of spinal fusion is not too different from the steps of bone healing after fracture. Techniques of spinal arthrodesis are varied and ever-changing with more and more research ongoing to increase the success rates of fusion. Spinal stabilization with metallic or polymeric implants incorporated with bone grafts as well as augmentation of fusion with biologic agents like Demineralized bone matrices (DBMs) or ceramic scaffolds has been successfully used by spine surgeons. Bone grafts used can be autologous or allogenic wherein DBMs are made by removing the mineral content while maintaining a cell population to promote fusion. Iliac crest autografts form the gold standard of spinal fusion to date due to their ability to avoid immune rejection, low to negligible infection rates, and also the fact they combine the three pillars of bone healing - osteogenic, osteoinductive, and osteoconductive capabilities. Allogenic grafts have the advantage of avoiding graft site morbidities in the patient. DBMs comprise the organic matrix of acid-extracted allografts rich in growth factors which render it with osteoinductive potential. Synthetic biologics like ceramic or bioactive

*Corresponding Author's Email:dibyendukray@gmail.com

In: Neurosurgery Research
Editors: Amit Agrawal, Pradeep Chouksey, Adesh Shrivastava et al.
ISBN: 978-1-68507-837-9

glass are cheap and easily manufactured, have a long shelf life with potent osteoconductive capabilities. Recombinant growth factors, most commonly used being Bone Morphogenetic Proteins, have potent osteogenic capacity but are costly, have a significant risk profile, and are potentially oncogenic. Autologous growth factors, Mesenchymal stem cells, synthetic peptides are also currently being utilized and research is underway to develop genetic therapies using viral transduction to optimize the rates of spinal fusion. This chapter provides an overview of the biologics currently in use for spinal arthrodesis, the risks, and benefits of each as well as the role of growth factors, stem cells as per presently available literature, and potential future directions including genetic therapy.

Keywords: spinal fusion, bone grafts, iliac crest autografts, allogenic grafts, demineralized bone matrices, ceramic, bone morphogenetic proteins, mesenchymal stem cells, genetic therapy

Introduction

Excessive motion due to spinal instability can lead to neural compression frequently causing back pain and radiculopathy. In such patients, neural decompression needs to be supplemented with spinal fusion to limit abnormal motion. A variety of pathologies like degenerative conditions, spinal deformity, tumors, or traumatic conditions of the spine may lead to spinal instability thereby requiring spinal fusion [1]. Approaches may be posterior spinal instrumentation alone, anterior interbody fusion alone, or a combination of both also referred to as a 360-degree fusion. The choice of approach is largely dictated by the pathology being tackled. Surgery aims to provide a solid, stable arthrodesis of the spinal segments for maintenance of sagittal plane balance, prevent loss of disc height, and therefore help the spinal column to sustain loads [2-6]. This usually involves the placement of an interbody device such as a cage, spacer, or structural graft to replenish the dead space created by a discectomy or a corpectomy and to promote bony ingrowth [7]. A variety of grafts can be used including autografts, allografts, demineralized bone matrices (DBM), graft substitutes such as ceramic scaffolding products. For further optimization of fusion rates mesenchymal stem cells (MSCs), growth factors, and synthetic peptides are being utilized and further research on gene therapies using viral vectors is ongoing [8]. Autogenous iliac crest graft has been the gold standard for spinal fusion to date with reported fusion rates of approximately 85% (ranging 35% to 100%) depending on various studies. Our chapter explores the wide variety of biologics currently being used for spinal fusion including the specific indications, advantages, and disadvantages of each as well as the role of growth factors, stem cells, genetic, and other emerging therapies [8-12].

Bone Healing – An Overview

Before we proceed with selecting one of the wide variety of biologics currently in use for our surgical patient, we must understand the physiology of bone healing. Bone regeneration broadly involves three mechanisms –

1) Osteogenesis, which involves the synthesis of new bone cells derived from the graft or the host. The ability of a graft to provide a suitable micro-environment for the osteoprogenitor cells to proliferate and differentiate into osteoblasts and osteocytes is defined as its "osteogenic" potential [13].

2) Osteoinduction, which includes the recruitment of immature mesenchymal stem cells and their differentiation into bone-forming cells [14]

3) Osteoconduction i,e the formation of a scaffold by the capillaries, perivascular tissue, and the Mesenchymal stem cells that provides the bone cells with the structural framework to form viable bone [14, 15].

The osteoblasts formed during osteoinduction are responsible for new bone formation whereas the scaffolding formed during osteoconduction is responsible for host-graft bony fusion. Bone formation and spinal fusion are all but an interplay of these three underlying mechanisms of orthobiologics. An ideal graft incorporates these three properties in the right proportions to promote optimum bony regeneration and thereby provide the spine with stable arthrodesis [16,17].

Bony regeneration via the above-mentioned mechanisms follows a definite timeline involving three distinct stages which include the inflammatory stage, the repair stage, and the late remodeling stage. The progression through these stages involves a series of systemic and local interactions between the graft and the host bed. The inflammatory stage which ranges from hours to the first few days post-operatively is characterized by prostaglandin-mediated chemotaxis of inflammatory cells and fibroblasts into the graft leading to the formation of granulation and vascular tissues. Osteoinductive differentiation of osteoprogenitor cells and the formation of osteoblasts also take place in this stage. The repair stage ranging from weeks to months post-operatively is characterized by the fibroblast-mediated formation of a stroma which supports ingrowth of vascular tissue and collagen matrix deposition which provides the framework for secretion of osteoid and bone mineralization. Eventually, the late remodeling stage which takes months to years after surgery leads to the restoration of the newly formed bone to its original structural strength. The integrity of the newly remodeled bone depends on the osteoconductive properties of the bone graft wherein the mechanical stress placed on the construct over time leads to resorption of the graft tissue and its replacement with new bone, a process also called "Creeping substitution". Successful temporal progression through these three stages forms the cornerstone of achieving successful fusion [15,18].

Bone Grafts

Autologous Bone Grafts

Autologous bone grafts which involve transplantation of bone from one anatomical site to another in the same patient currently form the gold standard for spinal grafting. One of the major advantages of autologous bone grafts is that they combine all the three properties of bone healing i,e osteogenic, osteoinductive and osteoconductive potential, a capability few other grafts can offer. Also, risks of infection are low to nil, and chances of hypersensitivity are absent as there is complete histocompatibility. The most common site of harvest is the iliac crest. However, grafts can also be taken from the proximal tibia, ribs, distal radius as well as the bony spinal elements including the lamina, spinous process, or the body of the vertebra that might be removed in course of surgery [19].

Autografts can be broadly classified into two types – Cortical and Cancellous. Cortical bone is characterized by high density which helps in providing early stability to the construct. However, due to low porosity, the osteoinductive potential of cortical bone grafts is less which means that there is poor early revascularization. In fact, in such grafts, there has to be an initial phase of osteoclastic resorption of the graft which would form cavities in the graft to make a pathway for the osteoblasts to reach and begin to form new bone. A cortical bone graft is more often than not completely resorbed and replaced with new bone [17]. Cancellous bone grafts have properties quite the opposite of cortical grafts. They are highly porous which means they usually have a larger surface area, a property that contributes to their high osteogenic potential. Although the lower density of the construct means early mechanical strength is lesser when compared to cortical grafts, this is largely offset by the fact that rapid osteoblastic infiltration coupled with early revascularization leads to faster new bone formation [17].

Autografts form the cheapest, most readily available grafts whilst also being able to promote strong bony fusion with low rates of infection and without histocompatibility issues. However, they are limited by the fact that the quality of such grafts varies according to age, metabolic activity, pre-existing disease in the individual patient and might not be a feasible option in all patients. Also, the fact that a separate donor site on the same surgical patient needs to be explored in certain patients carries with it the additional risks of blood loss, pain, and wound complications [20,21]. These factors have led to the need for the development of autograft substitutes.

Iliac Crest Bone Grafts

Although the iliac crest forms the most common site of autograft harvest to date, it is not without its fair share of complications [22]. A few of the reported complications include infections, seromas, hematomas, iliac spine fractures, graft site hernias. Iatrogenic nerve injuries most commonly involve the lateral femoral cutaneous nerve often leading to chronic pain at the donor site and/or sensory disturbances [23,24]. Some studies have reported complication rates as high as 19.37% following iliac crest bone graft harvest with several patients requiring further operative intervention [19]. It is because of these complications iliac crest bone grafting is increasingly being replaced with other modalities. However, in cases of a lumbar fusion wound where iliac crest exposure is part of the surgical field, it may continue to have a role.

To circumvent the donor site complications and morbidities associated with iliac crest autografting, some surgeons have utilized Bone Marrow Aspirates (BMA) harvested from the hosts' posterior iliac bone using large-bore Bone Marrow Aspiration needles. These Bone Marrow Aspirates when used along with a scaffolding have reported fusion rates comparable to autografts used in isolation, with Khashan et al. reporting fusion rates of 100% for BMA with scaffolding [25,26]. BMAs although rich in osteoprogenitor and haematoprogenitor cells are limited in their osteoconductive potential and frequently need to be combined with allografts or a scaffold for ensuring optimum fusion [27].

Additionally, novel methods are being developed for harvesting autografts from local bone sources such as the Reamer/Irrigator/Aspirator which have reported lower complication rates [19].

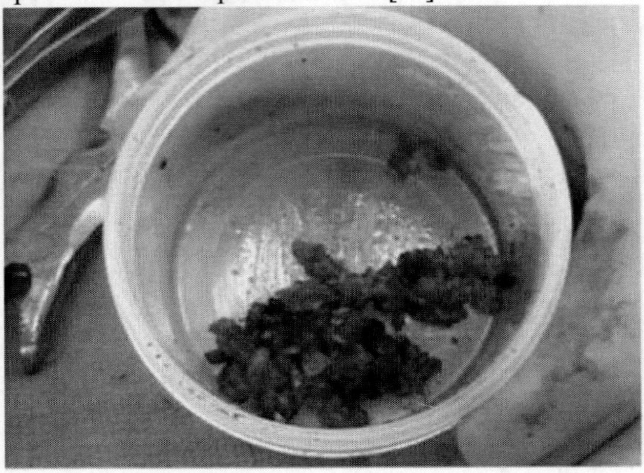

Figure 1. Autograft for spinal fusion.

Allografts

An allograft is a bone transplanted from one individual to another. The donor may be a cadaver or a living individual. Allografts similar to autografts may be cortical or cancellous [17]. An allograft scores over an autograft in that it avoids additional incisions on the patient needed for harvesting an autograft [28]. Allografts when incorporated with Mesenchymal stem cells have shown higher fusion rates [20].

Allografts carry a limited risk of disease transmission from the donor especially HBV or HCV infection and hence they require sterilization. The standard method used for sterilization of allografts is Gamma radiation which apart from being able to neutralize the disease-causing pathogens due to their higher penetration, more certainty of sterilization notwithstanding the temperature and pressure, is also largely able to preserve the structural integrity of the tissues [29,30]. However, the process of sterilization can alter the more fragile biological microenvironment such as the bone matrix composition, the cytokines, chemokines, the growth factors which are essential for adequate bony regeneration [30,31]. Also, these allografts lack osteogenic potential due to the loss of viable cells as a result of the sterilization process [32].

Liao et al. conducted a systemic review to compare the efficacy of allografts to autografts in patients of lumbar fusion and found no significant difference in fusion rates between the two (OR = 0.567, 95% CI = 0.15-2.17; $p > 0.05$). They also found good outcomes in terms of Oswestry Disability Index scores (ODI) and Visual Analogue scale (VAS) scores with allografts and suggested the same as a suitable alternative to autografts [33]. Suchomel et al. conducted a large retrospective case-controlled study of 113 patients of posterolateral fusion and found comparable fusion rates between allografts (93.4%) and autografts (94.6%) [34]. Despite multiple comparative studies having demonstrated similar fusion rates between autografts and allografts, autografts continue to be the gold standard for spinal arthrodesis chiefly due to their ability to achieve complete fusion at a faster pace [35,36].

Demineralized Bone Matrices (DBMs)

Demineralized Bone Matrices (DBMs), derived from human allografts were first introduced in 1991 to replace or act as an adjunct to autologous bone grafts [37]. Derived from human cadaveric bone, acid treatment extracts the mineralized portion while preserving the collagens (mostly type I), the noncollagenous proteins, and growth factors (GF) [38]. DBMs although lacking in osteogenic potential, have osteoconductive properties incorporated by the scaffolding of collagens and noncollagenous proteins as well as osteoinductive properties provided by a variety of growth factors such as bone morphogenetic proteins (BMP), Fibroblast growth factors, and Transforming growth factor-β [39]. DBMs are widely available as well as have the advantage of avoiding additional donor site morbidity when compared to autografts. However, due to the wide variety of manufacturers and their differing methods of preparation, there is significant variability in composition especially the levels of the critically important Bone Morphogenetic proteins. Therefore, the efficacy of DBMs as a whole is difficult to analyze in clinical studies with significant variations observed between different manufacturers [40,41].

Even though after initial processing DBMs are usually in the particulate powder or fiber forms, for ease of clinical application as far as surgeries are concerned DBMs are commercially also available as injectable gels, putties, pastes, flexible sheets, or blocks. These rather moldable forms are achieved by combining them with biocompatible carriers such as sodium hyaluronate, carboxymethylcellulose, or glycerol [9,38].

Due to their poor inherent mechanical strength and lack of structural integrity, DBMs have a greater risk of graft collapse when used alone as compared to autografts. Therefore, more often than not, they are used in conjunction with local autografts. A large number of studies have been carried out to analyze outcomes of DBM use as an extender in spinal fusion. Kang et al. performed a randomized clinical trial in patients undergoing single-level posterior lumbar fusion and found comparable fusion rates between commercial DBM graft (Grafton™) with local autograft (86%) and Iliac Crest Bone Grafting (92%) at 24 months postoperatively [42]. The above trial also found that the DBM group had significantly lower mean intraoperative blood loss and higher physical outcome scores (though not statistically significant) at two years follow up [42]. Cammisa et al. conducted another study involving 120 patients who received DBM/autograft composite on one side of the spine and Iliac crest autograft only on the other side in the same patient. Radiologic evidence of fusion at two years follow up was 54% for autologous iliac crest graft versus 52% for DBM suggesting DBMs to be almost equally as efficacious as a bone graft extender as autologous grafts. Chang et al. identified 5 studies involving a total of 264 patients where DBMs were used as a graft extender in MIS posterior interbody fusions and calculated mean fusion rates of 85% (77–97%) [11]. They also analyzed studies for minimally invasive anterior and lateral interbody fusions and recorded that DBMs when added to other biologics achieved a fusion rate of 98% (97-98%) which was significantly higher than any other bone graft material except for BMA as extender and rhBMP-2 in isolation [11].

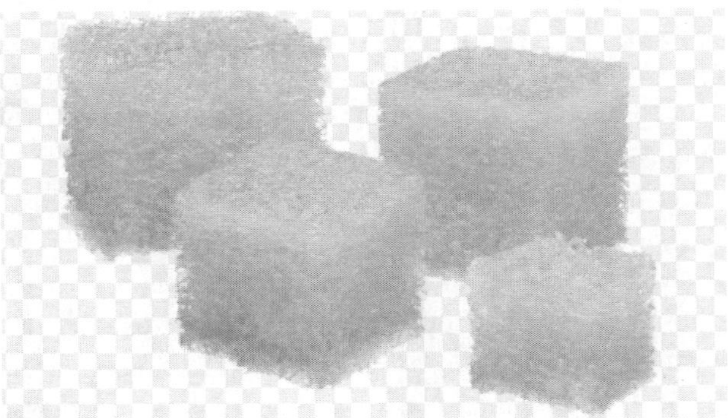

Figure 2. DBM blocks.

DBMs have their limitations as they can rarely be used alone due to their inferior structural composition as well as they carry a risk of contaminants, one such being ethylene glycol known to cause Acute tubular necrosis [43,44]. However as stated earlier, various studies have found DBMs used as an additive to autografts to achieve high rates of spinal fusion and further scope of research is there involving the use of DBMs with various growth factors [38].

Graft Substitutes and Supplements

Ceramics

Ceramics are synthetic bone grafts based upon calcium salts and hydroxyapatite found in normal human bone. The fact they possess only osteoconductive properties and lack any osteogenic or osteoinductive potential means they can only be used as bone graft extenders [32]. The addition of osteogenic cells and growth factors to ceramic scaffolds imparts them with both osteoinductive and osteogenic capabilities [45]. Ceramics are manufactured by "sintering," a process whereby chemical compounds are forced to bond together using high temperatures [46]. Certain properties of ceramics like shapes, compositions, porosities, biodegradability, etc can be tailored to individual patients by controlling the chemical environment in which they are manufactured. Additional advantages include virtually zero risk of disease transmission, longer shelf life, ease of manufacturing, and therefore widespread availability. However, a lack of cortical stability means ceramics are usually brittle. [40,32].

Ceramics may include hydroxyapatite (HA), tricalcium phosphate (TCP), calcium sulfate, or calcium phosphate. The biomechanical strength of a ceramic scaffold may vary depending upon the respective porosity of the particular type. TCP has lower compressive strength due to its higher porosity when compared to HA but provides for a better biologic response and faster bone formation. HA being denser provides better biomechanical strength to the construct [13]. Because of their unique individual strengths and varied functionality HA and TCP may often be combined for better outcomes [13,47].

Chang et al. analyzed 4 studies that utilized ceramics in isolation or as bone graft extenders. They found a mean fusion rate of 86% (83-88%) in the 3 studies which used ceramics as local autograft extenders [11]. In the other remaining study by Alimi et al. where silicate substituted calcium phosphate was used alone, an overall fusion rate of 82.9% was observed [48]. In retroperitoneal approaches, studies showed fusion rates of about 95% (80–100%) when ceramics were being used as extenders and 88% (80–100%) when used alone [11]. The lack of osteoinductive components may be responsible for the lower fusion rates of ceramics when used alone. For better results, ceramics may be combined with different growth factors [9].

Polyetheretherketone

Acromed first introduced polyether ether ketone (PEEK) in the 1990s in the form of a spinal cage for aiding spinal fusion [49]. PEEK is a biocompatible polymer and the fact that PEEK cages have lower elastic modulus and are radiolucent mean they form a viable alternative to autografts. However, they are not without their fair share of complications like graft migration, subsidence, and pseudoarthrosis [50]. One meta-analysis of six studies comparing PEEK cages and titanium cages in anterior cervical discectomy and transforaminal interbody fusion found similar fusion rates between the two implants but reported higher subsidence rates with titanium cages when compared to PEEK cages [51]. Another systematic review comparing PEEK cages to bone grafts for cervical spine fusion found minimal evidence for better clinico-radiological outcomes with PEEK [50].

Ceramics when used along with PEEK cages may provide additional osteoconductive benefits. One study found the combination of PEEK cages with ceramics to be comparable to autografts in anterior cervical discectomy and fusion [52]. PEEK cages may be used with both allografts and autografts. One study comparing allografts vs autografts in combination with PEEK cages for single-level lumbar instrumented fusion found no significant difference in fusion rates [35]. Although the use of PEEK cages in spinal fusion is widespread with outcomes comparable to the existing alternatives, further randomized studies are required to establish their effectiveness.

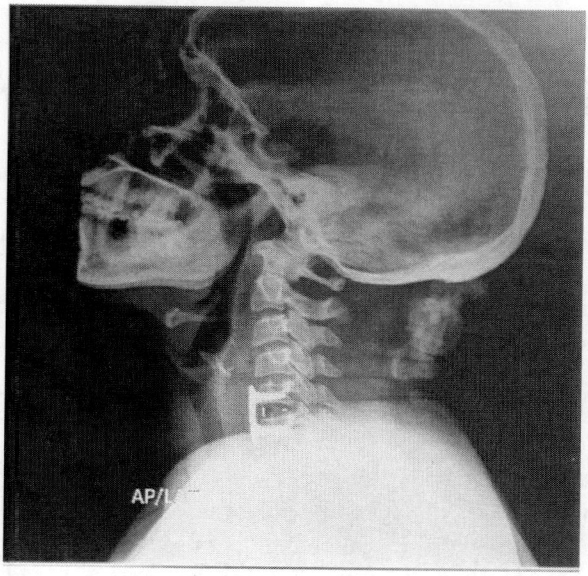

Figure 3. Post-op radiograph showing PEEK interbody spacer at C5-6.

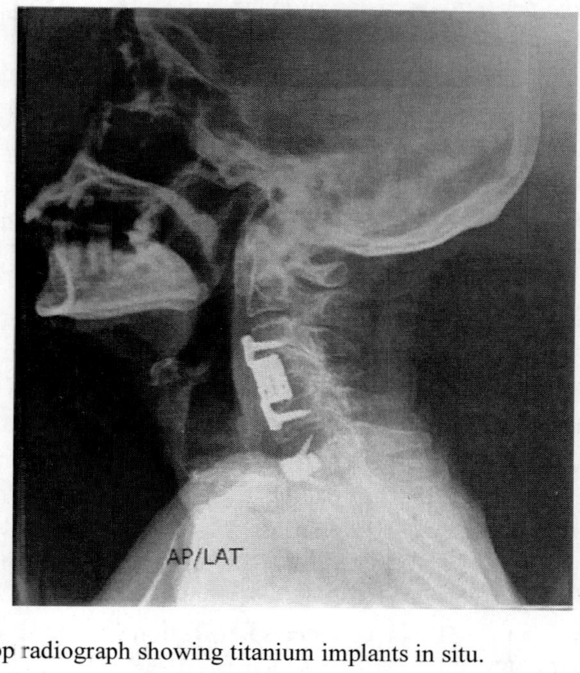

Figure 4. Post-op radiograph showing titanium implants in situ.

Bone Morphogenetic Proteins

First isolated by Robert Urist in 1965, Bone morphogenic proteins (BMPs) cover an array of 20 different cytokines and growth factors belonging to the TGF-β family. BMPs are endowed with osteogenic potential and their role in spinal fusion has been subject to extensive clinical studies especially BMP-2, BMP-4, and BMP-7 (osteogenic protein-1) [11,53,54].

BMPs are capable of inducing endochondral ossification due to their osteoinductive properties. Downstream signaling involves the SMAD pathway which once stimulated by Type I and II BMP receptors act by modulation of cytoplasmic transcription regulators and the expression of tissue-specific transcription factors [53]. The ability to produce large quantities of BMPs with the advent of genetic cloning has made it possible to ensure more effective bony fusion [11].

The efficacy of BMPs in aiding spinal fusion has been subject to multiple comparative studies. They can either be used in isolation along with a synthetic collagen carrier or may be added to other autografts or allografts. Furthermore, studies have also shown enhanced rates of spinal fusion when BMPs have been augmented with additional factors like FK506, elcatonin, hyperbaric oxygen, and/or basic fibroblast growth factor [55].

Parajón et al. conducted a meta-analysis of 40 studies and found that the use of recombinant human bone morphogenetic protein (rhBMP) leads to higher fusions rates (96.6%) as against those where rhBMP was not being used (92.5%) [10]. The highest rate of fusion (99.1%) was observed in cases where rhBMP was used as an additive to local bone autograft.

Studies have shown BMP antagonists expressed by mesenchymal stem cells to have increased activity in intervertebral discs and cartilaginous endplate cells [56, 57]. In one study by Chan et al, the authors suggest that better spinal fusion can be ensured if therapeutic modalities can be directed to target BMP antagonists such as ghrelin, chordin, follistatin, and noggin [58].

Complications like dysphagia and airway compromise have been reported with the use of rhBMP [59]. Another significant limitation of BMPs is their potential to induce oncogenesis [60]. In vitro studies by Kokorina et al. found that rhBMP-2 to adversely impacts the invasiveness of human oral squamous cell carcinoma cell lines [61]. Certain studies seem to implicate high doses of rhBMP-2 with increased incidence of deep infections, arrhythmias, and pseudarthrosis [62,63].

The use of rhBMPs in cervical spine fusion has been associated with certain adverse effects which have led the FDA to issue a warning [64].

Khajavi and Shen in a study of 38 patients who underwent multi-level Anterior cervical fusion using rhBMP, found two patients with dysphagia and major airway complications requiring readmission and steroids. Excessive bone formation leading to neural compression was also correlated with rhBMP use, especially in cases where the transforaminal approach was adopted [65,66].

Some animal studies seem to suggest a reduction in BMP dose by adding parathyroid hormone may be an effective way to reduce certain side effects related to high BMP dosage [67,68,69].

Finally, one of the major limitations of rhBMP is its high cost which makes it a non-viable fusion tool for a large number of patients [70].

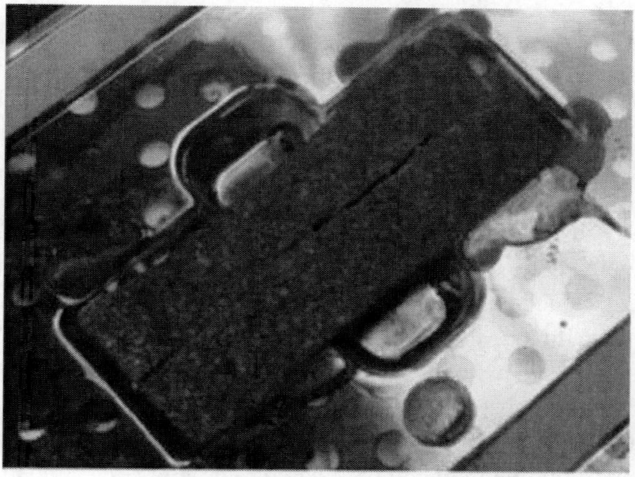

Figure 5. BMP with collagen sponge.

Autologous Growth Factors (AGFs)

Autologous growth factors play a vital role in bone and wound healing due to their ability to stimulate the proliferation of osteoblasts, fibroblasts, and mesenchymal stem cells [71]. Commercially these growth factors can be extracted from ultra-concentration of platelets. Of the numerous growth factors active in the human body, Platelet-derived growth factors (PDGF) and TGF-β have been the focus of most extensive research. PDGF has been found to stimulate osteogenesis and bone remodeling by increasing the synthesis of bone matrix proteins whereas, TGF-β has angiogenic properties as well as the ability to regulate the synthesis of extracellular bone matrix [15,71].

Although basic scientific research data suggests autologous growth factors could be a very useful tool for aiding spinal fusion when used in conjunction with autograft, allografts, or ceramics, clinical studies to date are yet to provide sufficient evidence on the usefulness of AGFs in spinal fusion, especially when compared to traditional autograft [9,72,73]. Another significant drawback with AGFs is the increased financial costs attributed to the manufacturing processes involved [74]. In comparing allografts with AGFs and autografts alone, Jenis et al. reported almost identical fusion rates and recommended the use of AGFs with allografts as an alternative to iliac graft harvesting [75].

Mesenchymal Stem Cells (MSCs)

Adult mesenchymal stem cells (MSCs) have the capability of differentiating into various cell lines including bone precursors making them an attractive tool for promoting spinal fusion [76]. Stem cells can be harvested from a variety of sites, the most common being the iliac crest. Usually, the needle puncture technique is used wherein the needle with the trochar is drilled into the cortical bone and the bone marrow is aspirated. Thereafter the aspirate is filtered, centrifuged, and placed in platelet deficient plasma. The final product is further verified with a hemoanalysis and a complete blood count with differential before being placed within the grafts to stimulate the formation of new bone [77].

A graft comprising of stem cells, ceramics, and allografts, incorporates all the three aspects of bone regeneration i,e osteogenesis, osteoinduction, and osteoconduction, something only autografts seem to possess in isolation [78].

Studies have shown MSCs to be as effective as a combination of rhBMP and grafts in ensuring bony fusion. One study of patients undergoing MIS-TLIF showed comparable rates of fusion and redo surgery in those undergoing fusion with MSCs versus those with rhBMP-2 and allograft [79].

Chronic pain at the harvesting site is one of the common side effects of using MSCs. One way to alleviate this would be to harvest local surgical site grafts. Furthermore, local harvests seem to be richer in fibroblastic colony-forming units when compared to iliac crest grafts making them a viable alternative [22,23].

Synthetic Peptides

One of the newer additions to graft substitutes is i-FACTORTM (Cerapedic Inc, Westminster, CO) made up of two components: 1) Anorganic bone mineral (ABM), a collection of calcium phosphate granules and 2) P-15, a synthetic peptide, both incorporated in a hydrogel carrier [81]. P-15 derived from the alpha-1 chain of type I collagen, has biomimetic potential and is therefore capable of promoting mineralization of bone when used in combination with ABMs which act as the scaffolding as well as the principal calcium source for bone formation [8,80,81].

i-FACTOR being a relatively recent addition to the pool of graft substitutes, comparative studies with conventional grafts are relatively few. Comparable fusion rates have been noticed between PEEK interbody cages packed with i-FACTOR versus those filled with autologous bone. Compared to autograft, i-FACTOR seems to show slightly better fusion rates in anterior cervical fusion as well as faster intra-cage bridging in posterior lumbar fusions [82,83,84]. Mobbs et al. in a study focussing on isolated i-FACTOR outcomes could demonstrate radiological evidence of fusion in 97.5% of one-level, 81% of two-level, and 100% of three-level fusions at two-year follow up as well as a statistically significant improvement of the postoperative disability index [85].

However, it is worthwhile mentioning that further evidence is required to mandate the use of i-FACTOR over autograft in spinal fusion procedures.

Gene Therapy

Therapeutic modulation of genes encoding osteoinductive and osteogenic factors forms one of the most promising avenues of modern research as far as spinal biologics is concerned. Animal studies with BMP-2 and BMP-9 have shown encouraging results whereby genes are induced via viral vectors to promote the release of growth factors and therefore enhance bone formation [53,83,86].

The limitation as of date with gene therapy is to reproduce the theoretical benefit in clinical efficacy studies as successful in vivo gene transduction is difficult to ascertain [83,87]. To circumvent this issue, ex vivo gene transduction is being tried and has been found to be effective in rat models [83,88]. In this method, donor cells cultured on laboratory media are transduced with a viral vector. This is followed by quantification of the amount of protein expressed and once optimum levels of the growth factor are reached, the autogenous cells are transplanted back into the donor. The ex vivo approach allows for a very generous production of growth factors due to the ease of isolation and expansion of transduced cells [89].

Most clinical trials of bone healing to date have utilized adenoviral vectors because of their high transfection capacity [86,90]. However, the adenoviral vectors cannot integrate into the host genome and hence are limited in their protein production capabilities. Also, they carry a significant risk of an immune response [91].

Though gene therapy with viral vectors forms one of the more exciting ventures for the future of spine biologics, further long-term safety and efficacy studies are mandated before they could be safely applied in clinical practice.

Conclusion

The field of spine biologics and grafts is ever-changing with a continually expanding array of options to choose from. Whilst Iliac crest autografts remain the gold standard for spinal fusion, donor site complications remain a significant limiting factor. This has led to the increasing use of alternatives like allografts, DBMs, and synthetic ceramics. Graft supplements like proteins and growth factors are also increasingly being used with improved results in patients. Another novel emerging domain of spinal biologics is genetic therapy to stimulate growth factor synthesis which has shown promising results in preliminary animal studies. The scientific boundaries need to be pushed further to develop even better grafting techniques and biologics to achieve the best rates of spinal fusion and ensure optimum clinical outcomes for our patients.

References

Ahn, J., Jorgensen, A. Y., Bohl, D. D., Tabaraee, E., Rossi, V. J., Aboushaala, K., Singh, K. Neuroforaminal bone growth following minimally invasive transforaminal lumbar interbody fusion with BMP : A computed tomographic analysis. *Clin. Spine Surg.* 2017, 30, E754–E758.

Albrektsson, T., and C. Johansson, "Osteoinduction, osteoconduction and osseointegration," *European Spine Journal*, vol. 10, no. 2, pp. S96–S101, 2001.

Alden, T. D., Beres, E. J., Laurent, J. S., Engh, J. A., Das, S., London, S. D., Jane, J. A., Hudson, S. B., Helm, G. A. The use of bone morphogenetic protein gene therapy in craniofacial bone repair. *J. Craniofac. Surg.* 2000, 11, 24–30.

Alimi, M., et al. "Radiographic and clinical outcome of silicate-substituted calcium phosphate (si-cap) ceramic bone graft in spinal fusion procedures," *Clinical Spine Surgery,* vol. 30, no. 6, pp. E845–e852, 2017.

An, H. S., Lynch, K., Toth, J. Prospective Comparison of Autograft vs. Allograft for Adult Posterolateral Lumbar Spine Fusion : Differences Among Freeze-Dried, Frozen, and Mixed Grafts. *J. Spinal Disord.* 1995, 8, 131–135.

Arrington, E. D., Smith, W. J., Chambers, H. G., Bucknell, A. L., Davino, N. A. Complications of iliac crest bone graft harvesting. *Clin. Orthop. Relat. Res.* 1996, 329, 300–309.

Bae, H. W., L. Zhao, L. E. A. Kanim, P. Wong, R. B. Delamarter, and E. G. Dawson, "Intervariability and intravariability of bone morphogenetic proteins in commercially available demineralized bone matrix products," *The Spine Journal,* vol. 31, no. 12, pp. 1299–1306, 2006.

Bansal, S., Chauhan, V., Sharma, S., Maheshwari, R., Juyal, A., Raghuvanshi, S. Evaluation of hydroxyapatite and beta-tricalcium phosphate mixed with bone marrow aspirate as a bone graft substitute for posterolateral spinal fusion. *Indian J. Orthop.* 2009, 43, 234–239.

Bhatnagar, R. S., Qian, J. J., Wedrychowska, A., Sadeghi, M., Wu, Y. M., Smith, N. Design of biomimetic habitats for tissue engineering with P-15, a synthetic peptide analogue of collagen. *Tissue Eng.* 1999, 5, 53–65.

Brown, M. D., Malinin, T. I., Davis, P. B. A roentgenographic evaluation of frozen allografts versus autografts in anterior cervical spine fusions. *Clin. Orthop. Relat. Res.* 1976, 119, 231–236.

Bruder, S., Fink, D. Mesenchymal stem cells. *J. Cell. Biochem.* 1994, 56, 283–294.

Buser, Z., Brodke, D. S., Youssef, J. A., Rometsch, E., Park, J. B., Yoon, S. T., Wang, J. C., Meisel, H. J. Allograft Versus Demineralized Bone Matrix in Instrumented and Noninstrumented Lumbar Fusion : A Systematic Review. *Glob. Spine J.* 2018, 8, 396–412.

Campana, V., Milano, G., Pagano, E., Barba, M., Cicione, C., Salonna, G., Lattanzi, W., Logroscino, G. Bone substitutes in orthopaedic surgery : From basic science to clinical practice. *J. Mater. Sci. Mater. M.* 2014, 25, 2445–2461.

Carragee, E. J., Hurwitz, E. L., Weiner, B. K. A critical review of recombinant human bone morphogenetic protein-2 trials in spinal surgery : Emerging safety concerns and lessons learned. *Spine J.* 2011, 11, 471–491.

Carreon, L. Y., Glassman, S. D., Anekstein, Y., Puno, R. M. Platelet gel (AGF) fails to increase fusion rates in instrumented posterolateral fusions. *Spine* 2005, 30, E243–E246.

Centrella, M., McCarthy, T., Canalis, E. Platelet-derived growth factor enhances deoxyribonucleic acid and collagen synthesis in osteoblast-enriched cultures from fetal rat parietal bone. *Endocrinology* 1989, 125, 13–20.

Chahla, J., Mannava, S., Cinque, M. E., Geeslin, A. G., Codina, D., LaPrade, R. F. Bone marrow aspirate concentrate harvesting and processing technique. *Arthrosc. Tech.* 2017, 6, e441–e445.

Chan, S. C. W., Tekari, A., Benneker, L. M., Heini, P. F., Gantenbein, B. Osteogenic differentiation of bone marrow stromal cells is hindered by the presence of intervertebral disc cells. *Arthritis Res.* 2015, 18, 29.

Chang, K. Y., Hsu, W. K. Spinal Biologics in Minimally Invasive Lumbar Surgery. *Minim. Invasive Surg*. 2018, 2018.

Delawi, D., Dhert, W. J. A., Castelein, R. M., Verbout, A. J., Oner, F. C. The incidence of donor site pain after bone graft harvesting from the posterior iliac crest may be overestimated : A study on spine fracture patients. *Spine* 2007, 32, 1865–1868.

Dimitriou, R., Mataliotakis, G. I., Angoules, A. G., Kanakaris, N. K., Giannoudis, P. V. Complications following autologous bone graft harvesting fr om the iliac crest and using the RIA : A systematic review. *Injury* 2011, 42, S3–S15.

Duarte, R. M., P. Varanda, R. L. Reis, A. R. Duarte, and J. Correia-Pinto, "Biomaterials and Bioactive Agents in Spinal Fusion," *Tissue Engineering Part B: Reviews,* vol. 23, no. 6, pp. 540–551, 2017.

Dutta, S. R., Passi, D., Singh, P., Bhuibhar, A. Ceramic and non-ceramic hydroxyapatite as a bone graft material : A brief review. *Ir. J. Med. Sci.* 2015, 184, 101–106.

Garrison, K. R., Donell, S., Ryder, J., Shemilt, I., Mugford, M., Harvey, I., Song, F. Clinical effectiveness and cost-effectiveness of bone morphogenetic proteins in the non-healing of fractures and spinal fusion : A systematic review. *Health Technol. Assess.* 2007, 11, 1–150.

Giannoudis, P. V., H. Dinopoulos, and E. Tsiridis, "Bone substitutes : an update," *Injury,* vol. 36, supplement 3, pp. S20–S27, 2005.

Glowacki, J., Mulliken, J. Demineralized Bone Implants. *Clin. Plast. Surg*. 1985, 12, 233–241.

Goldberg, V. M., and S. Akhavan, "Biology of Bone Grafts," in in *Bone Regeneration and Repair : Biology and Clinical Applications,* J. R. Lieberman and and G. E. Friedlaender, Eds., pp. 57–65, Humana Press, 2005.

Grabowski, G., and C. A. Cornett, "Bone graft and bone graft substitutes in spine surgery : Current concepts and controversies," *Journal of the American Academy of OrthopaedicSurgeons,* vol. 21, no. 1, pp. 51–60, 2013.

Grabowski, G., Robertson, R. Bone allograft with mesenchymal stem cells : A critical review of the literature. *Hard Tissue* 2012, 2, 1–8.

Gruskin, E., B. A. Doll, F. W. Futrell, J. P. Schmitz, and J. O. Hollinger, "Demineralized bone matrix in bone repair : history and use," *Advanced Drug Delivery Reviews,* vol. 64, no. 12, pp. 1063–1077, 2012.

Hanley E. N. The indications for lumbar spinal fusion with and without instrumentation. *Spine* 1995; 20(suppl 24) : S143–S153.

Harrell, C. R., Djonov, V., Fellabaum, C., Volarevic, V. Risks of using sterilization by gamma radiation : The other side of the coin. *Int. J. Med. Sci.* 2018, 15, 274–279.

Heldin, C. H., Miyazono, K., Ten Dijke, P. TGF-β signalling from cell membrane to nucleus through SMAD proteins. *Nature* 1997, 390, 465–471.

Hsu, W. K., M. S. Nickoli, J. C. Wang et al. "Improving the Clinical Evidence of Bone Graft Substitute Technology in Lumbar Spine Surgery," *Global Spine Journal,* vol. 2, no. 4, pp. 239–248, 2012.

Humphreys S. C., Hodges S. D., Patwardham A. G., et al. Comparison of posterior and transforaminal approaches to lumbar interbody fusion. *Spine* 2001; 26 : 567–571.

Jenis, L. G., Blanco, R. J., Kwon, B. A prospective study of Autologous Growth Factors (AGF) in lumbar interbody fusion. *Spine J.* 2006, 6, 14–20.

Kadam, A., Millhouse, P., Kepler, C., Radcliff, K., Fehlings, M., Janssen, M., Sasso, R., Benedict, J., Vaccaro, A. Bone substitutes and expanders in Spine Surgery : A review of their fusion efficacies. *Int. J. Spine Surg.* 2016, 10, 1–29.

Kaito, T., Morimoto, T., Kanayama, S., Otsuru, S., Kashii, M., Makino, T., Kitaguchi, K., Furuya, M., Chijimatsu, R., Ebina, K., et al. Modeling and remodeling effects of intermittent administration of teriparatide (parathyroid hormone 1–34) on bone morphogenetic protein-induced bone in a rat spinal fusion model. *Bone Rep.* 2016, 5, 173–180.

Kalfas, I. H., "Principles of bone healing," *Neurosurgical Focus,* vol. 10, no. 4, p. E1, 2001.

Kang, J., H. An, A. Hilibrand, S. T. Yoon, E. Kavanagh, and S. Boden, "Grafton and local bone have comparable outcomes to iliac crest bone in instrumented single-level lumbar fusions," *The Spine Journal,* vol. 37, no. 12, pp. 1083–1091, 2012.

Kannan, A., S. N. M. Dodwad, and W. K. Hsu, "Biologics in spine arthrodesis," *Journal of Spinal Disorders & Techniques,* vol. 28, no. 5, pp. 163–170, 2015.

Kersten, R. F. M. R., Van Gaalen, S. M., De Gast, A., Öner, F. C. Polyetheretherketone (PEEK) cages in cervical applications : A systematic review. *Spine J.* 2015, 15, 1446–1460.

Khashan, M., Inoue, S., Berven, S. H. Cell based therapies as compared to autologous bone grafts for spinal arthrodesis. *Spine* 2013, 38, 1885–1891.

Kok, D., Peeters, C. M. M., Mardina, Z., Oterdoom, D. L. M., Bulstra, S. K., Veldhuizen, A. G., Kuijer, R., Wapstra, F. H. Is remaining intervertebral disc tissue interfering with bone generation during fusion of two vertebrae ? *PloS One* 2019, 14, 1–10.

Kokorina, N. A., Zakharkin, S. O., Krebsbach, P. H., Nussenbaum, B. Treatment effects of rhBMP-2 on invasiveness of oral carcinoma cell lines. *Laryngoscope* 2011, 12, 1876–1880.

Kurz, L., Garfin, S. Harvesting autogenous Iliac Bone Graft : A review of complications and techniques. *Spine* 1989, 14, 1324–1331.

Lauweryns, P., Raskin, Y. Prospective analysis of a new bone graft in lumbar interbody fusion : results of a 2-year prospective clinical and radiological study. *Int. J. Spine Surg.* 2015, 9, 2.

Li, X., Ghavidel Mehr, N., Guzmán-Morales, J., Favis, B. D., De Crescenzo, G., Yakandawala, N., Hoemann, C. D. Cationic osteogenic peptide P15-CSP coatings promote 3-D osteogenesis in poly(epsilon-caprolactone) scaffolds of distinct pore size. *J. Biomed. Mater. Res. A* 2017, 105, 2171–2181.

Liao, Z., Wang, C. H., Cui, W. L. Comparison of Allograft and Autograft in Lumbar Fusion for Lumbar Degenerative Diseases : A Systematic Review. *J. Investig. Surg.* 2016, 29, 373–382.

Lieberman, J. R., Daluiski, A., Stevenson, S., Jolla, L., Wu, L., Mcallister, P., Lee, Y. P., Kabo, J. M., Finerman, G. A. M., Berk, A. J., et al. The Effect of Regional Gene Therapy with Bone Morphogenetic Protein-2-Producing Bone-Marrow Cells on the Repair of Segmental Femoral Defects in Rats*. *J. Bone Jt. Surg.* 1999, 81, 905–917.

Lou, J., Xu, F., Merkel, K., Manske, P. Gene therapy : Adenovirus-mediated human bone morphogenetic protein-2 gene transfer induces mesenchymal progenitor cell proliferation and differentiation in vitro and bone formation in vivo. *J. Orthop. Res.* 1999, 17, 43–50.

Louis-Ugbo, J., Kim, H. S., Boden, S. D., Mayr, M. T., Li, R. C., Seeherman, H., D'Augusta, D., Blake, C., Jiao, A., Peckham, S. Retention of 125I-labeled recombinant human bone morphogenetic protein-2 by biphasic calcium phosphate or a composite sponge in a rabbit posterolateral spine arthrodesis model. *J. Orthop. Res.* 2002, 20, 1050–1059.

Lowery, G. L., Kulkarni, S., Pennisi, A. E. Use of autologous growth factors in lumbar spinal fusion. *Bone* 1999, 25, 47S–50S.

Mack, C. A., Song, W. R., Carpenter, H., Wickham, T. J., Kovesdi, I., Harvey, B. G., Magovern, C. J., Isom, O. W., Rosengart, T., Falck-Pedersen, E., et al. Circumvention of anti-adenovirus neutralizing immunity by administration of an adenoviral vector of an alternate serotype. *Hum. Gene* 2008, 8, 99–109.

Majidinia, M., Sadeghpour, A., Yousefi, B. The roles of signaling pathways in bone repair and regeneration. *J. Cell. Physiol.* 2018, 233, 2937–2948.

Makino, T., Tsukazaki, H., Ukon, Y., Tateiwa, D., Yoshikawa, H., Kaito, T. The biological enhancement of spinal fusion for spinal degenerative disease. *Int. J. Mol. Sci.* 2018, 19, 2430.

Manyalich, M., Navarro, A., Koller, J., Loty, B., de Guerra, A., Cornu, O., Vabels, G., Fornasari, P. M., Costa, A. N., Siska, I., et al. European Quality System for Tissue Banking. *Transpl. P.* 2009, 41, 2035–2043.

May, R. D., Frauchiger, D. A., Albers, C. E., Benneker, L. M., Kohl, S., Gantenbein, B. Inhibitory effects of human primary intervertebral disc cells on human primary osteoblasts in a co-culture system. *Int. J. Mol. Sci.* 2018, 19, 1195.

Mesfin, A. High-dose rhBMP-2 for adults : Major and minor complications : A study of 502 spine cases. *Bone Jt. J.* 2013, 95, 1546–1553.

Mobbs, R. J., Maharaj, M., Rao, P. J. Clinical outcomes and fusion rates following anterior lumbar interbody fusion with bone graft substitute i-FACTOR, an anorganic bone matrix/P-15 composite. *J. Neurosurg. Spine* 2014, 21, 867–876.

Mobbs, R., Phan, K., Malham, G., Seex, K., Rao, P. J. Lumbar interbody fusion : Techniques, indications and comparison of interbody fusion options including PLIF, TLIF, MI-TLIF, OLIF/ATP, LLIF and ALIF. *J. Spine Surg* 2015, *1*, 2–18.

Mohr, J., Germain, M., Winters, M., Fraser, S., Duong, A., Garibaldi, A., Simunovic, N., Alsop, D., Dao, D., Bessemer, R., et al. Disinfection of human musculoskeletal allografts in tissue banking : A systematic review. *Cell Tissue Bank.* 2016, 17, 573–584.

Morimoto, T., Kaito, T., Kashii, M., Matsuo, Y., Sugiura, T., Iwasaki, M., Yoshikawa, H. Effect of intermittent administration of teriparatide (parathyroid hormone 1–34) on bone morphogenetic protein-induced bone formation in a rat model of spinal fusion. *J. Bone Jt. Surg. Am.* 2014, 96, e107.

Musgrave, D. S., Pruchnic, R., Bosch, P., Ziran, B. H., Whalen, J., Huard, J. Human skeletal muscle cells in ex vivo gene therapy to deliver bone morphogenetic protein-2. *J. Bone Jt. Surg.* 2003, 84, 120–127.

Okubo, Y., Kusumoto, K., Bessho, K. Accelerators of osteogenesis by recombinant human bone morphogenetic protein-2. *Drug Target. Insights* 2007, 2, 55–60.

Overley, S. C., Mcanany, S. J., Anwar, M. A., Merrill, R. K., Lovy, A., Guzman, J. Z., Zhadanov, S., Doshi, A., Rothenberg, E., Vaishnav, A., et al. Predictive Factors and Rates of Fusion in Minimally Invasive Transforaminal Lumbar Interbody Fusion Utilizing rhBMP-2 or Mesenchymal Stem Cells. *Int. J. Spine Surg.* 2019, 13, 46–52.

Owens, K., Glassman, S. D., Howard, J. M., Djurasovic, M., Witten, J. L., Carreon, L. Y. Perioperative complications with rhBMP-2 in transforaminal lumbar interbody fusion. *Eur. Spine J.* 2011, 20, 612–617.

Parajón, A., Alimi, M., Navarro-Ramirez, R., Christos, P., Torres-Campa, J. M., Moriguchi, Y., Lang, G., Härtl, R. Minimally invasive transforaminal lumbar interbody fusion : Meta-analysis of the fusion rates. What is the optimal graft material ? *Clin. Neurosurg.* 2017, 81, 958–971.

Poon, B., Kha, T., Tran, S., Dass, C. R. Bone morphogenetic protein-2 and bone therapy : Successes and pitfalls. *J. Pharm. Pharm.* 2016, 68, 139–147.

Putzier, M., Strube, P., Funk, J. F., Gross, C., Mönig, H. J., Perka, C., Pruss, A. Allogenic versus autologous cancellous bone in lumbar segmental spondylodesis : A randomized prospective study. *Eur. Spine J.* 2009, 18, 687–695.

Rao, P. J., Pelletier, M. H., Walsh, W. R., Mobbs, R. J. Spine Interbody Implants : Material Selection andModification, Functionalization and Bioactivation of Surfaces to Improve Osseointegration. *Orthop. Surg.* 2014.

Resnick, D. K., Watters, W. C., Mummaneni, P. V., Dailey, A. T., Choudhri, T. F., Eck, J. C., Sharan, A., Groff, M. W., Wang, J. C., Ghogawala, Z., et al. Guideline update for the performance of fusion procedures for degenerative disease of the lumbar spine. Part 10 : Lumbar fusion for stenosis without spondylolisthesis. *J. Neurosurg. Spine* 2014, 21, 62–66.

Risbud, M. V., Shapiro, I. M., Guttapalli, A., Di Martino, A., Danielson, K. G., Beiner, J. M., Hillibrand, A., Albert, T. J., Anderson, D. G., Vaccaro, A. R. Osteogenic potential of adult human stem cells of the lumbar vertebral body and the iliac crest. *Spine* 2006, 31, 83–89.

Roberto, C., Fernando, L. The Biology of Bone Grafts. *Recent Adv. Arthroplast.* 2012, 13, 77–86.

Salazar, V. S., Gamer, L. W., Rosen, V. BMP signalling in skeletal development, disease and repair. *Nat. Rev. Endocrinol.* 2016, 12, 203–221.

Seaman, S., Kerezoudis, P., Bydon, M., Torner, J. C., Hitchon, P. W. Titanium vs. Polyetheretherketone (PEEK) interbody fusion : Meta-analysis and review of the literature. *J. Clin. Neurosci.* 2017, 44, 23–29.

Sherman, B. P., Lindley, E. M., Turner, A. S., Seim, H. B., Benedict, J., Burger, E. L., Patel, V. V. Evaluation of ABM/P-15 versus autogenous bone in an ovine lumbar interbody fusion model. *Eur. Spine J.* 2010, 19, 2156–2163.

Shields, L. B. E., Raque, G. H., Glassman, S. D., Campbell, M., Vitaz, T., Harpring, J., Shields, C. B. Adverse effects associated with high-dose recombinant human bone morphogenetic protein-2 use in anterior cervical spine fusion. *Spine* 2006, 31, 542–547.

Skovrlj, B., Guzman, J. Z., Al Maaieh, M., Cho, S. K., Iatridis, J. C., Qureshi, S. A. Cellular bone matrices : Viable stem cell-containing bone graft substitutes. *Spine J.* 2014, 14, 2763–2772.

Sonntag V. K., Marciano F. F. Is fusion indicated for lumbar spinal disorders ? *Spine* 1995; 20(suppl24) : S138 – S142.

Stonecipher T., Wright S. Posterior lumbar interbody fusion with facet screw fixation. *Spine* 1989;14 : 468 – 471.

Suchomel, P., Barsa, P., Buchvald, P., Svobodnik, A., Vanickova, E. Autologous versus allogenic bone grafts in instrumented anterior cervical discectomy and fusion : A prospective study with respect to bone union pattern. *Eur. Spine J.* 2004, 13, 510–515.

Summary of safety and effectiveness data (Ssed) 2008, 1–18. Available online : https://www.accessdata.fda. gov/cdrh_docs/pdf/P010031S232b.pdf (accessed on 26 September 2019).

Tilkeridis, K., P. Touzopoulos, A. Ververidis, S. Christodoulou, K. Kazakos, and G. I. Drosos, "Use of demineralized bone matrix in spinal fusion," *World Journal of Orthopedics,* vol. 5, no. 1, pp. 30–37, 2014.

Tohmeh, A. G., Watson, B., Tohmeh, M., Zielinski, X. J. Allograft cellular bone matrix in extreme lateral interbody fusion : Preliminary radiographic and clinical outcomes. *Sci. World J.* 2012, 2012, 30–32.

Velchuru, V. R., Satish, S. G., John Petri, G., Sturzaker, H. G. Hernia through an iliac crest bone graft site : Report of a case and review of the literature. *Bull. Hosp. Jt. Dis.* 2006, 63, 166.

Walker, B., Koerner, J., Sankarayanaryanan, S., Radcliff, K. A consensus statement regarding the utilization of BMP in spine surgery. *Curr. Rev. Musculoskelet. Med.* 2014, 7, 208–219.

Yoon, S. T., Boden, S. D. Spine fusion by gene therapy. Gene Ther. 2004, 11, 360.

Zadegan, S. A., Abedi, A., Jazayeri, S. B., Bonaki, H. N., Vaccaro, A. R., Rahimi-Movaghar, V., Rao, P. J., Pelletier, M. H., Walsh, W. R., Mobbs, R. J., et al. Titanium vs. Polyetheretherketone (PEEK) interbody fusion : Meta-analysis and review of the literature. *Eur. Spine J.* 2017, 15, 364–377.

Zdeblick T. A. A prospective randomized study of lumbar fusion. *Spine* 1993; 18 : 983–991.

Zimmermann, G., Moghaddam, A. Allograft bone matrix versus synthetic bone graft substitutes. *Injury* 2011, 42, 16–21.

Chapter 14

Endoscopic Third Ventriculostomy for Hydrocephalus Associated with Tubercular Meningitis

Kaushik Sil, Siddharth Mistri and Sandip Chatterjee*
Park Clinic, Kolkata, India

Abstract

Tuberculosis is one of the deadliest endemic diseases known to mankind, with the World Health Organisation declaring it as a public health emergency in 2018. In 2019 itself, 10 million people in the world have fallen victim to this disease, out of whom some 1.4 million had died [1]. The disease and death burden is more severe in patients with HIV [2]. More than one fourth of the tuberculosis patients of the world are from India with an incidence rate of 159 per 100000 population. Multidrug resistant (MDR) and Extreme drug resistant (XDR) cases are steadily rising in the affected population. A vast majority of the cases occurs in the pediatric age group. Amongst the lethal complications in children, tuberculous meningitis (TBM) ranks first with a death rate of 10 per 100000 affected. The most common sequel of TBM is hydrocephalus with an incidence of almost 70% – majority of which are communicating while a significant number may also be of the non communicating type. The non – communicating hydrocephalus usually requires surgical intervention while the communicating hydrocephalus usually responds to medical therapy in 70-92% cases. However surgical intervention is required only when level of consciousness deteriorates or CT scan shows progressive enlargement of the ventricular system or when the CSF

*Corresponding Author's Email: sandipchat@gmail.com.

In: Neurosurgery Research
Editors: Amit Agrawal, Pradeep Chouksey, Adesh Shrivastava et al.
ISBN: 978-1-68507-837-9

pressure increases progressively [3]. Early shunt surgery increases chances of good recovery [4].

Pathophysiology

Tuberculosis spreads into the nervous system from the lung focus created by inhalation of tuberculous bacilli. Children, immunocompromised people, HIV affected host are the most susceptible to develop this disease. The infection spreads to the nervous system through the bloodstream. Inside the brain, the relative hypoxic zones served by the end arteries act as the main nidus of infection. As the lymphocytes rush in to surround this zone, the exudates start forming. Rupture of such a focus leads to spread of caseous material around the subarachnoid cisterns, encasing the great vessels and nerves. Meningitis is associated with the neuro-inflammatory cascade triggered by the interaction of the bacteria with the host immune response [5]. The progressive encasement of arteries and resultant perivascular inflammation leads to ischaemia and downstream infarction. Multiple cranial nerve involvement at the cisterns leads to cranial polyneuropathy. The body manages to localize the infection in some cases as tuberculomas, while in others the disease remains virulent, The child accordingly gets progressively drowsy and develops vasculitis symptoms and infarctions, along with multiple cranial neuropathies especially involving the sixth, fourth and third nerves . Exudates block the fourth ventricular outlets, narrow the aqueduct and prevent reabsorption of CSF across the arachnoid granulations – all of which singly or combination cause hydrocephalus [6]. Hydrocephalus further results in deterioration of the consciousness level and the child becomes comatose. Progressive hydrocephalus leads to transependymal seepage of cerebrospinal fluid in the brain already softened by infarction. The greatly compliant "wet" brain leads to further increase of hydrocephalus and vasculitis symptoms.

In TBM, a thick gelatinous exudate develops around the basal cisterns, the sylvian fissure and the brainstem. As this may cause obstruction to the outflow from the fourth ventricle or indeed from the cerebral aqueduct, hydrocephalus frequently develops in these children, and this further exacerbates the clinical condition by raising the intracranial pressure (ICP). The brain itself shows edema, perivascular infiltration with lymphocytes and mononuclear cells, and a microglial reaction. Indeed, a vasculitis-like syndrome may result, where inflammatory changes may be seen in the vessel wall, and the lumen of these vessels may be narrowed or even occluded by formation of the thrombi, and this may result in small areas of infarction. In the majority of patients, the location of the infarctions is in the distribution of the medial striate and thalamoperforating arteries. Rarely, hemorrhagic transformation of these infarcts may occur.

Clinical Stages

The clinical progress has been variously described in different stages – described eloquently in the Palur grading [7] system. Grade I patients have headaches, vomiting, fever with normal sensorium; Grade II patients present with neurodeficit, patients in grade III have altered sensorium but are easily arousable and grade IV patients are deeply comatose . Vasculitis gives rise to hemiparesis and cranial neuropathies result in various opthalmoplegias and facio-vestibulocochlear paresis. Hydrocephalus compounds this picture with headache, nausea, vomiting and papilledema - all hallmarks of the primary disease itself. Many a times symptoms of hydrocephalus are overshadowed by the obtundation caused by fever and meningitis.

Diagnosis

Clinical suspicion may be confirmed by doing contrast CT or MRI scan of the brain which show enhancement of the cisterns, hydrocephalus and infarctions. MR spectroscopy can suggest lipid lactate peaks in tuberculoma distinguishing them from other granulomas. Lumbar puncture may be useful in communicating hydrocephalus both as a diagnostic and a therapeutic measure. Hallmarks of Tuberculosis in CSF are golden yellowish exudates, high protein count with relatively preserved sugar count with lymphocytosis. Rarely are quantitative measurements like TB Gold or TB PCR of any value in endemic zones. Gram stain and culture isolation of Mycobacterium is definitive but delayed by 6-8 weeks.

Hydrocephalus is TBM is usually communicating to start with but may become non communicating in later stages. Unlike pyogenic meningitis, septations and multiloculations are less. The ventricular wall becomes thick after being studded with exudates and the expansion is slow but precipitous after some time. Transependymal seepage is also late. So, there is a period when the child is preserved (grades I & II) only to drop precipitously later.

Management of TBM Hydrocephalus

The management is dictated by the clinical grading. In grades 3 and 4, where the child is obtunded, quick external ventricular drainage is the game changer. Definitive management is deferred till the sensorium improves and the "wet" brain appears dry. The definitive treatment of choice is Ventriculo-peritoneal (VP) shunt – it is done in good grade patients and those who have recovered from obtundation and done early gives good result [8]. However, the highly protineaceous CSF, non compliant ventricular walls and soft brain – all result in a high incidence of shunt failure. Shunt dysfunction rates may be as high as 43% in various published series [9]. Herein comes the role of endoscopic third ventriculostomy (ETV) as an alternative – first suggested and described by Figagai et al. in 2003 [10].

ETV in TBM

In spite of the hydrocephalus in TBM being of non communicating variety in some patients, it is theoretically possible that ETV will be successful [11]. With experience, ETV can be offered as a safe, long-lasting and ideal solution for hydrocephalus associated with TBM [12]. However the intraoperative hurdles are many. The ventricular walls are stiff and studded with tubercles (Figure 1) which often bleed on touch. The local inflammation does not allow the foramen of Munro to dilate as much as in a normal hydrocephalus – so injury to the foraminal wall and fornix by the endoscope is possible. The third ventricle, its walls and its floor are layered by tubercles and exudates leading to difficulty in identifying the landmarks for perforation. Inflammation often leads to very thick floor and adhesion of the basilar artery or the perforators to the floor on the cisternal side – this may result in inadvertent bleeding. There may be multiple layers of thick adhesions between the floor and the basal cistern. (Figure 2) Most importantly if the cistern is opened at a focal point, the circulation may not be adequate in the other part of the cistern. Similarly, the reabsorption across the arachnoid villi may be suboptimal due to exudates [13, 14, 15].

Endoscopic third ventriculostomy is still preferred as first choice effective treatment [16, 17, 18] as it, if successful, gives shunt independence relieving the child of nightmares of shunt revision.

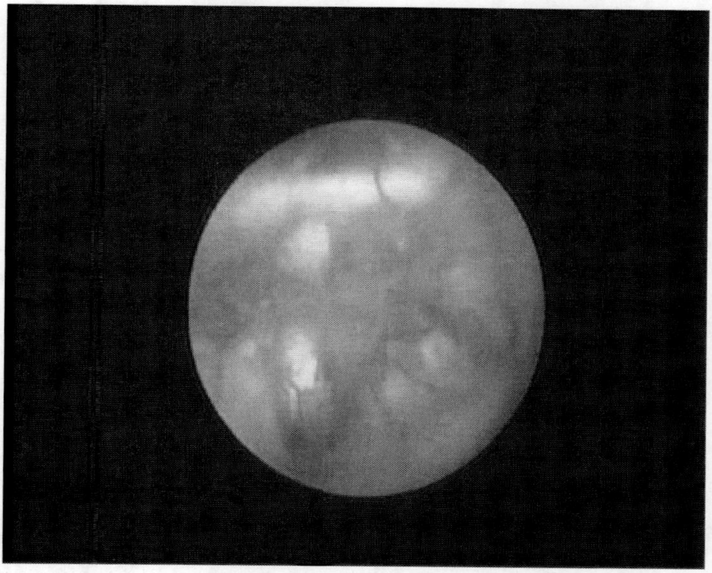

Figure 1. tubercles on the floor of the third ventricle.

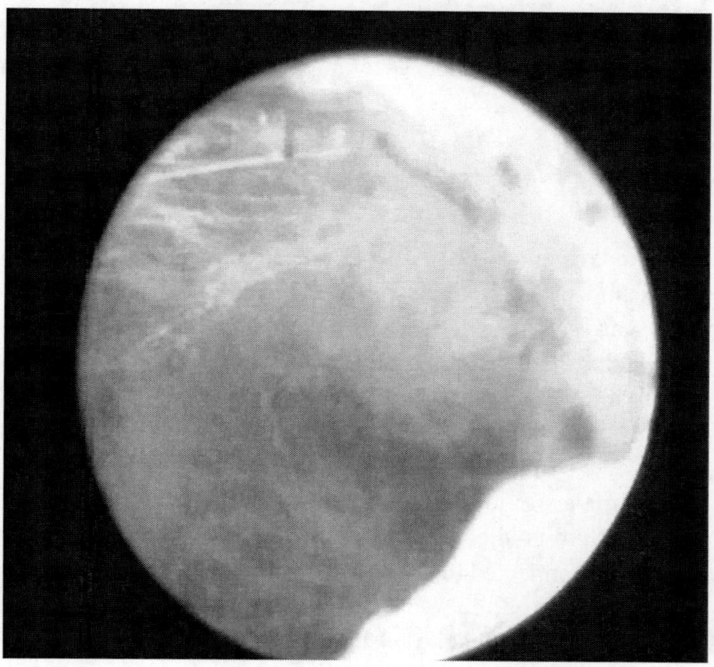

Figure 2. Multiple leayers at the ETV site.

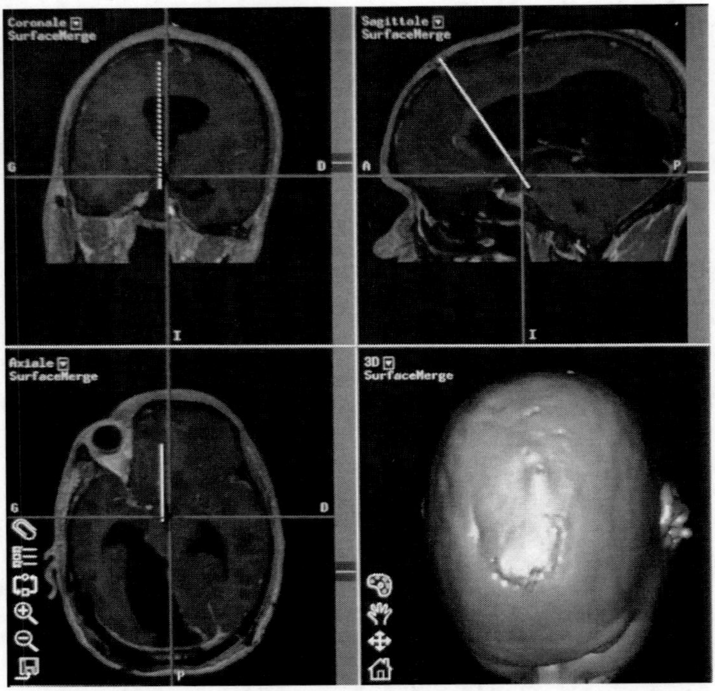

Figure 3. Neuronavigated ETV.

Techniques of ETV in Hydrocephalus Associated with TBM

1. NeuroNavigation – Intraoperative neuronavigation has opened a new vista for safe ETV surgery in TBM. (Figure 3) The narrow foramen of Munro can be negotiated by placing the burrhole strategically with the help of neuronavigation. Navigation also aids in adjuvant procedures like septostomy [19].
2. Water jet technique - The non visualisation issue of the floor can be overcome by waterjet technique [20]. An initial tentative hole is made with bipolar tip just behind the dorsum sellae after feeling it. Warm Ringer fluid is injected through this with a 2 mm catheter (10ml per 4-8 secs) connected to a syringe through which aspiration of cisternal content is also done. A stoma is established within 2 to 5 minutes, which is then dilated in the standard fashion.
3. Intraoperative Doppler: A 2- MHz pulse – waved Doppler transducer with 1.8 mm diameter can be inserted through the working channel of

the rigid endoscope with its head sticking out. Once the floor is touched, the sonometer pinpoints the location of the basilar artery complex and perforators. Fenestration is then made in the appropriate portion of the floor [21, 22].

4. Using blunt probe only to open the floor when no Doppler guidance is available – avoiding sharp bipolar tip or graspers.
5. Lumbar puncture in first few postoperative days – a cycle of lumbar punctures in first 3-4 days can help in maintaining a gradient for opening of stoma, unless the spinal arachnoid space is blocked [17].

Conclusion

- ETV must be offered as an option in third week of the disease after the acute phase is over
- ETV is useful in non communicating hydrocephalus following TB meningitis.
- ETV must be done by the most experienced team.
- Intraoperative adjuncts like navigation and Doppler must be used if available
- Patience and persistence are the key to success.
- Backup plan for intraoperative complications must always be kept handy.
- Close follow up is necessary for detecting early failure.
- In selected patients of TBM, ETV renders the child a shunt free life.

References

Aranha A, Choudhary A, Bhaskar S, Gupta L. A randomized study comparing endoscopic third ventriculostomy versus ventriculoperitoneal shunt in the management of hydrocephalus due to tuberculous meningitis. *Asian J. Neurosurg.* 2018;13(4):1140.

Bhagwati S, Mehta N, Shah S. Use of endoscopic third ventriculostomy in hydrocephalus of tubercular origin. *Child's Nerv. Syst.* 2010;26(12):1675–82.

Chatterjee S. Review Article Brain tuberculomas, tubercular meningitis, and post-tubercular hydrocephalus in children. *J. Pediatr. Neurosci.* 2011;6:96–100.

Chugh A P, Husain M, Gupta R K, Ojha B K, Chandra A, Rastogi M. Surgical outcome of tuberculous meningitis hydrocephalus treated by endoscopic third ventriculostomy: Prognostic factors and postoperative neuroimaging for functional assessment of ventriculostomy - Clinical article. *J. Neurosurg. Pediatr.* 2009;3 (5):371–7.

Donovan J, Thwaites G E, Huynh J. Tuberculous meningitis: Where to from here? *Curr. Opin. Infect. Dis.* 2020;33(3):259–66.

Eguchi S, Aihara Y, Tsuzuki S et al. A modified method to enhance the safety of ETV-transendoscopic pulse –waved microvascular Doppler –assisted ETV, technical note . *Childs Nerv. Syst.* 2014;30(3): 515-9.

Feng H, Huang G, Liao X, Fu K, Tan H, Pu H, et al. Endoscopic third ventriculostomy in the management of obstructive hydrocephalus: An outcome analysis. *J. Neurosurg.* 2004;100(4):626–33.

Figaji A A, Fieggen A G, Peter J C. Endoscopic third ventriculostomy in tuberculous meningitis. *Child's Nerv. Syst.* 2003;19(4):217–25.

Global Tuberculosis report- 2020. Geneva: World Health Organisation: 2020.

Jha D K, Mishra V, Choudhary A, Khatri P, Tiwari R, Sural A, et al. Factors affecting the outcome of neuroendoscopy in patients with tuberculous meningitis hydrocephalus: a preliminary study. *Surg. Neurol.* 2007;68(1):35–41.

Jha D, Khatri P, Choudhary A, Sethi R, Kumar S. Endoscopic third ventriculostomy in prepontine-suprasellar tuberculoma with tuberculous meningitis hydrocephalus: A case report. Pediatr. *Neurosurg.* 2006;43(1):42–6.

Jonathan A, Rajshekhar V. Endoscopic third ventriculostomy for chronic hydrocephalus after tuberculous meningitis. *Surg. Neurol.* 2005;63(1):32–5.

Kemaloglu S, Özkan Ü, Bukte Y, Ceviz A, Özates M. Timing of shunt surgery in childhood tuberculous meningitis with hydrocephalus. *Pediatr. Neurosurg.* 2002;37(4):194–8.

Kemaloglu S, Özkan Ü, Bukte Y,et al. Timing of shunt surgery in childhood tuberculous meningitis with hydrocephalus. *Pediatr. Neurosurg.* 2002;37(4):194–8.

Marais S, Thwaites G, Schoeman J F, et al. Tuberculous meningitis: a uniform case definition for use in clinical research. *Lancet Infect Dis [Internet].* 2010;10 (11):803–12.

Martinez –Moreno M, Widhalm G, Mert A et al. A novel protocol of continuos navigation guidance for ETV. *Neurosurgery* 2014 Dec;10 Suppl 4:514-23.

Palur R, Rajsekhar V, Chandy M J, Joseph T et al. Shunt surgery for hydrocephalus in tuberculous meningitis : a long term follow up study. *J. Neurosurg.* 1991;74:64-9.

Sil K, Chatterjee S. Shunting in tuberculous meningitis: A neurosurgeon's nightmare. *Child's Nerv. Syst.* 2008;24(9):1029–32.

Singh D, Sachdev V, Singh A K, Sinha S. Endoscopic third ventriculostomy in post-tubercular meningitic hydrocephalus: A preliminary report. *Minim Invasive Neurosurg.* 2005;48(1):47–52.

Yadav Y R, Parihar V, Agrawal M, Bhatele P R. Endoscopic third ventriculostomy in tubercular meningitis with hydrocephalus. *Neurol. India.* 2011;59(6):855–60.

Yadav Y R, Shenoy R, Mukerji G, Parihar V. Water jet dissection technique for endoscopic third ventriculostomy minimises the risk of bleeding and neurological complications in obstructive hydrocephalus with a thick and opaque third ventricle floor. *Minim Invasive Neurosurg.* 2010;53(4):155–8.

Yadav Y, Parihar V, Todorov M, Kher Y, Chaurasia I, Pande S, et al. Role of endoscopic third ventriculostomy in tuberculous meningitis with hydrocephalus. *Asian J. Neurosurg.* 2016;11(4):325.

Chapter 15

Recent Evidence for Decompressive Craniectomy

Gustavo Adolfo Gaitán-Herrera[1,2], Laura Marcela Acevedo-Aguilar[1,2] and Iván David Lozada-Martínez[1,2,*]

[1]School of Medicine, Universidad de Cartagena, Cartagena, Colombia
[2]Colombian Clinical Research Group in Neurocritical Care, Latin American Council of Neurocritical Care, Cartagena, Colombia

Abstract

Multiple pathologies give rise to brain injuries that cause one or more of the components of the cranial vault to suffer an increase in their usual volume, resulting in an excessive increase in pressure inside the skull, a condition known as intracranial hypertension (ICH), which is the main cause of disability and mortality in patients with brain injury. Because of this, decompressive craniectomy (DC) has emerged as a therapeutic alternative in patients with this condition who do not respond satisfactorily to medical management. This surgical procedure, which aims to increase the capacity of the intracranial space, consists in the resection of the cranial bone together with a dura mater plasty, thus allowing a decompression of such space. This chapter will deal with its clinical utility, inquiring about relevant aspects to consider, such as its indications, the different surgical techniques and possible complications, in order to provide an adequate knowledge about this procedure.

---

[*]Corresponding Author's Email: ilozadam@unicartagena.edu.co.

In: Neurosurgery Research
Editors: Amit Agrawal, Pradeep Chouksey, Adesh Shrivastava et al.
ISBN: 978-1-68507-837-9

Introduction

Numerous types of brain injuries, particularly traumatic brain injury (TBI), are important causes of ICH (Ban et al., 2010). In addition, they are a major source of disability in survivors of these types of injuries, leading to a significant loss of potential years of active life, as well as very high socioeconomic costs to the health care system (Grille and Tommasino 2015). Intracranial pressure (ICP) may be elevated due to increased mass effect from hematomas and contusions, diffuse cerebral edema formation, or hydrocephalus (Kolias et al., 2016). This increased volume within the skull can lead to ischemia due to reduced cerebral perfusion pressure (CPP), ultimately resulting in disability or death (Hawryluk et al., 2020; Kolias et al., 2016).

Based on the above, management of brain inflammation and ICH are a key component of care in brain injury (Hutchinson et al., 2019). Elevated ICP and reduced CPP are associated with an increased burden of cerebral ischemia and worsening clinical outcomes, therefore, the goal of treatment will be to maintain these two variables at optimal levels and thus maintain adequate cerebral blood flow (CBF) and prevent ischemia (Smith 2017).

On the other hand, refractory ICH, defined as ICH that is not controlled with conventional therapeutic measures, occurs in 10-15% of patients and is associated with high mortality; in this type of patient, DC is an alternative to the usual medical treatment (Ban et al., 2010; Grille and Tommasino 2015). Until now, the paucity of high-quality outcome data from randomized controlled trials has led to uncertainty about the efficacy of such a procedure (Hutchinson et al., 2019). Because of this, technical aspects of surgery, timing and patient selection continue to be debated, and there has even been disagreement as to whether this procedure should be performed at all (Hawryluk et al., 2020). The present chapter will detail and review based on the most recent evidence, focusing on the most important aspects of DC.

Decompressive Craniectomy

CD is a surgical procedure that has gained great interest in recent years (Zhang et al., 2017). It consists of removing a large part of the skull and opening the underlying dura mater (Hutchinson et al., 2016; Kolias et al., 2016), with the aim of providing a wider space in which the injured or ischemic brain can expand (Honeybul and Ho 2014), thus reducing ICP and improving CPP (Viruez-Soto et al., 2018). This procedure is based on the Monroe-Kellie doctrine, which determines that an increase in intracranial volume by any of its components requires a simultaneous decrease in another of them as a compensatory mechanism to maintain adequate ICP levels (Brown and Wijdicks 2017), which is why this procedure could be an important therapeutic tool in different clinical settings (Grille and Tommasino 2015). However, DC remains a controversial procedure due to the significant risks it may entail (Brown and Wijdicks 2017). For this reason, several randomized controlled trials have emerged in order to provide adequate guidance on the appropriate indications for this procedure, including DECRA (Decompressive Craniectomy in Patients with Severe Traumatic Brain Injury) and RescueICP (Trial of Decompressive Craniectomy for Traumatic Intracranial Hypertension), who, in spite of the study carried out, concluded that to perform or not to perform this procedure is a complex decision, being of great importance to evaluate individually in each patient if the potential benefits outweigh the possible complications that may occur (Hawryluk et al., 2020).

Types of Surgical Decompression

DC can be performed in different clinical contexts (Sahuquillo and Dennis 2019). According to the time at which it is performed, it can be categorized into two types: primary and secondary (Godoy et al., 2017).

Prophylactic Decompression or Primary Decompressive Craniectomy (P-DC)

Primary DC consists of the removal of a bone flap subsequent to the evacuation of intracranial lesions (Hutchinson et al., 2019), with the aim of avoiding potential increases in ICP following surgery (Sahuquillo and Dennis 2019). Thus, this type of decompression is mainly employed in the context of a subsequent evacuation of an acute subdural hematoma, on which a lower mortality rate has been demonstrated in patients undergoing this procedure (Smith 2017). However, it does not constitute a standard line of treatment, so proper evaluation and selection of patients by a qualified specialist is necessary (Wettervi et al., 2018).

Secondary Decompressive Craniectomy

Secondary DC is performed to control late increases in intracranial pressures, generally in patients who are under constant monitoring of intracranial pressures (Hawryluk et al., 2020; Hutchinson et al., 2016). However, it is used only as a last resort when medical treatment does not provide favorable results (Smith 2017; Zhang et al., 2017).

Surgical Techniques

DC can be performed with different surgical techniques according to the requirements of each patient (Sahuquillo and Dennis 2019). However, each of them must comply with certain requirements that have evidenced more satisfactory results; the most important of them is that the extension of the extracted bone must be greater than 12 or 15 cm in diameter exceeding the margins of the lesion to be treated, in order to avoid herniation through the craniectomy space and the consequent development of infarcts (Hawryluk et al., 2020; Lacerda 2013).

There are mainly two surgical variants to develop DC: bifrontal craniectomy and frontotemporo-parietal craniectomy, the latter can be performed unilaterally or bilaterally (Lacerda 2013).

Bifrontal: It is performed especially in the context of diffuse cerebral edema and in the presence of bilateral frontal contusions evidenced on diagnostic imaging (Brown and Wijdicks 2017; Grindlinger et al., 2016), contributing to the decrease of ICP in such cases, as well as to the reduction of patients' stay in intensive care unit (UCI) (Hawryluk et al., 2020).

Fronto-temporo-parietal: It is mainly performed in clinical scenarios where the intracranial lesion affects only one cerebral hemisphere, either focally or diffusely (Beez et al., 2019). However, it can also be employed bilaterally in the context of diffuse axonal lesions with compressed or absent cisterns along with a maximum 5 mm deviation of midline structures with an ICP greater than 25 mmHg that is unresponsive to medical management (Lacerda 2013).

Additionally, it has been shown that at the time of performing the duroplasty required in this procedure, it can be performed safely and effectively without suture technique, providing a decrease in operating time and generating less blood loss compared to the context of duroplasty with suture technique (Jeong et al., 2020).

On the other hand, with respect to cranial reconstruction, it is recommended to perform it in the shortest possible time, as long as the patient is in an adequate clinical condition, generally within three months (Grindlinger et al., 2016).

Indications

The exact indications for DC remain uncertain, as there is no standard guideline established for its performance (Jeong et al., 2020; Kolias et al., 2016). However, in the present chapter we will mention some of the recommendations presented by different guidelines and updated studies, without neglecting the importance of performing an individualized evaluation and selection of each patient (Hawryluk et al., 2020).

- Severe TBI: It has been recommended that the use of DC in patients with refractory ICH as a consequence of TBI constitutes a last-level therapeutic procedure because it has not demonstrated efficacy as an early intervention in this clinical scenario (Smith 2017). On the other hand, the most significant mass lesion in these patients corresponds to acute subdural hematoma, for which the Brain Trauma Foundation guidelines suggest the immediate execution of DC if its thickness exceeds 10 millimeters or if the displacement caused from the midline is greater than 5 millimeters, or in patients with a score lower than 9 on the Glasgow scale, or even if the score decreases 2 or more points with respect to that presented at the time of injury, since its effectiveness has been demonstrated in these different situations (Hutchinson et al., 2019; Phan et al., 2017).
- Malignant middle cerebral artery infarction: It has been shown that performing DC early (before the first 48 hours) and in patients aged less than or equal to 60 years, reduces mortality in the context of malignant middle cerebral artery infarction (Rajwani et al., 2017; Viruez-Soto et al., 2018). However, it continues to be a major concern that post-procedure there is an increase in patients with some major disability and, therefore, with poor quality of life (Rajwani et al., 2017).
- Cerebral venous thrombosis: It is suggested to take into account the performance of DC in patients with cerebral venous thrombosis who present neurological deterioration and who have a significant mass effect (Smith 2017).
- Cerebral empyema: DC has been proposed as initial therapy in patients with cerebral empyema in whom the collection expands to the pontocerebellar angle (Feo and Patiño-Ladino 2019).

Complications

Although DC is an uncomplicated procedure for most neurosurgeons to perform, it has been associated with the development of a number of significant complications with great impact on both quality of life and overall cost-effectiveness of the procedure (Kurland et al., 2015). Following the removal of a major portion of the skull, a series of pathophysiological changes occur that are the basis for various complications, which tend to occur over different periods of time (Castelluccio et al., 2017). These changes include increased intracranial volume to ICP ratio with rightward deviation of the pressure-volume curve, alterations in cerebrospinal fluid (CSF) circulation dynamics, increased CSF and cerebral metabolism, and a loss of cerebral autoregulation that tends to normalize around 72 hours after the procedure (Castelluccio et al., 2017; Honeybul and Ho 2014).

Thus, each of the complications that can occur following DC show a tendency to occur within a specific time window (Casteluccio et al., 2017). In the following, each complication will be detailed and divided into one of three groups according to the time of occurrence after surgery; early (≤ 1 week), late (from day 8 to 30) and delayed (> 1 month) (Ban et al., 2010) (Table 1):

– Early (≤ 1 week)

Hemorrhagic progression of a contusion has been reported only in trauma cases and occurs in 12.6% of patients after DC (Ban et al., 2010). A new intracranial hematoma may develop after DC, and may occur ipsilaterally in approximately 10.2% of patients undergoing the procedure for any indication, and contralaterally in 8.6% of cases, but only in patients undergoing DC after traumatic brain injury (Huang et al., 2011; Kurland et al., 2015). From the pathophysiological point of view, it is believed that the occurrence of these complications occurs as a result of the changing pressure dynamics that occur in the context of the opening of the skull, with a reduction or loss of the tamponade effect (Gopalakrishnan et al., 2018).

On the other hand, with respect to seizures, the mechanism of postoperative epilepsy is not yet fully understood, but gradual increases in hyperexcitability and a reduced epileptogenic threshold have been suggested as possible causes (Chen et al., 2009).

With respect to external cerebral herniation, its main causative mechanism is cerebral edema; this complication can cause compression of the cortical vein, resulting in cortical laceration that will subsequently cause venous infarction of the herniated brain tissue and cortical damage (Brown and Wijdicks 2017). However, the herniation is unlikely to affect the postoperative outcome, especially when a large craniectomy is performed as it allows the brain to expand outward without constriction and therefore minimizes the risk of venous infarction (Gopalakrishnan et al., 2018).

Finally, CSF leaks occur in situations where the integrity of the arachnoid and dura mater is compromised, allowing CSF to escape into the extradural space; this complication usually occurs in 6.3% of patients (Kurland et al., 2015). It occurs in few patients through minor wound dehiscence and is usually resolved by placement of a simple suture (Ban et al., 2010).

- Late (from day 8 to 30)

Subdural hygroma is caused by traumatic rupture of the dura-arachnoid interface and resulting changes in the dynamics of CSF circulation; it usually appears at 13.3 ± 9 days postoperatively, being the most common complication after Dc (Ban et al., 2010; Honeybul 2010). Its incidence after DC in patients with TBI has been reported to be about 27.4%, while in patients undergoing DC for stroke it is about 12.5% (Ki et al., 2015; Kurland et al., 2015). Additionally, it has been evidenced that they frequently appear on the ipsilateral side of the craniectomy; however, they can occur on the contralateral side or bilaterally (Jeong et al., 2020). Although most resolve spontaneously, they are associated with longer hospitalization and rehabilitation and worse neurological outcome (Paredes et al., 2011).

On the other hand, another complication is postoperative infection, commonly caused by S. epidermidis, which can increase patient morbidity and mortality (Ban et al., 2010; Zunt 2010). Superficial infections (flap necrosis, poor wound healing, subgaleal and skin wound infections) occur in approximately 8.1% of all patients undergoing DC; while deep infections (abscesses and empyemas) occur in 5.1% of patients with TBI and 5.9% of patients with ischemic stroke undergoing DC; in addition, other infections such as meningitis and ventriculitis occur in 6.1% of patients, with a greater predilection in patients undergoing DC for trauma (Brown and Wijdicks 2017).

- Delayed (> 1 month)

Post-traumatic hydrocephalus develops when CSF flow and circulation is altered, thus giving rise to malabsorption and subsequent obstruction (Ding et al., 2014; Honeybul 2010). It is a common post-DC complication and occurs in 16.4% and 25.5% of patients undergoing DC for TBI and stroke, respectively (Brown and Wijdicks 2017).

On the other hand, tremor syndrome has an overall prevalence of 10% and is characterized by presenting with headache, seizures, mood swings and behavioral disturbances (Gopalakrishnan et al., 2018). After DC, the scalp above the bony defect sinks due to lack of bony support, transmitting atmospheric pressure directly to the brain resulting in a complex constellation of symptoms attributed to reduced cerebral perfusion and altered CSF flow (Brown and Wijdicks 2017). Because of this, cranioplasty is beneficial in improving the symptoms of this syndrome and therefore early cranioplasty after DC has been recommended (Gopalakrishnan et al., 2018; Honeybul 2010; Yan et al., 2008).

Finally, in addition to the complications related to DC, we must take into account the complications derived from a second intervention; cranioplasty, which is required for brain protection, restoration of the original contour of the skull for cosmetic reasons and, in some cases, as mentioned above, to alleviate neurological symptoms attributable to trephination syndrome (Castelluccio et al., 2017; Smith 2017). Among its complications, infections with the need for bone flap removal, bone resorption and extracerebral hematomas stand out (Grindlinger et al., 2016; Honeybul and Ho 2011). These complications can develop in the immediate postoperative course or months and even years later (Hutchinson et al., 2019).

Table 1. Approximate time of onset of complications after CD

TIME OF ONSET	COMPLICATIONS
Early (≤ 1 week)	Hemorrhagic progression of a contusion
	New intracranial hematoma
	Postoperative epilepsy
	External brain herniation
	CSF leakage
Late (day 8 to 30)	Subdural hygroma
	Postoperative infection
Delayed (>1 month)	Post-traumatic hydrocephalus
	Trephine syndrome

Post-Procedure Quality of Life

DC is a surgical intervention based on pathophysiologic principles that when performed in some clinical scenarios can improve the likelihood of survival and overall functional outcome (Brown and Wijdicks 2017). However, there is concern that it may also prolong poor quality of life by increasing the number of survivors with severe disabilities (Rajwani et al., 2017; Smith 2017). In this context, the RescueICP trial showed that DC does not provide an absolute risk reduction (ARR) for an unfavorable outcome compared to medical treatment (RR 0.95, 95% CI 0.83 to 1.09) (Hutchinson et al., 2016; Sahuquillo and Dennis 2019). Therefore, such results should be carefully evaluated, since, although medical therapy has a lower probability of survival, patients who survive tend to do so with a low level of disability, while surgical decompression provides a higher probability of survival, but with a higher risk of severe disability (Honeybul et al., 2017).

While perceptions towards different degrees of disability vary from one individual to another, it is the overall quality of life that is probably most important to many people, as they seem to adapt to life-changing events and even accept a degree of disability that they would have previously considered unacceptable (Smith 2017). As evidence of the above, in a study investigating outcomes after severe TBI, the majority of patients who had survived with severe disability 3 years after DC indicated that they would have accepted surgery even if they had been aware of what the final outcome would be (Honeybul et al., 2013).

Because of the above, the degree of disability that should be considered a "bad outcome" is a matter of great debate in the context of performing a DC and is a variable to be decided by the patients and caregivers, not solely by the health care professional (Sahuquillo and Dennis 2019). Therefore, shared decision-making in discussions about the possible outcomes of therapeutic options, prolonged recovery times and possible post-procedure quality of life is of vital importance in order to make a decision that respects the patient's expectations, preferences and principles (Smith 2017).

Conclusion

DC is a surgical procedure for which multiple studies have demonstrated its high efficacy in reducing ICP. However, its precise usefulness in the treatment of various neurological emergencies continues to be a matter of debate, as there are numerous significant risks associated with it. Because of this, it is of utmost importance to perform an individual evaluation of each patient in order to select those for whom the benefit is greater than the possible complications that may occur, without neglecting that further research is required to address the issue in order to resolve the doubts that currently exist about the appropriate indications for DC.

References

Ban, S. P., Son, Y. J., Yang, H. J., Chung, Y. S., Lee, S. H. and Han, D. H. (2010). Analysis of complications following decompressive craniectomy for traumatic brain injury. *J. Korean Neurosurg. Soc.*, 48(3):244-50.

Beez, T., Munoz-Bendix, C., Steiger, H. J. and Beseoglu, K. (2019). Decompressive craniectomy for acute ischemic stroke. *Critical care*, 23:209.

Brown, D. A. and Wijdicks, E. F. M. (2017). Decompressive craniectomy in acute brain injury. *Handbook of Clinical Neurology*, 140(3rd series).

Castelluccio, G., Bertullo, G., Fernández, M. and Spagnuolo, E. (2017). Complicaciones de la craniectomía descompresiva. Reporte de caso y revisión de la literatura. Rev Argent de Neuroc. 31(1): 54-62. [Complications of decompressive craniectomy. Case report and literature review. *Rev. Argent de Neuroc.* 31(1): 54-62].

Chen, J. W., Ruff, R. L., Eavery, R. and Wasterlain, C. G. (2009). Posttraumatic epilepsy and treatment. *J. Rehavil. Res. Dev.*, 46: 685-696.

Ding, J., Guo, Y. and Tian, H. (2014). The influence of decompressive craniectomy on the development of hydrocephalus: a review. *Arq. Neuropsiquiatr.*, 72(9):715-20.

Feo-Lee, O. and Patiño-Ladino, S. (2019). *Decompressive Craniectomy for Empyema by Aggregatibacter aphrophilus: Literature Review and Case Report.* Univ Med, 60(1).

Godoy, D. A., Moscote-Salazar, L. R., Rubiano, A., Muñoz-Sánchez, Á., Lubillo, S. and Murillo-Cabezas, F. (2017). Secondary decompressive Craniectomy for the management of refractory endocraneal hypertension in severe traumatic brain injury. Lights and shadows from recent studies. *Med. Intensiva.,* 41(8):487-490.

Gopalakrishnan, M. S., Shanbhag, N. C., Shukla, D. P., Konar, S. K., Bhat, D. I. and Devi, B. I. (2018). Complications of Decompressive Craniectomy. *Front. Neurol*., 9:977.

Grille, P. and Tommasino, N. (2015). Decompressive craniectomy in severe traumatic brain injury: prognostic factors and complications. *Rev. Bras. Ter. Intensiva.,* 27(2):113-118.

Grindlinger, G. A., Skavdahl, D. H., Ecker, R. D. and Sanborn, M. R. (2016). *Decompressive craniectomy for severe traumatic brain injury: clinical study, literature review and meta-analysis.* SpringerPlus, 5:1605.

Hawryluk, G. W. J., Rubiano, A. M., Totten, A. M., O'Reilly, C., Ullman, J. S., Bratton, S. L., Chesnut, R., Harris, O. A., Kissoon N., Shutter, L., Tasker, R. C., Vavilala, M. S., Wilberger, J., Wright, D. W., Lumba-Brown, A. and Ghajar J. (2020). Guidelines for the Management of Severe Traumatic Brain Injury: 2020 Update of the Decompressive Craniectomy Recommendations. *Neurosurgery*, 87(3).

Honeybul S. (2010). Complications of decompressive craniectomy for head injury. *J. Clin. Neurosci.*, 17(4):430-5.

Honeybul, S. and Ho, K. M. (2011). Long-term complications of decompressive craniectomy for head injury. *J. Neurotrauma*, 28(6):929-35.

Honeybul, S., Janzen, C., Kruger, K. and Ho, K. M. (2013). Decompressive craniectomy for severe traumatic brain injury: is life worth living? *J. Neurosurg.*, 119:1566–1575.

Honeybul, S. and Ho, K. M. (2014). Decompressive Craniectomy – A narrative review and discussion. *Aust. Crit. Care*, 27(2):85-91.

Honeybul, S., Ho, K. M., Lind, C. R. P. and Gillett, G. R. (2017). The current role of decompressive craniectomy for severe traumatic brain injury. *J. Clin. Neurosci.*, 43:11-15.

Huang, Y. H., Lee, T. C., Chen, W. F. and Wang, Y. M. (2011). Safety of the non-absorbable dural substitute in decompressive craniectomy for severe traumatic brain injury. *J. Trauma*, 71(3):533–7.

Hutchinson, P. J., Kolias, A. G., Tajsic, T., Adeleye, A., Aklilu, A. T., Apriawan, T., Bajamal, A. H., Barthélemy, E. J., Devi, B. I., Bhat, D., Bulters, D., Chesnut, R., Citerio, G., Cooper, D. J., Czosnyka, M., Edem, I., El-Ghandour, N. M. F., Figaji, A., Fountas, K. N., Gallagher, C., Hawryluk, G. W. J., Iacaarino, C., Joseph, M., Khan, T., Laeke, T., Levchenko, O., Liu, B., Liu, W., Maas, A., Manley, G. T., Manson, P., Mazzeo, A. T., Menon, D. K., Michael, D. B., Muehlschlegel, S., Okonkwo, D. O., Park, K. B., Rosenfeld, J. V., Rosseau, G., Rubiano, A. M., Shabani, H. K., Stocchetti, N., Timmons, S. D., Timofeev, I., Uff, C., Ullman, J. S., Valadka, A., Waran, V., Wells, A., Wilson, M. H. and Servadei, F. (2019). Consensus statement from the International Consensus Meeting on the Role of Decompressive Craniectomy in the Management of Traumatic Brain Injury. *Acta Neurochir.*, 161:1261-1274.

Hutchinson, P. J., Kolias, A. G., Timofeev, I. S., Corteen, E. A., Czosnyka, M., Timothy, J., Anderson, I., Bulters, D. O., Belli, A., Eynon, C. A., Wadley, J., Mendelow, A. D., Mitchel, P. M., Wilson, M. H., Critchley, G., Sahuquillo, J., Unterberg, A., Servadei, F., Teasdale, G. M., Pickard, J. D., Menon, D. K., Murray, G. D. and Kirkpatrick, P. J. (2016). Trial of Decompressive Craniectomy for Traumatic Intracranial Hypertension. *N. Engl. J. Med.*, 375(12):1119-30.

Jeong, T. S., Yee, G. T., Lim, T. G., Kim, W. K. and Yoo, C. J. (2020). Efficacy and safety of decompressive craniectomy with non-suture duraplasty in patients with traumatic brain injury. *PLoS ONE*, 15(10): e0232561.

Ki, H. J, Lee, H. J., Lee, H. J., Yi, J. S., Yang, J. H. and Lee I. W. (2015). The risk factors for hydrocephalus and subdural hygroma after decompressive craniectomy in head injured patients. *J. Korean Neurosurg. Soc.*, 58 (3):254.

Kolias, A. G., Adams, H., Timofeev, I., Czosnyka, M., Corteen, E. A., Pickard, J. D., Turner, C., Gregson, B. A., Kirkpatrick, P, J., Murray, G. D., Menon, D. K. and Hutchinson, P. J. (2016). Decompressive craniectomy following traumatic brain injury: developing the evidence base. *British Journal of Neurosurgery*, 30:2,246-250.

Kurland, D. B., Khaladj-Ghom, A., Stokum, J. A., et al., (2015). Complications associated with decompressive craniectomy: a systematic review. *Neurocrit. Care*, 23 (2): 292-304.

Lacerda-Gallardo, A. J. (2013). Decompressive craniectomy in the treatment of severe traumatic brain injury. *Rev. Cubana Neurol. Neurocir.*, 3(1):93-100.

Paredes, I., Cicuendez, M., Delgado, M. A., Martinez-Pérez, R., Munarriz, P. M. and Lagares, A. (2011). Normal pressure subdural hygroma with mass effect as a complication of decompressive craniectomy. *Surg. Neurol. Int.* 2.

Phan, K., Moore, J. M., Griessenauer, C., Dmytriw, A. A., Scherman, D. B., Sheik-Ali, S., Adeeb, N., Ogilvy, C. S., Thomas, A. and Rosenfeld, J. V. (2017). Craniotomy versus decompressive craniectomy for acute subdural hematoma: systematic review and meta-analysis. *World Neurosurgery.*

Rajwani, K. M., Crocker, M. and Moynihan, B. (2017). Decompressive craniectomy for the treatment of malignant middle cerebral artery infarction. *British Journal of Neurosurgery.*

Sahuquillo, J. and Dennis, J. A. (2019). Decompressive craniectomy for the treatment of high intracranial pressure in closed traumatic brain injury (Review). *Cochrane Database of Systematic Reviews*, 12: CD003983.

Smith, M. (2017). Refractory Intracranial Hypertension: The Role of Decompressive Craniectomy. *Anesth. Analg.*, 125:1999-2008.

Viruez-Soto, J. A., Alí-Yucra, N., Chuquimia-Rodríguez, G. N., Re-Gutiérrez, S. D., Vargas-Ordoñez, P., Videtta, W. and Vera-Carrasco, O. (2018). Decompressive craniectomy, current recommendations. *Rev. Med. La Paz.,* 24(2).

Wettervi, T. S., Lenell, S., Nyholm, L., Howells, T., Lewén, A. and Enblad, P. (2018). Decompressive craniectomy in traumatic brain injury: usage and clinical outcome in a single centre. *Acta Neurochir.*, 160:229-237.

Zhang, D., Xue, O., Chen, J., Dong, Y., Hou, L., Jiang, Y. and Wang, J. (2017). Decompressive craniectomy in the management of intracranial hypertension after traumatic brain injury: a systematic review and meta-analysis. *Scientific Reports*, 7:8800.

Zunt, J. R. (2010). Infections of the central nervous system in the neurosurgical patient. *Handb. Clin. Neurol.*, 96: 125-14.

Chapter 16

Neuro-Endovascular Device Research

Mariana Hurtado-Pinillos[1,2],
Ivan David Lozada-Martínez[1,2]
and Yelson Alejandro Picón-Jaimes[1,2]
[1]Colombian Clinical Research Group in Neurocritical Care, Colombian Chapter, Latin American Council in Neurocritical Care, Colombia
[2]Medical and Surgical Research Center, Future Surgeons Chapter, Colombian Surgery Association, Bogotá, Colombia

Abstract

The implementation of neuro-endovascular devices constitutes one of the fundamental pillars of contemporary neurosurgery worldwide, for which mechanisms are required that allow highly safe, effective, and efficient results to be obtained. At the end of the 20th century, flow-diverting clips, endovascular coils, and devices began to be used that have generated knowledge applied to different neurovascular disorders. This has led to improvement in the quality of life of patients. This allowed the development of studies that support the creation of instruments that reduce the complexity of this type of procedure, without overshadowing the capacity of conventional endovascular treatment methods.

Introduction

Endovascular devices appeared as a support mechanism, demonstrating their effectiveness against different pathologies. With the progressive refinement of medical practice, little by little these devices have been coupled to specialties

In: Neurosurgery Research
Editors: Amit Agrawal, Pradeep Chouksey, Adesh Shrivastava et al.
ISBN: 978-1-68507-837-9

such as radiology and diagnostic imaging (Bilbao et al., 2005). These have become protagonists for the therapeutic innovation they represent, as well as for the use of various materials and extensive research development, which has generated a greater impact on the outcome of the operated patients.

The development of endovascular technology began in 1964, through the work of two neurosurgeons, Luessenhop and Velásquez from Georgetown University Hospital in Washington (Guglielmi, 2007), who came up with a plan to design a small catheter, using a glass chamber that was surgically connected to a blood vessel, specifically an external carotid artery. With the presentation of their results, they published the first exploration of the circle of Willis and the adjacent arterial tree, showing how these blood vessels perfectly tolerated intraluminal manipulation (Guglielmi, 2007). Years later, the experience of these neurosurgeons began to produce changes in medicine and thus gave way to endovascular field of neurosurgery. This allowed the recognition of devices, including the use of coils and flow diverters, to reduce the flow inside the aneurysms (Goubergrits et al., 2014).

This chapter is intended to be a tool for future research and academic field, which provides information regarding the outcome of endovascular devices, knowing its process, implementation, and progress in the field of neuro-endovascular surgery.

History of Endovascular Occlusion of Cerebral Aneurysms

During the 1960s, in the electronics department of the Institute of Israel, an instrument known as a microcatheter was designed (Guglielmi, 2007). This was further improved by two neurosurgeons of the University hospital of Georgetown. This device was given the name of Paraoperative Device (POD) in 1966. It was shown that this catheter was "submerged" inside the blood vessels, reducing the friction between the tip of the catheter and the inner wall of the vessel. This device used a guide in the extracranial vasculature for the POD, and a lateral arm that was for bridging to introduce the microcatheter, and at the same time added saline solution to perform cleaning.

In 1967, a group of doctors belonging to the Neurosurgery program at Massachusetts General Hospital created a magnetic system (Guglielmi, 2007) for the treatment of aneurysms and endovascular malformations. The system featured a 1.3mm magnet embedded in the tip of the microcatheter and another magnet with a heating coil at the back that allowed connection to a power source.

This device was created to have these applications: 1) Block the feeding vessels of certain intracranial vascular malformations, uncovering the detachable tip or injecting freezable plastic; 2) Administer chemotherapeutic drugs in high concentrations for the treatment of gliomas; and, 3) Achieving the destruction of the aneurysm through the separation of the sac by utilizing one of its magnetic tips. This would be followed by injecting iron particles through the catheter that would adhere to the detachable tip.

In the years of 1969 and 1970, several experiences with this type of device were published. Among publications, there was the first report of magnetically guided intracranial navigation, in which POD catheter was used (developed in 1967). This major advancement was thanks to the skills and techniques acquired through studies carried out years ago. This catheter was introduced by a percutaneous carotid puncture, being known as the first catheterization of the middle cerebral artery carried out in a patient. In 1970, a physician named Montgomery and his working group described a new version of the POD (Guglielmi, 2007), which incorporated a balloon that could be inflated and was detachable, giving rise to the first report of a detachable balloon for endovascular use.

In 1973, through a joint effort between the Department of Neurology, Massachusetts General Hospital, and the Massachusetts Institute of Technology, brief reports were published related to the management of aneurysm occlusion through endovascular balloons (Cares, Hale, Montgomery, Richter and Sweet, 1973). This experimental research allowed a microcatheter to be magnetically driven, being able to administer iron and using detachable balloons to seal the conduit of arteriovenous malformations and aneurysm locations. This device was directed by the flux and the magnetic field located on the outside to deflect its tip in the arterial unions of the great complex.

In 1974, (Hilal, Michelsen, Driller, & Leonard, 1974) at Columbia University, the clinical use of the modified version of the POD microcatheter was reported in 120 patients. Different processes derived from the use of this device were recorded, including percutaneous catheterization of vessels in the basilar and middle cerebral arteries, and the administration of certain medications. The use of this device for the treatment of arteriovenous malformations was also studied. At that time, the records of the investigations were carried out promptly, with great contributions and success for the information of the time, giving fame to the POD.

“The tracer microcatheter” was the term that put aside the previous devices and passed as the new system. Debrún, a well-known neuroradiologist, applied a coaxial microcatheter system with a detachable latex balloon (Debrun et al., 1975), but its stiffness only allowed it to reach the cavernous portion of the internal carotid artery. This procedure became the gold standard for endovascular balloon treatment of carotid fistulas, reducing the involvement of the carotid artery and large intracavernous aneurysms.

Following his process, Hieshima, a neuroradiologist, created a thin soft polyethylene catheter (Hieshima, Grinnell, & Mehringer, 1981) for the treatment of endovascular occlusion of intracranial aneurysms through an elastic balloon. It became a powerful element, used by many specialists in the medical field for the intervention of brain aneurysms. The new "Tracker" was released on the market, a micro-wire device with a non-rigid tip, which allowed adequate movement in vascular curves; this became known for allowing intracranial navigation by pushing the catheter over the guidewire. The catheter was first used in patients in 1986 in the external carotid artery and intracranial vessels.

However, high rates of morbidity and mortality were reported after balloon occlusion, leading to the rejection of these devices by most neurosurgeons (Guglielmi, 2007). One of the main complications was the late rupture of the aneurysm. This caused these devices to be only used in certain groups. Interventional neuroradiology remove this device since its use was more in line with genuine ideas that sought to develop a better future for patients with risk pathologies, with history and comorbidities, but forgetting the high cost that is generated including serious complications and death of many patients.

In 2006, the use of treatments with detachable coil techniques was published and in 2007, a high impact was generated in the development of the detachable coils for endovascular intervention. The technology revealed an implementation that enabled safe intracranial access, producing access that uses the arteries as fluid channels to reach the aneurysm. According to the literature, 40 years later, tools were developed for ~~some~~ systems that are still being used.

The contribution from different parts of the world has continued to be significantly in the field of vascular interventionism, mainly the treatment of endovascular aortic aneurysm repair (EVAR: Endovascular Aneurysm Repair) (Hurtado et al., 2020). This technique was initially used in a patient with an abdominal aortic aneurysm, to access the vascular section affected by the widening of the vessel and, through a fabric graft and metallic components, to seal the affected area.

The historical review of the different devices developed during previous times allows the opportune knowledge of elements, investigations, and analyses in different patients. This led to recognizing the step-by-step of vascular interventionism and generating greater strategies that are coupled to the collective and individual need and the proper functioning of this type of system, from current technology. This would allow the design and implementation of new categories in the field of neurosurgery, serving as a solid foundation for future generations interested in research.

Hemodynamic Effect in the Endovascular Treatment of Patients with the Presence of a Cerebral Aneurysm

The hemodynamic stability of patients with cerebral aneurysm is a challenge that must be focused on long-term success, directly related to an adequate set of parameters that establish the functioning of the endovascular devices used.

A cerebral aneurysm is recognized as a dilation located in the wall of the arterial vessel, frequently located at bifurcation points (Santana et al., 2020). It is a condition that presents a high-risk index due to the potential for rupture and hence catastrophic subarachnoid hemorrhage. Technological devices that allow early recognition of its development play an important role; since it allows visualizing the integrity of the compromised arterial tree. This can be done through MRA, CT scans with contrast, and cerebral subtraction digital angiography.

Various classifications of unruptured aneurysms are identified, including symptomatic, asymptomatic, and incidental unruptured aneurysms (Milet, 2006). The fatal outcome that abnormal blood vessel dilation could lead to is a biomechanical issue (Goubergrits et al., 2014) because the parameters are related to wall resistance, the radius of curvature, intraaneurysmal pressure, and wall thickness. It is estimated that the prevalence of cerebral aneurysms is 5% to 8% of the general population, considering that most people with the presence of a cerebral aneurysm are unaware of it until the end of their life (Goubergrits et al., 2014).

The treatment decision is directly related to the timely outcome of each patient, and the hemodynamic parameters that describe the forces of blood flow on the blood vessel wall (Goubergrits et al., 2014) since they are more closely related to the onset and increased risk of rupture of cerebral aneurysms. On the other hand, studies have revealed modern imaging modalities, such as 3D rotational angiography (3DRA) (Goubergrits et al., 2014), presenting a greater possibility of incidentally detecting asymptomatic aneurysms, a purpose that has been desired since the beginning of the studies on this discipline.

After analyzing the importance of timely recognition of aneurysms; it is considered that the patient should be diagnosed promptly through neuroimaging studies such as computed tomography of the brain, angiotomography, and magnetic resonance imaging (Santana et al., 2020). The main aim is to detect and stratify the risk according to size, morphology, and injury location.

Types of Endovascular Devices

There is a considerable number of studies in which it is sought to determine the most efficient device according to the anatomy of the aneurysm, and hemodynamic characteristics. The methods recorded in studies of the 20th century were included for clinical use, using metallic, polymeric, or hybrid devices, administered through a catheter at the site of widening of the blood vessels. Endovascular devices can be divided into three categories: metal, polymer, or a fusion between the two (hybrids) (Rodriguez et al., 2015).

Metallic Devices

Coils

These spirals, made of soft metal, can adapt to the geometry or current condition of the blood vessels, coiling around themselves and allowing the packing of the aneurysms. The use of these devices for the endovascular approach has proven to be effective, with low rates of complications in the procedure and a reduction in the hospital stay.

According to their biomechanical function, these coils guarantee a volumetric occlusion between 20% and 31%. Also, those coils are 0.012mm (305μm) diameter with complex geometry, allowing greater volumetric occlusion of the aneurysm, compared to 0.010 mm (254 μm) helical coils (Rodriguez et al., 2015).

Flow Diverters

These devices have a geometry similar to stents, with the difference that, due to their structure, these can generate a fine mesh (Rodriguez et al., 2015). The use of this element is considered more advanced than the previous ones, due to the greater density of pores as compared to stents, producing a decrease in blood flow in the neck of the aneurysm, and thus, facilitating stagnation of blood in the previously formed dome of the aneurysm. Although it was presented as an effective device with one of the best performances, some studies have shown that there is difficulty in occluding curved aneurysms, with lateral walls and at the bifurcation, in medium-sized biological models (Darsaut, Bing, Salazkin, Gevry, & Raymond, 2012).

Polymer Devices

These devices were proposed much earlier, around the 1970s; It consists of a liquid polymer implant that uses cyanoacrylates and ethylene vinyl alcohol (Rodriguez et al., 2015). The liquid components are injected through a microcatheter. The solidification time is recorded and is controlled by the proportion of etiodinated oil in the liquid polymer mixture.

Within this category are devices like Onyx (Covidien, Irvine, CA) and Trufill® n-BCA (Codman Neurovascular, Raynham, MA); proposed as the first advanced liquid polymer embolic system by the FDA, for the treatment of some brain pathologies (Jordan, Doelker, & Rüfenacht, 2005). The last registry of this group was performed by cPax (NeuroVasx) for cerebral aneurysms with a diameter greater than 10 mm.

Hybrid Devices

Hybrid coils contain metal and polymer materials. The former is designed to generate interaction with the response of a foreign agent, producing thrombogenesis using biodegradable polymers at the same time. These hydrogel-coated coils aim to increase occlusion by expanding in the presence of blood compared to bare platinum coils (Rodriguez et al., 2015).

Advances in the early 2000s produced soft steerable microcatheters that allowed safe and less traumatic intracranial access to an aneurysm. On the other hand, coil technology developed in parallel (Guglielmi, 2007), allowed the endovascular approach for aneurysm treatment more safely and effectively.

Polymeric Devices an Appropriate Change?

These elements can share greater benefits such as bioactive advantages and behave as radiopaque devices, for the occlusion of filler materials (Rodriguez et al., 2012). Bioactive hybrid devices are recognized for having greater technical qualities (Yuki et al., 2007). Within the range of characteristics that a therapeutic element have, the coagulation process must be taken into account effectively, since it is directly associated with the healing of epithelia, stability, and organic interaction; the biomechanical, hemodynamic process, and the intracranial environment (Sforza, Putman, & Cebral, 2009). Therefore, these devices are postulated as the future generation of endovascular therapeutic tools.

Endovascular Neuromodulation

Endovascular neuromodulation is an emerging technology that represents a synthesis between interventional neurology and neural engineering (Raza et al., 2020). This technology has various applications, including epilepsy monitoring, neurostimulation, and robotic limb control. It is recognized that the brain may be a conduit for endovascular neuromodulation devices; Therefore, this intervention is expected to be non-destructive and reversible in the treatment of pain (Enrique, Iglesia López, & Camba Rodríguez, 2008), promising high rates of effectiveness both in the clinical outcome and in the specific management of symptoms associated with each patient.

Some observations were highlighted within the investigative explorations carried out to date, to weigh the risks of this new technology, such as the complications of Strentrode (Stents with electrodes), given the lack of experience with the use of intravenous cables in the brain; therefore, higher quality data is needed to observe the relationship between the factors that arise in this process (cable and vein diameter). Although endovascular neuromodulation is a promising field with many possible diagnostic and therapeutic applications (Raza et al., 2020), it needs to be covered by solid strategies to reduce the rates of complications after the intervention and to develop studies that allow adequate safety.

Endovascular deep brain stimulation has also been recognized as another strategy that is delivered by administering current through electrode stents and is a potential alternative to brain stimulation. So far, this technique has proven effective in a wide range of movement disorders (Neudorfer et al., 2020). In related studies, it was concluded that for neurostimulation to be an effective and feasible therapy, it must have electrodes that deploy effectively, being close to the neuroanatomical plane. The prevention of adverse effects produced by this type of intervention should be considered in future research.

Care of Post-Surgical Patients due to Cerebral Aneurysms

The family or social nucleus that is closest to the operated patient must recognize that their action is of great importance in recovery. Comprehensive care favors decision-making that meets the sole purpose of recovering the physical, mental, and social well-being of individuals (Santana et al., 2020). It is considered of great importance to combine various exercises that benefit the functioning of the patient's body, such as passive and active exercises and position changes, to reduce complications. This field is new and is known as neurorehabilitation, which is a joint work between a multidisciplinary team of experts in the recovery and maintenance of the functional neurological capacity of the patient and his family.

Interventions with Endovascular Repair in the Years 2019, 2020 and 2021

The records of previous research gave way to the construction of new studies that allow for greater efficacy in the endovascular treatment of these patients. Some cases have aroused interest in the field of neurointervention and endovascular surgery, such as that of a 78-year-old male patient with a saccular aneurysm in the aortic arch. This patient was treated with a flow-modulating multilayer stent. Three months later, complete closure of the aneurysm was demonstrated (Vignau Cano, Daroca Martínez, Gómez Vidal, Bermúdez García, & Macías Rubio, 2019). It is recognized that in that year there was the existence of an uncovered endoprosthesis known as a multilayer flow modulator. This layer allows to generate a thread intertwined in several layers to form a mesh, it acts as a stabilizer, allowing blood flow to go from turbulent to laminar, improving thrombosis and endothelialization of lesions.

Although at present these cases are not so novel, at the time they represented breaks in paradigms on the management of neurovascular disorders.

In 2020, a multicenter study of emergency endovascular repair of the abdominal aorta was carried out (López Espada et al., 2021), revealing its indications and results. The study included patients with ruptured aneurysms of the descending thoracic aorta, traumatic injury to the thoracic aorta, and acute aortic dissections. After recognizing the hemodynamic condition, the experience of the specialists, and the theoretical knowledge of the specific data recorded in the evolution of different treatments chosen for aneurysms, it was concluded that these conditions can be treated using endovascular techniques, obtaining better outcomes and low morbidity and mortality. It was observed with a postoperative stroke rate of 5.2% and aortic reinterventions required in 12 patients, corresponding to only 9% (Guglielmi, 2007).

Clinical simulation has become an indispensable tool in medical training, allowing an approach with the patient, their condition, and the response that would be generated in the face of the various cases in a situation similar to reality. Recently, in the face of the public health catastrophe caused by the COVID-19 pandemic, simulation has played a fundamental role, favoring the development of necessary skills in safe environments, for students and residents to learn technical skills. At the same time, technological simulation has allowed the development of breakthrough research, for example, the case of a computational dynamic simulation under the action of a magnetic field was known. The idealized three-dimensional computational model of a cerebral saccular aneurysm was used to study vascular hemodynamics under the effect of electromagnetic fields. The results showed that, under the magnetic field emitted by an open resonator, the liquid enters the aneurysm sac at a higher speed compared to a closed resonator (Cardona et al., 2021). This model intends to make known a greater acquisition in the compression of the magnetic field phenomena, related to vascular pathologies.

Knowing the process of recent years and those currently developed, it can be noted that what was established a few years ago, carried out through clinical practice and studies, has been taken as a cornerstone to providing patients with efficient relief from its symptomatology. In addition, some studies continue to support procedures that prove to be successful and more effective in treatments. The acknowledgment of the historical antecedents provided by the registry of research studies, analysis of the different types of devices used, and reported cases discussed, intends to be a support that allows the undergraduate student to acquire greater knowledge in the field of the neurological specialty.

In conclusion, a significant advance has been observed in the development of endovascular devices, highlighting those for the approach of cerebral aneurysms. Although the evidence supports its use due to its safety and efficacy performance, it is necessary to carry out studies in low- and middle-income countries, which have financial, structural, training and technology limitations. This is a field that can be combined with translational medicine in neurosciences, which can generate products of new knowledge and valuable evidence of the highest quality.

References

Bilbao, JI, Martínez de la Cuesta, A., Domínguez Echavarri, P., Cosín, O., Desloques, L., & Zudaire, B. (2005). Endovascular therapeutic techniques. *Annals of the Navarra Health System*, 28, 117-134.

Cares, HL, Hale, JR, Montgomery, DB, Richter, HA & Sweet, WH (1973). Laboratory experience with a magnetically guided intravascular catheter system. *J Neurosurg*, 38(2), 145-154. doi:10.3171/jns.1973.38.2.0145.

Darsaut, TE, Bing, F., Salazkin, I., Gevry, G., & Raymond, J. (2012). Flow diverters failing to occlude experimental bifurcation or curved sidewall aneurysms: an *in vivo* study in canines. *J Neurosurg*, 117(1), 37-44. doi:10.3171/2012.4.jns111916.

Debrun, G., Lacour, P., Caron, JP, Hurth, M., Comoy, J., & Keravel, Y. (1975). Inflatable and released balloon technique experimentation in dog -- application in man. *Neuroradiology*, 9(5), 267-271. doi:10.1007/bf00333741.

Enrique, FV, Iglesia López, A. dl, & Camba Rodríguez, A. (2008). Spinal Cord Stimulation (SEM) in the treatment of peripheral vascular disease: Part I. *Journal of the Spanish Society of Pain*, 15, 324-332.

Gallitto, E., Faggioli, G., Spath, P., Marrozzini, C., Pini, R., Bruno, AG, . . . Gargiulo, M. (2021). [Endovascular repair of an aortic aneurysm by a custom-made three-inner branched endograft]. *G Ital Cardiol* (Rome), 22(3 Suppl 1), 46s-50s. doi:10.1714/3578.35635.

Goubergrits, L., Schaller, J., Kertzscher, U., Woelken, T., Ringelstein, M., & Spuler, A. (2014). Hemodynamic impact of cerebral aneurysm endovascular treatment devices: coils and flow diverters. *Expert Rev Med Devices*, 11(4), 361-373. doi:10.1586/17434440.2014.925395.

Guglielmi, G. (2007). History of endovascular endosaccular occlusion of brain aneurysms: 1965-1990. *Interv Neuroradiol*, 13(3), 217-224. doi:10.1177/ 159101990701300301.

Hieshima, GB, Grinnell, VS, & Mehringer, CM (1981). A detachable balloon for therapeutic transcatheter occlusions. *Radiology*, 138(1), 227-228. doi:10.1148/ radiology.138.1.7455087.

Higashida, RT, Halbach, VV, Barnwell, SL, Dowd, C., Dormandy, B., Bell, J., & Hieshima, GB (1990). Treatment of intracranial aneurysms with preservation of the parent vessel: results of percutaneous balloon embolization in 84 patients. *AJNR Am J Neuroradiol*, 11(4), 633-640.

Hilal, S. K., Michelsen, W. J., Driller, J., & Leonard, E. (1974). Magnetically guided devices for vascular exploration and treatment. *Radiology*, 113(3), 529-540. doi:10.1148/113.3.529.

Jordan, O., Doelker, E., & Rüfenacht, DA (2005). Biomaterials used in injectable implants (liquid embolics) for percutaneous filling of vascular spaces. *Cardiovasc Intervent Radiol*, 28(5), 561-569. doi:10.1007/s00270-004-0238-7.

López Espada, C., Linares Palomino, JP, Domínguez González, JM, Iborra Ortega, E., Lozano Vilardell, P., Solanich Valldaura, T., . . . Miralles Hernandez, M. (2021). A multicenter study of emergency endovascular repair of the thoracic aorta: indications and outcomes. *Intensive Med* (Engl Ed), 45(5), 280-288. doi:10.1016/j.medin.2019.10.008.

Neudorfer C, Bhatia K, Boutet A, Germann J, Elias GJ, Loh A., . . . Lozano, A.M. (2020). Endovascular deep brain stimulation: Investigating the relationship between vascular structures and deep brain stimulation targets. *Brain Stimul*, 13(6), 1668-1677. doi:10.1016/j.brs.2020.09.016.

Raza, SA, Opie, NL, Morokoff, A., Sharma, RP, Mitchell, PJ, & Oxley, TJ (2020). Vascular Neuromodulation: Safety Profile and Future Directions. *Front Neurol*, 11, 351. doi:10.3389/fneur.2020.00351.

Rodriguez JN, Hwang W, Horn J, Landsman TL, Boyle A, Wierzbicki MA, . . . Maitland, DJ (2015). Design and biocompatibility of endovascular aneurysm filling devices. *J Biomed Mater Res A*, 103(4), 1577-1594. doi:10.1002/jbm.a.35271.

Rodriguez, JN, Yu, YJ, Miller, MW, Wilson, TS, Hartman, J., Clubb, FJ, . . . Maitland, DJ (2012). Opacification of shape memory polymer foam designed for treatment of intracranial aneurysms. *Ann Biomed Eng*, 40(4), 883-897. doi:10.1007/s10439-011-0468-1.

Sforza, DM, Putman, CM, & Cebral, JR (2009). Hemodynamics of Cerebral Aneurysms. *Annu Rev Fluid Mech*, 41, 91-107. doi:10.1146/annurev.fluid.40.111406.102126.

Vignau Cano, JM, Daroca Martínez, T., Gómez Vidal, M., Bermúdez García, A., & Macías Rubio, D. (2019). Endovascular treatment of aortic arch aneurysm using flow-modulating multilayer endoprosthesis. *Cardiovascular Surgery*, 26(1), 59-61. doi:https://doi.org/10.1016/j.circv.2018.08.004.

Yuki I, Lee D, Murayama Y, Chiang A, Vinters HV, Nismmura I., . . . Vinuela, F. (2007). Thrombus organization and healing in an experimental aneurysm model. Part II. The effect of various types of bioactive bioabsorbable polymeric coils. *J Neurosurg*, 107(1), 109-120. doi:10.3171/jns-07/07/0109.

Chapter 17

Key-Hole Approaches to Anterior Circulation Aneurysms

Kuntal Kanti Das, Kamlesh Rangari, Anant Mehrotra and Awadhesh Jaiswal
Department of Neurosurgery, Sanjay Gandhi Postgraduate Institute of Medical Sciences, Lucknow, India

Abstract

Surgical clipping still plays a major role in the management of intracranial aneurysms, particularly those affecting the anterior circulation. The traditional approach to these aneurysms includes a frontotemporal or more commonly the pterional approach. This approach is a very versatile and time-tested technique, considered the gold standard for approaching anterior circulation aneurysms. However, there are certain drawbacks with this approach pertaining to the incision size, facial nerve morbidity, temporalis muscle-related complications, longer than necessary operating times and "unnecessary" exposure of the normal brain. With an increasing surgical experience and better preoperative radiological planning, an era of minimally invasive approaches (MIA) has ushered in. An increasing number of publications in this field is a testament to the growing popularity of these techniques. This chapter gives an overview of the philosophy of these approaches, different technical variations, limitations, advantages, associated complications, with a short review of the published literature so far.

Keywords: mini craniotomy, aneurysm, subarachnoid haemorrhage, minipterional, lateral supraorbital, supraorbital, eyebrow, eyelid, cosmesis

In: Neurosurgery Research
Editors: Amit Agrawal, Pradeep Chouksey, Adesh Shrivastava et al.
ISBN: 978-1-68507-837-9

Introduction

Ruptured intracranial aneurysms are a significant cause of morbidity and mortality [1, 2]. Their treatment paradigm has immensely changed in recent years. Many of these aneurysms are now treated using endovascular methods with very good results. Improvements in hardware, advances in neuroimaging, and technical mastery of endovascular surgeons has resulted in further improvements of results following endovascular treatment (EVT) [3–5]. This is particularly applicable to the posterior circulation aneurysms where EVT has emerged as the first line of treatment. That said, microsurgical clipping remains an effective and preferred treatment modality in many anterior circulation aneurysms, particularly in developing countries where financial hindrances affect treatment choices [6, 7].

Dandy first proposed a frontotemporal craniotomy for the clipping of these aneurysms. His technique remained most widely used until Yasargil proposed the pterional approach (PA) for these aneurysms in the 1970s [8]. In no time, PA became popular not only for anterior circulation aneurysms but also for a host of other non-vascular lesions of the anterior and middle cranial fossa. This approach relied on a bony opening focussed on the intracranial exposure desired, i.e., the Sylvian fissure (SF). Subsequently, many authors have modified this technique with the addition of sphenoid ridge drilling to not only improve the exposure but also to reduce the need for brain retraction. This approach is time-tested, versatile, and considered the gold standard surgical approach for anterior circulation aneurysms. There are, however, certain drawbacks of this approach. The skin incision is usually large, the frontal branch of the facial nerve is at a risk during skin flap elevation, oftentimes extensive dissection of temporalis muscle with a risk of subsequent atrophy and difficulty in mastication, the craniotomy, despite being smaller than a traditional frontotemporal craniotomy, is still large with attendant exposure of normal brain that is truly not needed for aneurysm clipping. A combination of these factors often results in an increased hospital stay, increased postoperative pain, and oftentimes, sub-optimal cosmetic outcomes.

Modern-day surgery in general and neurosurgery, in particular, has become minimalistic in philosophy, without compromising the basic goals of the surgery. This has paralleled the desire to innovate, find simpler solutions to a given problem, and hence can be considered a natural evolution of the neurosurgical practice. Moreover, sustained pressure from the endovascular colleagues has motivated the next generation of micro neurosurgeons to innovate and find ways to reduce the morbidity of traditional surgical techniques. Concerning the anterior circulation aneurysms, a range of MIAs has been described to reduce surgical exposure, improve patient comfort and acceptance by dint of their better cosmetic outcomes, while at the same time retaining the primary efficacy of the standard PA. The concept of keyhole neurosurgery is not to reduce the craniotomy size to as small as a "keyhole," rather make the "minimum craniotomy" required to access deep intracranial pathologies at the end of the route.

That said, the surgeon's experience and meticulous case selection largely determine the success of MIAs and hence need to be understood by those who plan to take up these surgeries. This chapter gives an overview of these approaches, their advantages, limitations, technical subtilities, complications, and their avoidance. Appropriate literature review detailing the surgical results in also presented.

Underlying Concept

A craniotomy is necessary to expose the target of interest inside the cranium. The same holds for aneurysms too. Moreover, brain swelling secondary to rupture, accompanying intracranial hematoma and the prospect of intraoperative rupture are reasons why a conventional, large craniotomy is preferred for these lesions. However, in this process, many structures come in the way of approaching the aneurysm like the overlying scalp, temporalis muscle, the frontal branch of the facial nerve, a large piece of the cranium, and exposed surrounding normal brain take the brunt. Unruptured aneurysms or delayed presentation after a rupture do not pose similar concerns for acutely ruptured aneurysms and hence may not always require large exposures. Morbidities secondary to the handling of these structures sometimes adds to the overall complication of surgery. Hence, it is only natural, in the process of surgical evolution, to find ways of reducing these "modifiable" morbidities. The standard PA has been a major technique in the treatment of intracranial pathologies, but the introduction of modern neuroimaging technologies, endoscopic assistance, surgical techniques, and other developments have encouraged the adoption of less invasive techniques including keyhole approaches for a subset of patients. The intracranial keyhole approaches are innovative techniques to minimize approach-related injuries in the skull and soft tissues including the temporalis muscle. The concept of keyhole neurosurgery is to access deep intracranial lesions through a minimum yet adequate bony opening. The spatial relationship between the small cranial window and the relatively wide operative field provides a reverse funnel-shaped surgical corridor. This special corridor provides a wide operative field but limits the working angle, generally the major disadvantage of keyhole strategies, and limits the directions for observation and manipulation of the target pathologies.

Intracranial aneurysms are located at the base of the brain, located much deeper than the overlying cranium. Here, the concept of "reverse funnel cone" applies, similar to other deep intracranial lesions [9]. The overlying bony opening need not be larger but the exposure of the lesion must be wider (Figure 1). This is in contrast to a superficial lesion where a wide craniotomy is a prudent choice. The advent of neuroendoscopes, image guidance, and refinement in the skull base techniques can allow tailored exposures to be made for individual case situations.

Different MIAs Described for Anterior Circulation Aneurysms

1. Minipterional craniotomy (MPC) described by Nathal et al. [10] and popularized by Figueiredo et al. [11]
2. The supraorbital craniotomy (SOC) through an eyebrow skin incision described by Pernezcky et al. [12], and the SOC through an eyelid skin incision described by Andaluz et al. [13]
3. The lateral supraorbital variant of the SOC (LSO) described by Hernieshnemi et al. [14]

Before discussing each of these approaches, it is pertinent to review the basic craniometric points necessary for the conduct of a particular procedure. Considering the precision involved, it is very important to draw the following relevant lines and landmarks on the patient's head before proceeding with the draping of the patient.

The lines and points of interest are shown in Figure 2:

1. Superior and lateral orbital margin: Can be easily palpated and marked.
2. The supraorbital foramen: Palpation along the inferior border of the superior orbital rim leads to the palpation of the supraorbital nerve and vessels as they glide below the finger.

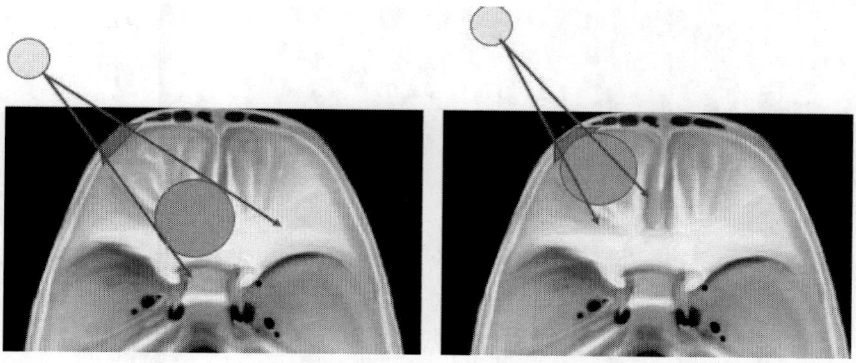

Figure 1. This figure explains the concept of utilising a keyhole approach in deep intracranial lesions. While appropriate angulation of the microscope can provide a circumferential view of a deep-seated lesion (A), the same is not possible in superficial lesions (B). Yellow circle = source of light, Red arrows = beam of light, Blue area = craniotomy, Orange circle = lesion of interest.

3. Superior temporal line (STL): It can be easily palpated above the bulk of the temporal muscle. It is particularly important to mark its junction with the superior orbital rim.
4. Zygomatic arch: It is easily palpated and its upper border is traced and marked from the base till it joins the lateral orbital margin.
5. The frontozygomatic point: This point is located on the orbital rim 2.5 cm above the level at which the upper edge of the zygomatic arch joins the orbital rim and just below the junction of the lateral and superior margins of the orbital rim. It can be easily palpated.
6. The Sylvian line: The Sylvian fissure is located along a line that extends backward from the frontozygomatic point across the lateral surface of the head to the three-quarter point (75% of the distance between the nasion and the inion on the midline). During surgery, it is often seen as a groove or depression on the bone. It can be felt through the temporalis muscle in thin individuals or those with reduce temporalis bulk.
7. The pterion: It represents the site on the external surface of the cranium approximating the lateral end of the sphenoid ridge, is located approximately 3 cm behind the frontozygomatic point, on the path of the Sylvian fissure line, and in close relationship with the hairline.

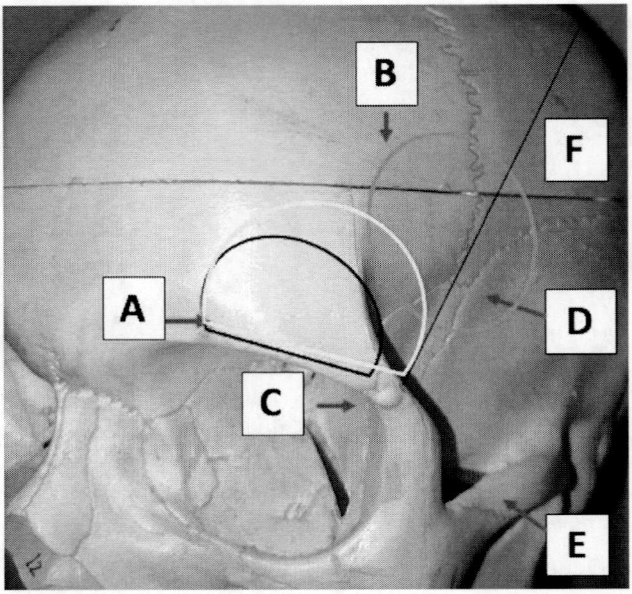

Figure 2. 3D printed skull specimen showing important craniometric points. A = supraorbital foramen, B = superior temporal line, C = fronto-zygomatic suture, D = pterion, E = zygomatic arch, F = Sylvian fissure line (junction between the point C and 75% point on the nasion to inion line). Areas encircled in black, yellow and blue represent craniotomy locations for SOA, LSO and MPA respectively.

With the above anatomical background, we discuss the technical details of each of these approaches:

Supraorbital Approach (SOA)

The supraorbital approach represents one of the commonest MIAs employed for anterior circulation aneurysms. There are a number of variations to this approach, depending on the placement of the incision. The eyebrow approach, where an incision is placed along the eyebrow, was proposed by Pernezcky [15] and remains the most commonly employed MIA. The eyelid variant involves an incision over the eyelid, described first by Andaluz et al. [13]. This approach provides an anterior sub-frontal trajectory unlike a trans Sylvian trajectory of the MPA. The basic steps of this technique are detailed below (Figure 3):

Table 1. Shows the basic differences between these procedures

	Supraorbital approach	Lateral supra orbital approach	Minipterional approach
Skin incision	Eyebrow or eyelid	Either hairline or forehead skin crease	Hairline
Bony opening	Above STL	2/3rd above and 1/3rd below STL	Below STL
Placement of key hole	Mc Carty's key point	Below STL beneath temporalis muscle	At pterion
Additional bony drilling	Bevelling of the inner table of bony opening and flattening of "juga".	Frontal base, part of sphenoid ridge	Sphenoid ridge is drilled till MOB; even anterior clinoidectomy is possible
Structures exposed	Frontal lobe	Frontal lobe and part of sylvian fissure on extreme posterior part	Sylvian fissure with fronto-temporal opercula
Corridor provided	Anterior sub frontal	Lateral sub frontal	Trans sylvian
Advantages	Cosmetically best, no or minimal TM atrophy	More lateral access and orienting than SOA, with some maneuver, SF may be approached	SF may be opened to allow CSF drainage, simulates PA most closely
Limitations	Late CSF release, unusual anatomy, cannot access lateral SF	Limited SF exposure, TM atrophy, limited exposure of posterior circulation	No sub frontal exposure, risk of frontal branch of 7th nerve and temporalis muscle atrophy
Suitable aneurysms	A-comm, ICA aneurysm, especially directed laterally	Posteriorly directed ICA, P-comm	MCA, located distally in SF, ICA bifurcation, p-comm

STL = superior temporal line, SF = Sylvian fissure, TM = Temporalis muscle, SOA = Supraorbital approach, LSO = Lateral Supraorbital approach, PA = Pterional approach, MPA = Minipterional approach, CSF = Cerebrospinal fluid, ICA = Internal carotid artery, MOB = Meningo-orbital band, COW = Circle of Willis

Eye Brow Variant

Skin Incision

The eyebrow variant is conducted through an incision over the ipsilateral eyebrow. Usually, the upper 3rd of the eyebrow is preferred as the resultant alopecia is cosmetically better. A supraciliary approach, often in a forehead skin crease is also described [16]. The medial end of the incision is at the supraorbital foramen and the lateral end typically extends just beyond the lateral end of the eyebrow. Pravadello group [17] proposed an extended SOA by extending the lateral end of the incision up to the zygomatic arch and 15 mm along its upper border to allow a larger bone flap elevation. The skin and subcutaneous tissue are resected along the line of the incision. It is important to preserve the insertion of the levator palpebrae muscle to avoid postoperative ptosis. A limited area of the temporalis muscle is disinserted to expose McCarty's point.

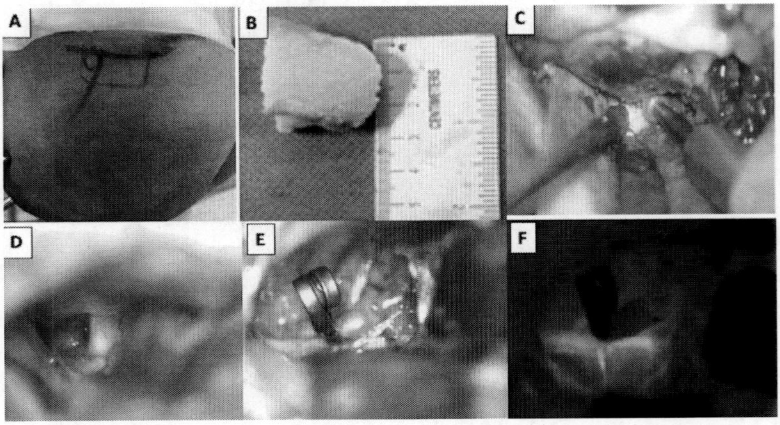

Figure 3. A-comm aneurysm clipping using SOA (eyebrow approach). Using a supine position with neck extension, an incision was marked on the upper third of the eyelid, starting just lateral to the supraorbital notch and extended laterally to the superior temporal line (A). With the help of a drill, a 3x2.5 bone flap is elevated (B). It is imperative to drill the frontal skull base before opening the dura (C). This step ensures an unhindered view flush with the skull base. The first intradural step is to drain CSF from the carotid-optic cistern (D). After aneurysm neck delineation, an appropriate sized clip was applied across the neck (E). Complete aneurysm occlusion was confirmed with intraoperative indocyanine green video angiography (F).

Craniotomy and Skull Base Drilling

The craniotomy is approximately 2.5 to 3 cm in width and around 2 cm in maximum height. The medial edge of craniotomy is just lateral to the supra orbital foramen while the lateral edge is just lateral to the superior temporal line. The initial burr hole is placed at the key point (just behind the fronto-zygomatic suture). After freeing a segment of duramater from the under surface of the bone, craniotomy is completed using a drill. Thereafter, the inner edge of the craniotomy is bevelled to widen the exposure. The duramater over the frontal lobe is elevated from the frontal skullbase in order to visualise and drill the bony elevations on the orbital plate, called "juga". This step is very important to widen the exposure, have an unhindered sub-frontal access to the basal cisterns.

Durotomy

Dura is opened in a C-shaped fashion, based inferiorly. Removal of the orbital rim can provide additional access and reduce the depth to the surgical target but it comes at the cost of orbital complications (discussed later). Since the Sylvian fissure is not opened in this approach, brain relaxation solely depends on the release of CSF from the carotid and chiasmatic cisterns. The rest of the steps are common and standard for microsurgical aneurysm clipping.

The extended SOA is a variation that allows a more lateral extension of the bony opening, thereby, bringing a part of the Sylvian fissure in view. This allows opening of the Sylvian fissure for early brain relaxation, gravity-assisted separation of the temporal lobe and a more lateral sub frontal corridor compared to the traditional SOA. Pravedello group [17] recently described this variation.

Advantages

The greatest advantage of the trans ciliary SOC is its excellent cosmetic outcome. As this technique requires minimal handling of the temporalis muscle, postoperative temporalis muscle atrophy is least or non-existent with this approach. Out of all MIAs, the bony opening is the least and this can be considered a true "keyhole" approach amongst the available choices. Exposure of the midline and contralateral structures is best among the available options.

Drawbacks

Despite the placement of the skin and bony opening lateral to the supraorbital foramen, forehead hypesthesia is not uncommon. A prominent frontal sinus is a contraindication for this approach. Moreover, the manoeuvrability of instruments is minimum with this approach, unless specific instruments are used. The line of sight through this approach is an anterior sub-frontal route and can be disorienting, especially for beginners.

Eyelid Variant

For the eyelid variant described by Andaluz et al. [13], the positioning and head rotation are the same. A temporary tarsorrhaphy is performed to protect the cornea. A 2.5 to 3.5 cm incision is placed on an eyelid crease or the supra tarsal fold and extended to the lateral orbital rim. The incision is at least 10 mm above the upper eyelid margin and 6 mm above the lateral canthus at its lateral extension. The skin and orbicularis oculi are divided as a single unit and elevated together. This layer is elevated and a plane is created below this myocutaneous flap on the orbital septum and with lateral and cranial dissection, the superior and lateral orbital rims are exposed. The periosteum over the orbital margin is divided horizontally and the periorbita is subperiosteally pushed down from the supraorbital foramen till 1-2 cm below the fronto-zygomatic suture. Care is taken to avoid opening the periorbita or the lacrimal gland. The temporalis muscle is sub-periosteally separated and pushed laterally, having preserved its insertion.

Bony Opening

Mc Carty's key point is exposed and a burr hole is placed to join the anterior cranial fossa with orbit. With the help of a drill, a craniotomy including the superior and lateral orbital rims and an orbital plate of the frontal bone is elevated. The rest of the steps are the same.

Advantages

The skin incision is cosmetically excellent as it remains hidden in the eye-lid crease. The craniotomy is most basal of all approaches and hence reduces the distance to the target while also minimising the brain retraction. A limited temporalis muscle dissection is a major advantage.

Disadvantages

The major disadvantage of this approach is a transient ocular swelling and ocular pseudo meningocele after surgery. Moreover, the angle of visualisation can be awkward. Supraorbital hypesthesia can occur similar to the trans-ciliary approach.

Lateral Supraorbital Approach (LSO)

LSO was described and popularised by the Hernieshnemi group from Helsinki, Finland [14]. It is a more lateral craniotomy compared to the SOA and has the advantage of providing lateral sub frontal view with additional provision to open the Sylvian fissure from the frontal side. This approach basically eliminates the temporal aspect of the PA. Therefore, amongst MIAs, it represents an intermediate approach between the SOA and the MPA. In comparison to the classic PA, the skin incision is smaller, the dissection of temporalis muscle is more limited and the craniotomy is smaller. Compared with the PA, the LSO offers equivalent access to the A-co A complex and sellar to para sellar regions, but much-restricted access to the retro sellar area [14, 18]. LSO provides a more median trajectory than the lateral viewing angle of the PA. Cha et al. [19] compared the LSO with PA and showed that with a significantly smaller craniotomy (1257.4 mm vs 2858.9 mm), equivalent outcomes can be obtained with a significantly shorter duration of hospital stay in LSO. **Figure 4** shows the steps involved in the exposure.

Technical Details

Skin Incision

The skin incision is similar to a traditional transcranial approach, starting 1 cm above the zygomatic arch, ascending along the hairline and reaching the midline. This incision allows a caudal reflection of the skin flap so that supraorbital margin is palpable. The temporalis muscle is incised along the same skin incision line and the myo-cutaneous flap is reflected together. This step not only ensures the safety of frontal branch of the facial nerve but also reduces the operating times.

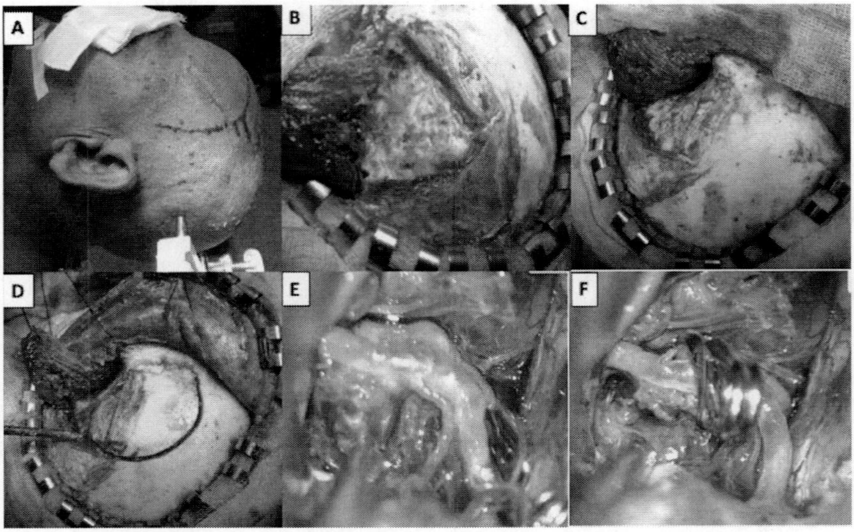

Figure 4. A-comm aneurysm clipping using the LSO approach. The incision starts at least 1 cm above the zygomatic arch and ends no further than the mid pupillary line (A). After leaving a cuff at the superior temporal line (B), the anterior part of the temporalis muscle is reflected anteriorly (c). A craniotomy of size 3.5x4 cm is elevated with the help of a drill, 2/3rd above and 1/3rd below the STL (D). A superiorly directed large A-comm artery aneurysm was dissected free of the A-comm perforators (E). Two straight fenestrated clips were used to obliterate the aneurysm neck, incorporating the ipsilateral A2 in the fenestration (F).

Craniotomy

The initial burr hole is placed just below the superior temporal line. The dura mater is freed from the edges of the burr hole and a craniotomy is created around 4x4 cm, two-thirds above and one third below the superior temporal line. The projections on the frontal skull base, called juga cerebri, are drilled flush with the craniotomy margin. Thereafter, dura mater is opened in a C-shaped fashion, based on the cranial base. The resultant exposure includes part that of the frontal lobe with the orbito-frontal surface, proximal Sylvian fissure on the extreme temporal side of the bony exposure.

Brain Relaxation

This approach provides a lateral sub-frontal corridor with the ability to enter the lateral Sylvian fissure by applying a gentle retraction over the frontal lobe. Here, the sphenoid ridge, which remains more or less intact, acts as a natural retractor. Once a small area of Sylvian fissure is opened, saline is insufflated inside the fissure to allow further opening. Thereafter, the optic, chiasmatic cistern and carotid-optic cistern are opened to let out CSF. This brings about significant brain relaxation.

Advantages

LSO can be performed very quickly, primarily because of a short incision, elevation of the myocutaneous flap and avoidance of sphenoid ridge drilling. Moreover, the trajectory is a more lateral sub frontal one making this approach more close to the orientation with which most neurosurgeons are well conversant. The ability to open the lateral end of the sylvian fissure, using a slight traction on the frontal lobe, also allows an early brain relaxation. The cosmetic outcome is good due to preservation of the bulkier posterior segment of the temporalis muscle and preservation of the frontal division of the facial nerve due to myocutaneous flap elevation. Moreover, this approach is akin to the MPA working angle, albeit without a trans-Sylvian working window.

Disadvantage

The disadvantage of this approach is a lack of temporal window, a non-existent trans-Sylvian corridor and the opportunity to drill the sphenoid ridge. One has to work predominantly using the sub frontal corridor. As stated earlier, exposure of the retro sellar area is very difficult. This limits working in certain aneurysms. Moreover, the anterior temporalis muscle atrophy can still happen with a resultant temporal fossa hollowing.

Minipterional Approach (MPA)

MPA is one of the most used approaches to these aneurysms. This is also the closest look-alike of the standard PA and therefore, the ideal keyhole approach to begin with. There are a few minor variations in the way it is performed. The first report on this approach emanated in 2005 when Nathan et al. [10] described this approach as the "sphenoid ridge keyhole approach". Subsequently, Figueiredo et al. [20] popularized this concept and named it a minipterional approach in 2007. Some other variations, mainly related to the placement of the burr-hole and opening of the temporalis muscle, have been reported. Figure 5 shows the basic steps involved.

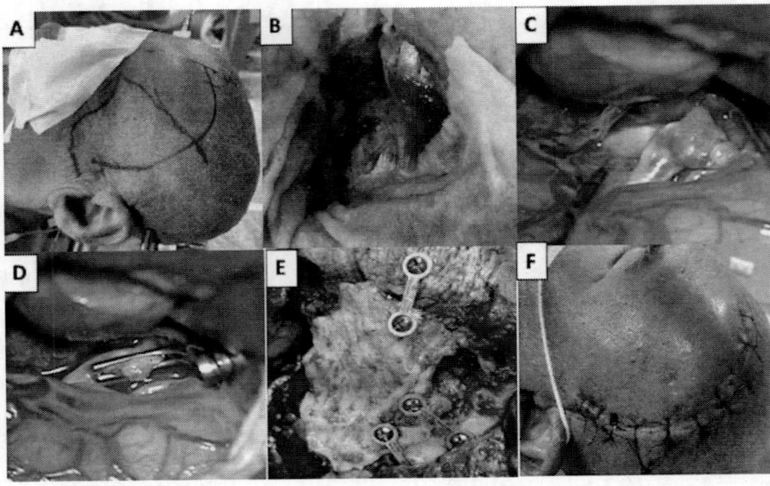

Figure 5. Shows MCA aneurysm clipping using MPA. After positioning, important landmarks like the orbital rim, zygomatic arch and the STL are drawn on the scalp. Then an incision, behind the hairline, is marked, starting 1 cm above the zygomatic arch and finishing no further than the mid pupillary line (A). After identification of the pterion, a bone flap of approximate size 3.5x3.5 cm was raised exposing the SF and adjoining operculum (B). Drilling of the sphenoid ridge increased the basal exposure. After durotomy, proximal Sylvian fissure is opened, the brain was made lax and MCA is exposed till the bifurcation (C). The aneurysm here was clipped with a right angled clip, applied across the neck and maintaining the patency of both M2 branches (D). The bone flap was secured with mini plates for better cosmesis (E). Skin is closed in the usual fashion using interrupted nylon sutures (F).

Technical Steps

Positioning and Incision

The positioning is the same as the classical PA. The head is typically fixed on pins, extended gently to bring in gravity assistance for the frontal lobe to separate away. The head is rotated contralaterally, the degree of which depends on the target on the circle of Willis. 15-20 degrees rotation generally exposes the A-Co A while 40-50 degrees of rotation brings MCA and its bifurcation into view.

The scalp incision follows the hairline, just behind it, starting 1 cm above the zygoma and reaching just above the superior temporal line, not crossing the mid-pupillary line. The incision is made in front of the STA trunk. The skin flap is elevated anteriorly and subfascial dissection ensures safety of the

7th nerve branch although in true sense, exposure of the Mc Carty's key point is barely needed in MPA. For the beginners, at least palpation of the lateral and superior orbital rim through the temporalis fascia is re-assuring.

Temporalis Muscle Exposure

After elevation of the skin flap, the temporalis muscle is exposed. There are slight variations in the way it is elevated. However, it is imperative to leave a cuff at the superior temporal line for a later approximation. Preservation of the muscle insertion ensures that the muscle functions normally after surgery. While Figueiredo et al. [20] advise reflecting the muscle en-masse in a posteroinferior direction, others advise a t-shaped opening, bifurcating the muscle while leaving a horizontal cuff of muscle for later re-approximation [20]. In our experience, the latter technique reduces the bony exposure and we prefer reflecting the muscle in toto.

Craniotomy

The initial burr-hole is placed either at the Mc Carty's point (Figueiredo et al.) or at the bony groove overlying the Sylvian vallecula. The very idea is to have the burr hole hidden either by a prominent bony edge of the bulk of the temporal muscle. The craniotomy is then completed in such a way that the pterion is included in the bone flap. It is imperative to drill the sphenoid ridge till the orbito-meningeal band. The bony opening in MPA is around 3x3 cm. Importantly, the bone flap is limited superiorly by the superior temporal line. This bony exposure gives access to the Sylvian fissure below the anterior ascending ramus and the adjoining frontotemporal opercula.

Making the Brain Lax

To be comfortable in aneurysm dissection and clipping, it is very important to have a slack brain. This is obtained by generously releasing CSF from the Sylvian fissure and then the basal cisterns before proceeding further. This step is essential to handle an intraoperative aneurysm rupture if so happens.

Advantages

The MPA provides lateral exposure to the suprasellar area and the COW. As the Sylvian fissure is exposed and frontotemporal lobes separate away, the basal cisterns can be approached allowing CSF drainage and dissection of the COW can be performed. Moreover, MPA resembles PA very closely and beginners find it easier to start with. Figueiredo et al. compared the MPA with the PA and demonstrated that the total area of exposure (PA, 1524.7x305 mm^2;

MPA 1469.7x 380.3 mm^2; $P < 0.05$), ipsilateral, lateral and contralateral zones of the circle of Willis as well as horizontal and vertical ranges of manoeuvrability were similar. The only limitation obtained in their study was an exposure of the distal Sylvian fissure.

Disadvantage

Apart from the inability to dissect distal Sylvian fissure, a lack of simultaneous sub-frontal access remains another major drawback of MPA. The possibility of temporalis muscle atrophy and possible injury to the frontal branch of the facial nerve still exist.

Anatomical Studies Showing their Differences with Respect to Manoeuvrability and Exposure Provided

Few studies have objectively compared the exposure and freedom of movement obtained with MIAs. Figueiredo et al. [20] compared the MPA with the traditional approach in their first publication. They chose 6 points on the circle of Willis as regions of interest, considering the normal exposure obtained with PA. 1) a point just lateral to the superior orbital fissure on the ipsilateral sphenoid ridge; 2) bifurcation of the ipsilateral MCA (middle cerebral artery); 3) the most distal point of the ipsilateral posterior cerebral artery (PCA); 4) the most distal point of the contralateral PCA; 5) the most distal point of the contralateral MCA; and 6) the most lateral point of the contralateral sphenoid ridge. The total area of this hexagon was further divided into: ipsilateral, middle, and contralateral areas. The ipsilateral area was formed between lateral superior orbital fissure, ipsilateral MCA bifurcation and the most distal exposable point on the ipsilateral PCA. The same points on the contralateral side formed the contralateral triangle. The middle area was formed between ipsilateral and contralateral points on the sphenoid ridge and the distal exposable point on the bilateral PCA.

For angular exposure, they used two planes, one longitudinal along the Sylvian fissure connecting the emergence of ICA to the distal Sylvian point and another perpendicular to the frontal base. They used three targets for this measurement. These were MCA bifurcation, ICA bifurcation and A -Co A on the ipsilateral side. They used robotic navigation, head fixation and a fixed retractor to keep the measurements uniform.

They did not find any statistical difference in the total area of surgical exposure between the MPA (1469.7 x 380.3 mm^2) and PT (1524.7 x 305 mm^2,

$P > 0.05$) craniotomies. Similarly, the smaller ipsilateral, middle and contralateral areas also did not differ between MPA and PA.

Maximum Allowable Transverse Working Angles

The transverse working angle to the targets did not vary significantly. The angle to the MCA bifurcation was 65.0 x 14.4 for the PA and 64.3 x 15.2 for the MPA opening ($P > 0.05$). Likewise, there were no statistical differences between the angles of approach to the ICA bifurcation (PA = 39.5 x 8.1; MPA = 37.6 x 10.7; $P > 0.05$) or A-CoA (PA = 19.8 x 9.6; MPA = 23.9 x 7.8; $P > 0.05$).

Maximum Allowable Longitudinal Working Angles

As far as the differences in the longitudinal angles of approach to the ipsilateral targets, the angle of approach to the MCA bifurcation was 70.1 x 20.3 for the PT and 68.4 x 18.3 for the MPA opening. The angle of approach to the ICA bifurcation was 60.3 x 12.6 for the PA and 62.9 x 15.5 for the MPA. The angle of approach to the A-CoA was 47.7 x 8.3 for the PA and 40.2 x 10.8 for the MPA. None of these differences reached statistical significance.

Therefore, this study objectively proves that MPA provides equivalent exposure of the areas of interest in the circle of Willis with a comparable angle of manoeuvrability.

Martinez-Perez et al. [21] recently compared the SOA with MPC using similar criteria proposed by Figueiredo et al. [20] and demonstrated that area of exposure was significantly larger in the MPA than in the SOA (1250 ± 223 mm^2 vs 939 ± 139 mm^2, p = 0.002). They observed that MPA provided larger areas of exposure in the ipsilateral and midline compartments, whereas no significant difference was observed for the contralateral compartment. All targets in the anterior circulation had significantly larger areas of surgical freedom when treated via the MPA than the SOA. They concluded that MPA provided greater surgical exposure and better manoeuvrability compared to SOA. However, it was noted that exposure of lesions on the contralateral side and anterior cranial fossa could be distinct advantages of SOA. The surgical exposure of the midline region was, however clearly better with MPA.

Technical Concerns and Solutions

While the concept of MIA is appalling, there are a number of concerns that need to be understood. The majority of the shortcomings result from the small size of the craniotomy, which cramps space and reduces angles of attack as well as instrument manoeuvrability. Conventional instruments have limited manoeuvrability in narrow deep corridors. Hence the aneurysm should be approached by the most direct route. In keyhole craniotomy, the approach is essentially a unidirectional one while in PA, it is multidirectional which facilitates aneurysm dissection from multiple directions and multidirectional clip application option.

For example, a trans ciliary supraorbital mini-craniotomy creates a very small cranial opening with a diameter ≤3 cm, this imposes many technical limitations. First, the viewing angles are narrow as the anterior sub-frontal view is the only available corridor and due to the light source being outside and partially blocked by the bony opening, there can be a reduction in the desired illumination at the site of interest. However, if hidden regions are problematic for microscopic visualization, an angled endoscope or surgical micro-mirror can be used to look around corners or behind structures.

Second, the small cranial opening reduces the manipulation of surgical instruments. While conventional aneurysm clip applicators, micro scissors, and bipolar coagulation forceps have limited manoeuvrability in a narrow corridor, new single-shaft slender-type instruments are now commercially available that can operate freely in such a narrow space. In the case of using the conventional type of instruments, one should use longer instruments, that provide better manoeuvrability. For example, longer bipolar coagulation forceps, when closed, have a narrower configuration at the apex. Furthermore, extra care must be taken to proceed with the surgery in a meticulous, step by step fashion. Thus, careful and clean arachnoid dissection is required to minimize venous bleeding, avoid a dim operative field, and facilitate surgical processes. On the positive side, the margin of the small cranial opening can be used to support the surgical instruments to reduce the surgeon's tremor, which is actually a critical advantage of keyhole surgery.

Third, the small cranial opening provides a uni-portal microsurgical procedure with essentially coaxial control of the surgical instruments. As the nature of the craniotomy allows only co-axial movement of the instruments, there can be additional difficulty in aneurysm clipping. One can overcome this with increasing experience.

Literature on Aneurysm Clipping Using MIAs

Rychen et al. [22] recently reviewed the published literature on aneurysm clipping using MIAs. They showed that SOA through the eyebrow remained the most frequently employed approach for aneurysms. The authors speculated that the preference for SOA could be reflective of the well-established nature of this approach. A total of 40 publications including 4004 surgically treated aneurysms were reported by the authors. Aneurysms of the anterior communicating artery (A-CoA) (33.2%; n = 1048) and MCA (27.6%; n = 871) were the most frequent aneurysms operated using this approach. Nearly a half of the reported aneurysm-clipping procedures were in the setting of an acute subarachnoid haemorrhage (a SAH, 45.8%; n = 1579). 15% of patients (n = 296) underwent clipping of multiple aneurysms in the same session demonstrating their feasibility. This approach was used even in the setting of giant aneurysms (2.5%, n = 50). Intraoperative aneurysm rupture was reported 5% (n = 51) patients with a postoperative infarction rate of 3.5% (n = 33). Complete aneurysm occlusion was achieved in 97.8% (n = 2338) patients indicating its durability. A temporary peri-orbital swelling (10.7%; n = 40) and transient frontal facial nerve palsy (6.6%; n = 121) were the most commonly reported direct approach-related complications. In a previous review by the same group, the incidence of periorbital swelling was higher in patients who underwent an additional orbital osteotomy. As far as the aesthetic outcome was concerned, Rychen et al. noted that 99.7% of the reported patients had an excellent or good outcome indicating an excellent cosmetic acceptance of this technique.

The supraorbital eyelid approach remains a less commonly employed SOA with only 5 previous studies available in the literature so far. Out of the 138 reported patients, the majority (n = 43, 31.2%) were operated for A-com artery aneurysms followed by P-comm aneurysms (23%). A vast majority of these patients had unruptured aneurysms while no patients with multiple or giant aneurysms were treated using this approach. A higher intraoperative aneurysm rupture (9%), postoperative infarction (7%) and a lower incidence of a complete aneurysm (90%) contrasted from the eyebrow variant of SOA. Understandably, periorbital swelling and orbital pseudo meningocele were the commonest complications reported with this approach. 80% of patients reported an excellent cosmetic outcome. The weighted average hospital stay (for both tumours and aneurysms) was 2.3 days.

The MPA has gained significant traction in recent years. Rychen et al. noted 28 publications dealing with 1628 patients who had undergone aneurysm clipping using this approach. The majority of these patients had MCA aneurysms (n = 772, 55%). 34.4% of the patients underwent MPA in the context of aSAH. A low intraoperative aneurysm rupture (3.6%), low rate of postoperative infarction (2.6%) and high aneurysm occlusion rates (98%) have been reported so far. Painful mastication remains the most frequently reported complication of MPA (3.4%). It has been considered that the rising popularity of MPA could be explained by an optimal balance in craniotomy size, temporalis muscle dissection, Sylvian fissure opening and the eventual microsurgical exposure.

Recently. Esposito et al. [23] published their experience of LSO and MPA for MCA aneurysms and they concluded that MCA aneurysms located 15 mm or more from the M1 origin are suitable for MPA while aneurysms in the proximal MCA, within 15 mm of the M1 origin can be clipped using a LSO.

Conclusion

Minimally invasive approaches or the so-called keyhole approaches to the anterior circulation aneurysms are certainly feasible, represent a technical advance of micro neurosurgery and these approaches are becoming increasingly popular. The three classic approaches, namely supraorbital approach, lateral supraorbital approach and minipterional approach have their own sets of advantages and disadvantages. The published experience is encouraging. Aneurysm location, direction, presence of aneurysm rupture, operator experience, etc. all come into play in the selection of surgical approach. The most important aspect determining the success of these approaches include a meticulous case selection and this point cannot be overemphasized. That said, the conventional approaches are still relevant and in the event of any doubt, it is prudent to be "safe than sorry" and PA must be favoured in these situations. Many modifications are being reported with the MIAs and with rapid progress in neuroimaging and preoperative planning, the clinical experience and the expanse of MIAs are only likely to increase in the future.

References

Andaluz N, Romano A, Reddy L v., Zuccarello M. Eyelid approach to the anterior cranial base: Technical note. *Journal of Neurosurgery.*, 2008 Aug; 109(2): 341–6.

Benitez RP, Silva MT, Klem J, Veznedaroglu E, Rosenwasser RH, Halbach V v., et al. Endovascular occlusion of wide-necked aneurysms with a new intracranial microstent (neuroform) and detachable coils. *Neurosurgery.*, 2004; 54(6): 1359–68.

Campos JK, Lien B v, Wang AS, Lin L-M. Advances in endovascular aneurysm management: coiling and adjunctive devices. *Stroke and Vascular Neurology* [Internet]. 2020 Mar 1 [cited 2021 Jul 13]; 5(1): 14. Available from: /pmc/articles/PMC7213502/.

Cha KC, Hong SC, Kim JS. Comparison between lateral supraorbital approach and pterional approach in the surgical treatment of unruptured intracranial aneurysms. Vol. 51, *Journal of Korean Neurosurgical Society.*, 2012. p. 334–7.

Czirják S, Szeifert T. Surgical Experience with Frontolateral Keyhole Craniotomy through a Superciliary Skin Incision.

da Costa MDS, Hardesty DA, Priddy B, Noiphithak R, Revuelta Barbero JM, Prevedello DM. Extended Supraorbital Approach with Modified Eyebrow Incision: Technical Note. *World Neurosurgery.*, 2019 Aug 1; 128: 354–9.

EG F, V D, P N, P D, MU C, N C, et al. An anatomical evaluation of the mini-supraorbital approach and comparison with standard craniotomies. *Neurosurgery* [Internet]., 2006 Oct [cited 2021 Jul 14]; 59(4 Suppl 2). Available from: https://pubmed.ncbi.nlm.nih.gov/17041490/.

Esposito G, Dias SF, Burkhardt JK, Fierstra J, Serra C, Bozinov O, et al. Selection Strategy for Optimal Keyhole Approaches for Middle Cerebral Artery Aneurysms: Lateral Supraorbital Versus Minipterional Craniotomy. *World Neurosurgery.*, 2019 Feb 1; 122: e349–57.

Figueiredo EG, Deshmukh P, Nakaji P, Crusius MU, Crawford N, Spetzler RF, et al. The Minipterional Craniotomy: Technical Description And Anatomic Assessment. *Operative Neurosurgery* [Internet]. 2007; 61. Available from: www.neurosurgery-online.comVASCULAR.

Figueiredo EG, Deshmukh P, Nakaji P, Crusius MU, Crawford N, Spetzler RF, et al. The minipterional craniotomy: technical description and anatomic assessment. *Operative neurosurgery* [Internet]., 2007; 61. Available from: www.neurosurgery-online.comvascular.

Hernesniemi1 J, Ishii1 K, Niemelä1 M, Smrcka3 M, Kivipelto1 L, Fujiki1 M, et al. Lateral supraorbital approach as an alternative to the classical pterional approach. Vol. 94, Acta Neurochir. Springer-Verlag; 2005.

M Wijdicks EF, Vermeulen M, ten Haaf JA, Hijdra A, Bakker WH, van Gijn J. Volume Depletion and Natriuresis in Patients with a Ruptured Intracranial Aneurysm.

Martinez-Perez R, Albonette-Felicio T, Hardesty DA, Carrau RL, Prevedello DM. Same viewing angle, minimal craniotomy enlargement, extreme exposure increase: the extended supraorbital eyebrow approach. *Neurosurgical Review.*, 2021 Apr 1; 44(2): 1141–50.

Millikan CH. Cerebral Vasospasm and Ruptured Intracranial Aneurysm [Internet]. Available from: http://archneur.jamanetwork.com/.

Mori K. Keyhole concept in cerebral aneurysm clipping and tumor removal by the supraciliary lateral supraorbital approach. *Asian Journal of Neurosurgery.*, 2014; 9(1): 14.

Nathal E, Gomez-Amador JL. Anatomic and surgical basis of the sphenoid ridge keyhole approach for cerebral aneurysms. *Neurosurgery.*, 2005 Jan; 56(1 SUPPL.).

Reisch R, Perneczky A, Filippi R. Surgical technique of the supraorbital key-hole craniotomy. *Surgical Neurology.*, 2003 Mar 1; 59(3): 223–7.

Reisch R, Perneczky A, Filippi R. Surgical technique of the supraorbital key-hole craniotomy. *Surgical Neurology.*, 2003 Mar 1; 59(3): 223–7.

RF S, CG M, JM Z, FC A, NK H, P N, et al. Ten-year analysis of saccular aneurysms in the Barrow Ruptured Aneurysm Trial. *Journal of neurosurgery* [Internet]., 2019 [cited 2021 Jul 13]; 132(3): 771–6. Available from: https://pubmed.ncbi.nlm.nih.gov/30849758/.

Rychen J, Croci D, Roethlisberger M, Nossek E, Potts M, Radovanovic I, et al. *Minimally Invasive Alternative Approaches to Pterional Craniotomy: A Systematic Review of the Literature.*, Vol. 113, World Neurosurgery. Elsevier Inc.; 2018. p. 163–79.

Spetzler RF, McDougall CG, Zabramski JM, Albuquerque FC, Hills NK, Russin JJ, et al. The Barrow Ruptured Aneurysm Trial: 6-year results. *Journal of Neurosurgery.*, 2015 Sep 1; 123(3): 609–17.

TM D, JL E, M M, GC S, EI L. Advances in endovascular approaches to cerebral aneurysms. *Neurosurgery* [Internet]. 2014 Feb [cited 2021 Jul 13]; 74 Suppl 1(2 SUPPL.). Available from: https://pubmed.ncbi.nlm.nih.gov/24402486/.

Yasargil MG, Antic J, Laciga R, Jain KK, Hodosh RM, Smith RD. Microsurgical pterional approach to aneurysms of the basilar bifurcation. *Surgical Neurology.*, 1976; 6(2): 83–91.

Chapter 18

3D Printing in Neurosurgery

M. S. Sridhar[1], Krishan K. Yadav[1] and S. Shashivadanan[2]
[1]Command Hospital Air Force Bangalore, Karnataka, India
[2]Military Hospital Bhatinda, Punjab, India

Abstract

3-Dimensional printing in neurosurgery is a technology which combines imaging and computer aided design to print a 3-dimensional object. This was adopted in neurosurgery initially for study of complex and intricate neurosurgical anatomy. Later as the 3D printing gained acceptance and its utility was recognized, it has been used in teaching complex neurosurgical procedures, simulation training of junior neurosurgeons and residents in neurosurgery. 3D printing is also now being used for intra operative assistance of screw placements in spine surgery, preoperative planning in aneurysm surgery, brain tumor surgery and precise kyphoscoliosis correction. Currently research is now focused on incorporating newer customizable implants and bioengineering for various neurosurgical ailments. This chapter focuses on the evolution of 3d printing, the amalgamation of this technology in neurosurgery, the current applications and the future prospects.

Introduction

3D printing, or *additive manufacturing,* is the construction of a 3-dimensional object from a CAD model or a digital 3D model [1]. The term "3D printing" can refer to a variety of processes in which material is deposited, joined or

In: Neurosurgery Research
Editors: Amit Agrawal, Pradeep Chouksey, Adesh Shrivastava et al.
ISBN: 978-1-68507-837-9

solidified under computer control to create a 3-dimensional object [2]. Variety of materials are used such as plastics, liquids or powder grains which are fused together, typically layer by layer. The 3D printing has been quickly adapted in routine neurosurgical practice from computer-aided designs quickly and inexpensively as the cost of 3D printing has come down drastically.

The earliest record of 3D printing was through a process of adding layer by layer, which was first performed by the Japanese inventor Hideo Kodama in 1981, he created a product that used ultraviolet lights to harden polymers (photopolymers - which are acrylic based substances that harden when they are exposed to UV light) and create solid objects. He unfortunately did not file a patent before the deadline. Charles W. "Chuck" Hull, later built a machine that used a UV laser to engrave layers of acrylic into shapes before stacking the layers to build objects. He patented the "apparatus for production of 3-dimensional objects by stereolithography" in 1984.

Initially in the 1980s, 3D printing techniques were considered suitable only for the production of functional or aesthetic prototypes. Since then, 3D printing has found applications across industries, including healthcare. As 3D printing becomes more advanced and more economically accessible, its medical applications continue to broaden. 3D printing can even be credited with some of medicine's most impressive recent advancements, including 3D-printed vascular tissue, prosthetic devices, and bones, as well as a slew of medical devices, including surgical guides, pacemakers, and more.

What Are Techniques Used in 3D Printing

There are various methods of 3D printing which is used today. Few which are used in neurosurgery are described below.

Stereolithography – (STL/SLA), a process where the object is printed layer by layer, rinsed with a solvent, and hardened with an ultraviolet light. The process uses computer-aided designs (CAD) to create the 3D models.

Selective Laser Sintering - (SLS) is another, more advanced, form of 3D printing. It uses additive manufacturing and a powder polymer—typically nylon—to create objects. SLS uses a laser to fuse the powder together, layer by layer, into more complex shapes than SLA is capable of creating. SLS is similar to SLM process in terms of material addition technique and the energy input it uses. The main difference in the SLS process compared to the SLM process is that the powder material is sintered instead of full melting.

Selective laser melting –[SLM], is powder based method like SLS and powder bed fusion methods contain at least one thermal resource to induce fusion between the powder particles. In SLM method, the part is created layer by layer out of a powder which is heated by a laser source. When the temperature decreases, the molten material begins to solidify. The molten material forms the object while the powder portion which has not melted, supports the structure. When the process is completed and part is built, the residual powder is removed. In the process, the powder layer is shaped by laser scanning, and the object is manufactured owing to laser energy.

Fused Deposition Modelling- (FDM), developed by Scott Crump, is the most common form of 3D printing today. It is known as the "desktop 3D printers" because it is the most commonly used form of the technology. To form an object, the printer heats a cable of thermoplastic into liquid form and extrudes it layer by layer.

3D printing technology can be applied to metal, ceramic, composite and polymer materials. The most commonly used metal materials are stainless steel, titanium, magnesium, aluminium, Chromium–Cobalt alloys. In addition to the benefits it provides, it is thought that the use of more metal alloys will increase in different applications. Metal materials, especially Titanium and Chromium–Cobalt alloys, are preferred in biomedical applications, mostly because of their mechanical properties, biocompatibility, thermal, magnetic and electrical conductivity and generally high temperature resistance. Although metals have many advantages compared to polymers and other materials due to their properties such as laser absorption power and stability at higher temperatures, it can be said that this method is new for metals, while polymer materials have been used for 3D printing for years.

How Has 3D Printing Transformed Neurosurgery?

Neuroimaging is an integral component of clinical practice as the entire neurosurgical planning and subsequent execution of the plan is based on 3D appreciation of the images acquired, which may be in 2D or a 3D volume in 2D slices. These images are usually acquired in X-ray, computed tomography (CT), and magnetic resonance imaging (MRI) [4]. Appreciation of the 3D orientation between structures in these images preoperatively and extrapolating it during surgery is often difficult, as the depth perception is absent, which is appreciated in the customized 3D models created by 3D printing. 3D printing technology is used to create a copy of the patient's special anatomy before complex operations or to understand the disease. In this way, the copy of the organ can be examined much more clearly than imaging methods such as tomography, neurosurgeons can practice the complex and delicate steps before performing the actual surgery, and the margin of error can be reduced.

In neurosurgery there has been substantial progress as a result of the use of 3D printing. 3D printing has taken the visualization and understanding of intricate neurosurgical anatomy and pathology to the next level. With 3D printing anatomy and structures can be appreciated and visualized noninvasively in intricate detail for both diagnosis and treatment. With this technology, anatomical structures can be reconstructed from various imaging modalities and then printed into 3D models. These can then be used for surgical planning and as teaching aids. In future this technology will be used for surgical simulations. Simulations provide a realistic experience of the surgical procedure safely. With 3D printing, high-resolution, customized simulators have been created which provide a realistic training environment.

3D printing can enable neurosurgeons to customize instruments and implants that correspond to individual patient, which can enable the neurosurgeon to adopt a personalized approach to treatment, tailor made to each individual patient.

Developments in 3D printing in neurosurgery

1. The creation of individualized patient-specific models for, preoperative planning, training.
2. 3D models to facilitate assessment and treatment of complex neurosurgical diseases
3. Research into bioengineered implants.
4. Future applications.

In this chapter, we will review these areas of application of 3D printing in neurosurgery.

The Creation of Individualized Patient-Specific Models for, Preoperative Planning, Training

Cerebrovascular Surgery

Cerebral aneurysm surgery requires an in-depth spatial orientation and understanding of the, individual aneurysms with relation to associated parent vessels, perforators, their orientation to the aneurysmal sac, where the aneurysm clip is likely to be applied and their possible compromise - if any, and surrounding anatomic structures. At present the neurosurgeons reconstructs mentally complicated anatomical vasculature from the 3D CT Angiography (3D-CTA) and Digital Subtraction Angiography (DSA) images, where a depth perception is lacking. 3D printed models can be held in hand and viewed from any angle, thus are a more advanced method of visualization. With the increased use of 3D printing, this approach has become a popular option, wherein physical 3D representations of vascular networks individualized to patient's anatomy can be reproduced as models (Figure 1) [5, 6, 7].

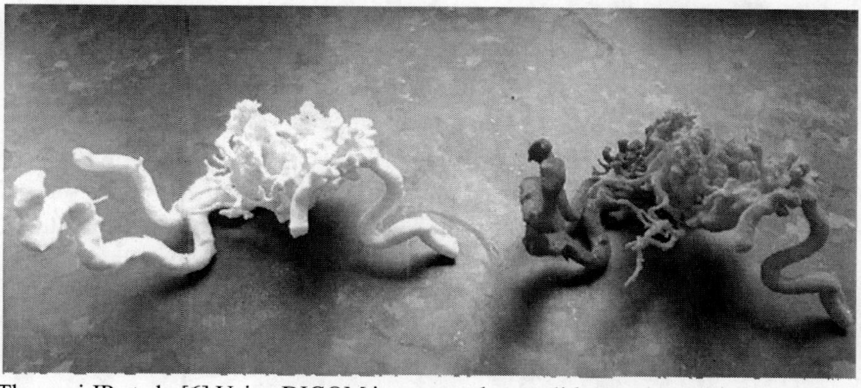

Thawani JP et al., [6] Using DICOM images and stereolithography (.STL), the authors have generated 3D models of a patient's complex vascular malformation.

Figure 1. Arteriovenous malformation.

Various studies have assessed the accuracy of the 3D printed models, of complex vasculature obtained from patient scans [8-12]. One study performed comparisons in the reproducibility of the length and thickness of the main arteries and the size of the aneurysm between a 3D-CTA and the printed model across 22 patients with unruptured aneurysms, [10] and concluded that that these models accurately represent patient anatomy. Using these anatomical models, surgical outcomes can be improved. Even clipping and the angle of approach to clipping can be practiced before the actual surgery.

Neuro-Oncology

Currently neurosurgeons use the images of MRI, CT scan in the pre-op planning for the resection of brain tumors. Even after adequate pre-op planning on imaging, it may be difficult for surgeons to appreciate the 3D spatial orientation during the surgery. 3D printing technology enables the surgeon to appreciate the relationship between the various structures such as tumor, skull, vasculature, non - pathologic brain tissue etc. (Figure 2) [13, 14]. Models can simulate realistic surgical approaches as visualized under microscope intraoperatively, this helps the surgeon to understand better the various relationships of the tumor to the surrounding structures and help in orienting the surgeon, this translates into improved surgical outcome, especially in those tumors which are close to eloquent cortex [13].

3D models have also been used in the research, planning and development of novel treatments for brain tumors (Figure 2). 3D printed models can be used as simulators, they can replicate the properties of the skull and cerebral tissue, they can also be used to evaluate the therapeutic potential of focused ultrasound, for non-invasive thermocoagulation of brain tumors [15]. Spottiswoode et al., reported the first 3D-printed brain tumor model [22]. These models were created for training and education purposes, surgical simulation, and surgical planning [23]. Tumors in various locations, including the cerebrum, cerebellum, brain stem and pituitary tumors, have thus far been 3D printed and used.

Spine

Understanding of anatomy of spine with respect to angulation, rotation and displacement of fragments and the adjacent vertebrae, is a fundamental component of planning the surgical treatment of spine fractures and complex Cervico Vertebral junction anomalies (CV junction). Neuroimaging techniques, such as CT and MRI, with 3D reconstruction and volume rendering have revolutionized the ability to recognize all these features in spinal fractures or complex CV junction anomalies. Li et al., investigated the efficacy of 3D models of complex spine anomalies, in understanding of pathology as compared to 2D CT and 3D images [17]. This large-scale study revealed that 3D printing of complex spine anomalies was extremely useful in identifying the fracture anatomy in comparison to the 2D CT images.

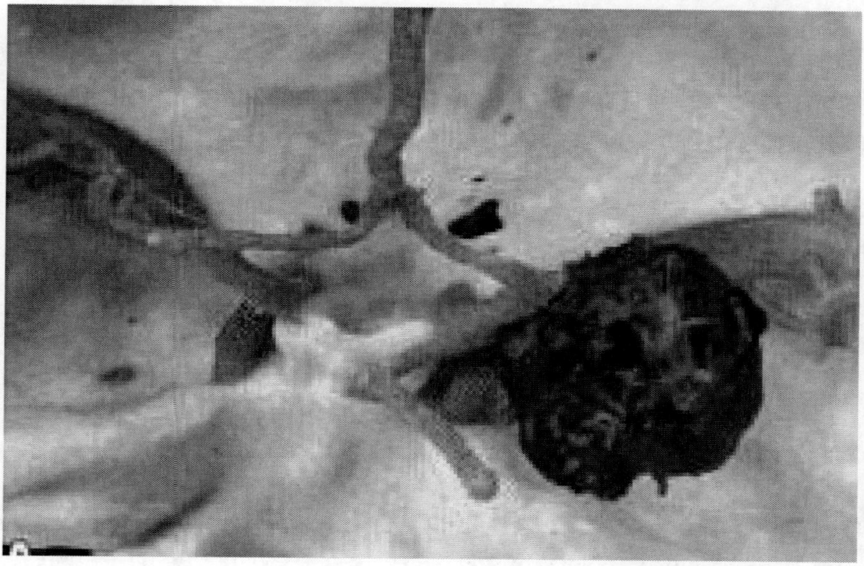

Figure 2. 3D printed models for greater sphenoid wing meningioma intervention training.

Simulators for spinal surgery have been developed with 3D printing technology. Bova et al., have developed a simulator where, a 3D spinal model is merged and enhanced with a virtual interface that also displays appropriate patient images [18].

Catheter and Endoscopic Applications - Surgical Training and Simulation

Simulators have been developed using 3D printing for ventriculostomy, which is virtual haptic-based system [18, 19]. These simulators consist of a reusable base segment representing, either the face or base of the skull and a disposable segment where users practice the procedure. Addition of a fluid-filled ventricular system enhances the haptic feedback, with variable ventricular pressures which can simulate any common pathological condition [19, 20].

Trans nasal trans sphenoid endoscopic surgery for pituitary tumors has been another area where 3D printing has helped in simulation development. Replicas of the face, skull and sphenoid sinus have been developed to practice endoscopic surgical approaches [21]. These simulators can also be used in conjunction with the surgical navigation system [20, 21].

3D Models to Facilitate Assessment and Treatment of Complex Neurosurgical Diseases

The application of 3D printing for planning and treatment was an extension of the use of 3D technology in teaching.

Cranioplasty Applications

Cranial defects which usually are encountered after surgery for trauma, like decompressive craniotomy, tumor resections with excessive brain bulge where the bone flap is not replaced, and in some congenital defects are areas where 3D printing is used extensively. The purpose of cranioplasty is to protect the underlying brain tissue, improve aesthetics and optimize function by improving the cerebral perfusion. 3D printed plates for cranioplasty are a safe and cost effective and accurate alternative than the conventional moulds which are created for preparation of cranioplasty plates. The materials used varies and this technology can be used to create plates using polymethyl-methacrylate (PMMA), PEEK (polyether ether ketone), hydroxyapatite, titanium meshes and Polylactic acid [24, 25, 26].

Spinal Surgery Applications

While 3D printing in spine surgery was initially limited to use as visual aids in preoperative planning for complex pathology, it has gained acceptance to create intraoperative patient-specific screw guides and templates. One of the initial surgical applications of 3D printing in spine surgery was creation of patient-specific drill guides and templates meant to address some of the drawbacks of early image-guided navigation systems (Figure 3), As patient-specific treatment and personalized medicine gained popularity in medicine, 3D printing provided a similar option for the surgical fields, particularly in the creation of customizable implants. Bova et al., have developed a 3D printed simulator that is paired with a neuronavigation system, that enables neurosurgeons to determine and practice the correct surgical trajectory for implant surgery preoperatively. Sugawara et al., have designed a patient specific 3D printed screw guide that is attached onto the lamina to further enhance the accuracy of the screw placement [18]. 3D guides have also been created to aid in osteotomies in both adult and paediatric patients undergoing corrections for kyphoscoliosis.

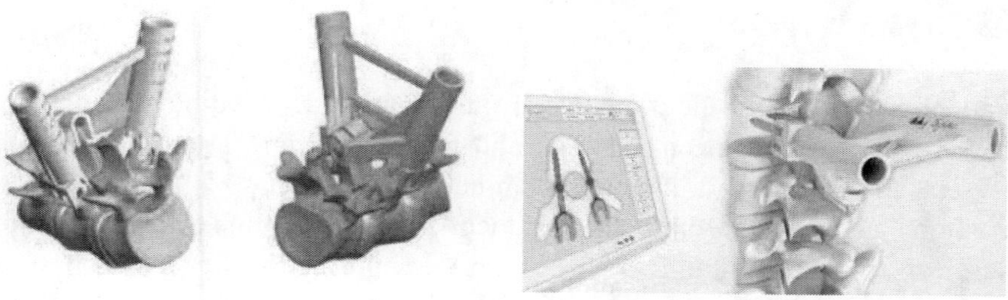

Figure 3. 3D printed surgical guides for screw trajectory.

3D printed vertebrae have been used in revision surgery after tumor recurrence in the lumbar spine. Chin BZ et al., used 3D reconstruction to create an implant which effectively filled the gap after an *en-bloc* spondylectomy of L1-L3, in a case report of recurrent giant cell tumor, after previous decompression and instrumented fusion of T12-L4, and achieved both osseointegration at the cranial and caudal levels of the construct, as well as fixation to posterior spinal instrumentation which may mitigate the risk of cage migration and subsidence [27].

3D printing has allowed for the creation of spinal implants with unique structures and surfaces for optimizing fusion, and in some cases may be used to augment biological deficiencies as well. In osteoporotic patients, 3D custom implants have been used to accommodate mismatch between the contour of the cage and the endplate which may be deformed as a result of previous insufficiency or fracture.

Brain Tumor Surgery

The Bragg peak enables proton therapy to deliver a high conformal target dose without exit dose. The passive scattering proton therapy employs patient-specific aperture and range compensator to shape the lateral and distal beam, and to deliver conformal dose to the target volume. 3D printed models have been used for the development of patient-specific proton range compensator, after brain tumor surgery, which provides an accurate conformal dose distribution during proton therapy in order to protect important structures near the target. Ju et al., have used a 3D printed range compensator which has optimized the dose distribution [16].

Aneurysm Surgery

Patient-specific 3D printed models are useful in understanding the anatomy and morphology of the aneurysms and the surrounding arterial branching pattern, perforators and, therefore, can help the interventional team to reach common ground regarding the treatment plan before the endovascular or surgical approach (Figure 4). It also enables the neurosurgeons to have a different and better perspective of the vessel's anatomy and a plan of the overall procedure.

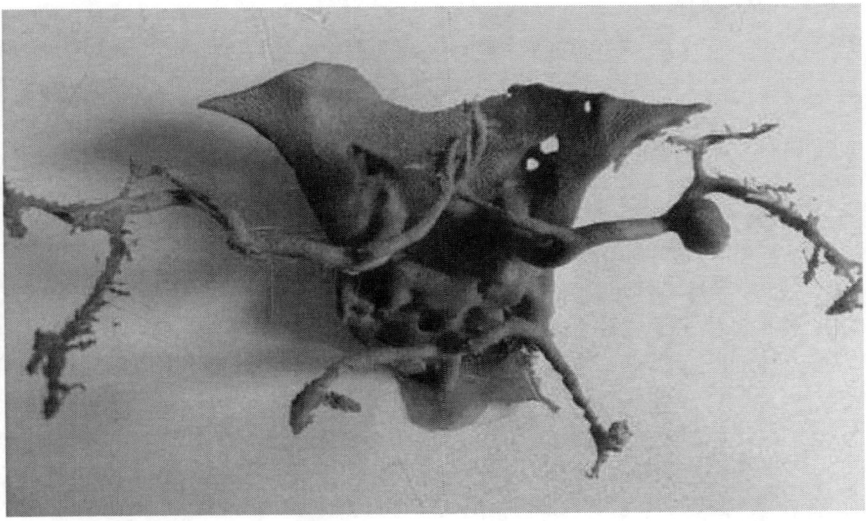

Figure 4. 3D printing in aneurysm surgery and planning treatment.

Research into Bioloengineered Implants

Artificial intervertebral discs based on tissue-engineered biodegradable scaffolds have been created which aims to replicate the viscoelastic nature of the disc [30, 31]. If successful this would revolutionize the treatment of degenerative disc disease.

Tissue-engineering is also being investigated for regenerating soft tissues by designing, and implanting a suitable matrix tissue and living cells using the 3D printing technology [32].

3D printed drug delivery systems are being investigated which can allow creation of implantable drug-delivery devices with complex drug release profiles. Using 3D printers, many innovative drug dosage delivery methods are being investigated such as: microcapsules, nanosuspensions, hyaluran-based synthetic extracellular matrices, mesoporous bioactive glass scaffolds, antibiotic printed micropatterns and multi-layered drug delivery devices [33]. Dong J et al., have successfully tested a novel drug delivery system for use in spinal tuberculosis in a laboratory setting. ATT drugs were mixed with Poly-DL-lactide (PDLLA) and nano-hydroxyapatite (nHA) and a unique porous 3D scaffold was created using 3D printing technology. Such a scaffold can be used individually or in combination with titanium mesh during reconstruction of defects in spinal stabilization surgery in spinal tuberculosis [34].

Conclusion

Future developments in 3D printing will include a wider range of biocompatible materials which will be more durable and realistic. Future improvements in the 3D printing technologies include, advances in layering process, fusion of multiple materials of different characteristics to create a single mould, which will result in greater product strength and accuracy in depicting intricate detail and improving the haptic feedback [35]. The cost and speed of 3D printers will improve, which will result in application of 3D printing in Neurosurgery to be more economical and readily acceptable for widespread usage, which should translate into better patient outcomes. 3D printed bioengineering should revolutionize replacement of organs and recovery in spinal cord injury patients.

References

"3D printing scales up". *The Economist*. 5 September 2013.

Abla A A, Lawton M T. 3-dimensional hollow intracranial aneurysm models and their potential role for teaching, simulation, and training. *World Neurosurg*. 2015;83:35-6.

Anderson J R, Thompson W L, Alkattan A K, Diaz O, Klucznik R, Zhang Y J, et al. 3-dimensional printing of anatomically accurate, patient specific intracranial aneurysm models. *J. Neurointerv. Surg*. 2016;8:517-20.

Berman, B. (2012). 3-D printing: the new industrial revolution. *Bus. Horizons* 55, 155–162.

Bova F J, Rajon D A, Friedman W A, Murad G J, Hoh D J, Jacob R P, et al. Mixed-reality simulation for neurosurgical procedures. *Neurosurgery* 2013;73:138-45.

Chin B Z, Ji T, Tang X, et al. 3-level lumbar en bloc spondylectomy with 3-dimensional-printed vertebrae reconstruction for recurrent giant cell tumor. *World Neurosurg*. 2019;129:531-7. 10.

Cranioplasty with 3-dimensional customised mould for polymethylmethacrylate implant: a series of 16 consecutive patients with cost-effectiveness consideration Erasmo Barros da Silva Júnior, Afonso Henrique de Aragão, Marcelo de Paula Loureiro, Caetano Silva Lobo, Ana Flávia Oliveti, Rafael Martinelli de Oliveira & Ricardo Ramina. *3D Printing in Medicine* (2021) 7:4.

de Beer N., van der Merwe A. Patient-specific intervertebral disc implants using rapid manufacturing technology. *Rapid. Prototyp. J.* 2013;19(2):126–139.

de Beer N., van der Merwe A. Patient-specific intervertebral disc implants using rapid manufacturing technology. *Rapid Prototyp. J.* 2013;19(2):126–139.

Dong J, Zhang S, Liu H, Li X, Liu Y, Du Y. Taylor & Francis; 2014. *Novel Alternative Therapy for Spinal Tuberculosis during Surgery: Reconstructing with Anti-tuberculosis Bioactivity Implants.*

Excell, Jon (23 May 2010). "The rise of additive manufacturing". *The Engineer*. Retrieved 30 October 2013.

Inoue D, Yoshimoto K, Uemura M, Yoshida M, Ohuchida K, Kenmotsu H, et al. 3-dimensional high-definition neuroendoscopic surgery: A controlled comparative laboratory study with two-dimensional endoscopy and clinical application. *J. Neurol. Surg. A Cent. Eur. Neurosurg.* 2013;74:357-65.

Ionita C N, Mokin M, Varble N, Bednarek D R, Xiang J, Snyder K V, et al. Challenges and limitations of patient-specific vascular phantom fabrication using 3D Polyjet printing. *Proc. SPIE Int. Soc. Opt. Eng*. 2014;9038:90380.

Ju S G, Kim M K, Hong C S, Kim J S, Han Y, Choi D H, et al. New technique for developing a proton range compensator with use of a 3-dimensional printer. *Int. J. Radiat. Oncol. Biol. Phys.* 2014;88:453-8.

Klein G T, Lu Y, Wang M Y. 3D Printing and Neurosurgery—Ready for Prime Time? *World Neurosurg*. 2013;80:233-5.

Kondo K1, Nemoto M, Masuda H, Okonogi S, Nomoto J, Harada N, et al. Anatomical Reproducibility of a Head Model Molded by a 3-dimensional Printer. *Neurol. Med. Chir*. 2015;55:592-8.

Li Z, Li Z, Xu R, Li M, Li J, Liu Y, et al. 3-dimensional printing models improve understanding of spinal fracture—A randomized controlled study in China. *Sci. Rep.* 2015;5:11570.

Lin, J. et al. Using 3-dimensional printing to create individualized cranial nerve models for skull base tumor surgery. *World Neurosurg.* 120, e142–e152 (2018).

Low-cost customized cranioplasty using a 3D digital printing model: a case report Abel De La Peña, Javier De La Peña-Brambila, Juan Pérez-De La Torre, Miguel Ochoa, and Guillermo J. Gallardo *3D Printing in Medicine* (2018) 4:4.

Mashiko T, Otani K, Kawano R, Konno T, Kaneko N, Ito Y, et al. Development of 3-dimensional hollow elastic model for cerebral aneurysm clipping simulation enabling rapid and low-cost prototyping. *World Neurosurg.* 2015;83:351-61.

Mashiko T, Otani K, Kawano R, Konno T, Kaneko N, Ito Y, et al. Development of 3-dimensional hollow elastic model for cerebral aneurysm clipping simulation enabling rapid and low cost prototyping. *World Neurosurg.* 2015;83:351-61.

Menikou G, Dadakova T, Pavlina M, Bock M, Damianou C. MRI compatible head phantom for ultrasound surgery. *Ultrasonics* 2015;57:144-52.

Oishi M, Fukuda M, Yajima N, Yoshida K, Takahashi M, Hiraishi T, et al. Interactive presurgical simulation applying advanced 3D imaging and modeling techniques for skull base and deep tumors. *J. Neurosurg.* 2013;119:94-105.

Pati F, Ha D-H, Jang J, Han H H, Rhie J-W, Cho D.-W. Biomimetic 3D tissue printing for soft tissue regeneration. *Biomaterials.* 2015;62:164–175.

Polylactic Acid Implant for Cranioplasty with 3-dimensional Printing Customization: A Case Report Tedy Apriawan, Khrisna Rangga Permana, Ditto Darlan, Muhammad Reza Arifianto, Fitra Fitra, Asra Alfauzi, Abdul Hafid Bajamal. *Macedonian Journal of Medical Sciences*. 2020 Nov 10; 8(C):151-155.

Spottiswoode B S, Van Den Heever D J, Chang Y, Engelhardt S, Du Plessis S, Nicolls F, et al. Preoperative 3-dimensional model creation of magnetic resonance brain images as a tool to assist neurosurgical planning. *Stereotact. Funct. Neurosurg.* 2013;91:162-9.

Spottiswoode, B. et al. Preoperative 3-dimensional model creation of magnetic resonance brain images as a tool to assist neurosurgical planning. *Stereotactic. Funct. Neurosurg.* 91, 162–169 (2013).

Sugawara T, Higashiyama N, Kaneyama S, Takabatake M, Watanabe N, Uchida F, et al. Multistep pedicle screw insertion procedure with patient-specific lamina fit-and-lock templates for the thoracic spine. *J. Neurosurg. Spine* 2013;19:185-90.

Thawani J P, Pisapia J M, Singh N, Petrov D, Schuster J M, Hurst R W, et al. 3D-Printed Modeling of an Arteriovenous Malformation Including Blood Flow. *World Neurosurg.* 2016;90:675-83.

Ursan I D, Chiu L, Pierce A. 3-dimensional drug printing: a structured review. *J. Am. Pharmaceut. Assoc.* 2013;53(2):136–144.

Waran V, Narayanan V, Karuppiah R, Thambynayagam H C, Muthusamy K A, Rahman Z A A, et al. Neurosurgical Endoscopic Training via a Realistic 3-Dimensional Model With Pathology. *Simul. Healthc* 2015;10:43-8.

Whatley B R, Kuo J, Shuai C, Damon B J, Wen X. Fabrication of a biomimetic elastic intervertebral disk scaffold using additive manufacturing. *Biofabrication*. 2011 3(1) 015004.
Whatley B R, Kuo J, Shuai C, Damon B J, Wen X. Fabrication of a biomimetic elastic intervertebral disk scaffold using additive manufacturing. *Biofabrication*. 2011;3(1) 015004.
Xu W H, Liu J, Li M L, Sun Z Y, Chen J, Wu J H. 3D printing of intracranial artery stenosis based on the source images of magnetic resonance angiograph. *Ann. Transl. Med*. 2014;2:74.
Xu W H, Liu J, Li M L, Sun Z Y, Chen J, Wu J H. 3D printing of intracranial artery stenosis based on the source images of magnetic resonance angiograph. *Ann. Transl. Med.* 2014;2:74.

Chapter 19

Dural Substitutes in Neurosurgery: Recent Advances

S. Shashivadhanan*

Military Hospital, Bathinda, Punjab, India

Abstract

Introduction: The duramater is a very important structure in the craniospinal cavity which maintains the internal milieu of the brain and protects the brain from external invasion. A good water tight closure of dura ensures an effective safe guard against cerebrospinal fluid (CSF) leak and subsequent infection. An ineffective dural closure leads to morbidity and mortality.

Materials & methods: A retrospective study was conducted in a single institute from September 2015 to Sept 2017 to evaluate the efficacy of the available dural substitutes. This included Fibrin sealants, collagen based dural substitutes, synthetic dural substitutes and synthetic sealants. They were used as standalone substitute or in combination with autologous dural substitutes. Their effectiveness was compared two weeks following surgery. Parameters checked postoperatively were, CSF leak, local infection/inflammation, seizures or systemic signs of hypersensitivity. Preoperatively the material was checked for user friendliness. Time taken to control CSF leak was evaluated and conclusions were drawn.

Observation: In this study 553 cases were included which required duroplasty. Of these 200 cases underwent auto graft duroplasty. Collagen based dural substitute was used in 135 cases, fibrin sealant in 177 cases, Tissue Patch (synthetic adhesive sealant) in 33 cases, Gore-Tex synthetic

*Corresponding Author's Email: drshashivadhanan@gamil.com.

In: Neurosurgery Research
Editors: Amit Agrawal, Pradeep Chouksey, Adesh Shrivastava et al.
ISBN: 978-1-68507-837-9

patch in 05 cases and PolyTetra FlorEthylene (PTFE) patch in 03 cases. In 43% of cases duroplasty was done using auto graft as a standalone substitute, while in 57% cases an additional supplementation was used.

Result: Collagen based dural substitutes had a success rate of 92.6% while autologous dural repair group showed a success rate of 91%. Although fibrin sealant group had a success rate of 95%, it was mostly used as an adjunct. In 15 cases fibrin sealant served well as a standalone substitute. The success rates with use of synthetic CSF sealant, Synthetic patch (G patch) and PTFE graft were 87.2%,80% and 66.7% respectively.

Conclusion: The present study suggests that Collagen based dural substitutes offer a definite advantage to the surgeon in effectively controlling postoperative CSF leak. Its use in appropriate setting offers a definite advantage in improving the postoperative outcomes.

Keywords: dural substitute, dural reconstruction, collagen based dural matrix

Introduction

Dura mater also called the "tough mother," is a protective meningeal covering of the neuraxis, serving as a barrier separating, the intra dural from extra dural contents of cranial cavity. Embryology of the meninges is complex as it has components of mesenchymal and neural crest origin. Sound knowledge of this covering is very important to the operating surgeon as this barrier needs to be invaded before one has to enter the brain or spinal cord. Closure of this layer is equally important as CSF leak and subsequent infection can lead to significant morbidity and mortality. In addition to a good closure technique the surgeon relies on dural substitutes which aid him in providing a satisfactory CSF barrier. Various dural substitutes are available in the market and each claims supremacy over the other. This is the first retrospective study which compares the efficacy of the currently available substitutes.

Materials and Methods

This was a retrospective study conducted in a single institute from September 2015 to Sept 2017. A total of 553 dural reconstruction procedures were performed in a single institute. Standalone auto grafts using the pericranium, temporalis fascia or tensor fascia lata (TFL) was the first choice offered for water tight dural closure. Where ever it was not possible or feasible, other biomaterials or synthetic substitutes were used. In majority they were used as adjuncts rather than as standalones. Efficacy was judged by monitoring for CSF Leak for a period of 7 days post operatively. Other factors evaluated were the ease of use and the operating time.

Observation

Table 1. Showing our experience of using the various dural substitutes

Our Institutional Experience(Sept 2016 till date)			
Technique of Duroplasty employed(Total 553 Cases)	Total cases	Complication	Success rate
Auto graft(Percrarium,Temp Fascia,TFL)	200	18	91 %
Collagen Based Graft(Duragen ,Durafoam)	135	10	92.6%
Tissue Patch	33	4	87.2%
Fibrin Sealant	177	9	95 %
PTFE	03	1	66.7%
G Patch	05	1	80 %

Results

1. Autologous Graft: This is the safest substitute as there is minimal risk of infection as its body's own. It was found ideal to cover large dural skull base defects. In most cases watertight duroplasty could be achieved with sutures. The undesirable effects included donor site morbidity which included pain and infection in 9% of the cases. Suturing and hemostasis increased the operating time by 10 to 15%. A 91% success rate was achieved in terms of prevention of CSF Leak within the first seven days following surgery.

Table 2. Showing the success rate with standalone versus supplemented techniques

Stand alone Vs Multiple methods		
Duroplasty Technique	Cases	Success Rate
Single stand alone	43%	94%
Two or more Methods employed	57%	96%

2. Collagen based graft: Amongst the collagen based grafts we used the standard collagen based dural substitute (Durafoam) and Ultra-pure type I collagen based dural substitute (Duragen).We found them to be immunologically well tolerated causing no foreign body reaction. We could achieve a 93% watertight closure rate. In most of the cases it was used as a standalone substitute. Unlike experience with other synthetic grafts, there was no encapsulation or graft rejection seen with Collagen based grafts. In the redo cases there were adhesion in areas with disruption of pia arachnoid. In all cases it was used as overlay graft thereby reducing duration of surgery. Infection was encountered in one case of traumatic brain injury. Although ultra-pure collagen has most of the properties required for an ideal dural substitute, its use is contraindicated in infection, neural tube defects and anterior dural defects of the spine. Its use should be avoided in patients with history of bovine allergy.
3. Fibrin Sealant: Fibrin serves as an adjunct when water tight dural closure is desired. In our series it was used in majority of cases as an additional reinforcement for watertight closure. When used, it helped in achieving 95% success rate. Fibrin offers the advantage of addressing intra as well as extradural bleed. Being a liquid sealant, it can reach to in accessible regions. It is of immense use in emergency situations where patient has coexisting coagulopathy. When used as a standalone substitute, CSF leak was higher. Fibrin Lacks

regenerative property, hence it does not contribute towards dural reconstruction.

4. PTFE: PTFE use in our series gave a success rate of 66%.We found it good for skull base dural reconstruction where mechanical support is desirable. It was not suited for infected cases. It has been found to reduce scalp vascularity, hence needs to be used with caution in redo cases and irradiated scalps where compromised vascularity may delay wound closure. We also found PTFE unsuitable for irregular dural surfaces as PTFE is non-conforming to uneven surface. It is unsuitable for infected cases.
5. Tissue Patch: Tissue patch can only be used as an adjunct in those cases where there is increased risk of CSF leak. It's known to cause an inflammatory reaction. One side of the material acts as a sealant while the other serves as a barrier. Use must be restricted when using near vital structures within closed space as it has a tendency to swell. In our series we achieved 88% success rate with use of Tissue patch. It was used as an adjunct. We did not use it in cases where CNS infection was present or suspected.
6. G Patch: G patch was used in 5 cases in our series and we achieved a success rate of 80%. Its use is restricted due to its rigid nature and propensity to cause mild to moderate inflammatory reaction. It is non-resorb able and causes encapsulation with dural thickening. The rigidness may help in cases of reconstruction of dural defects where mechanical support is also required to cover and protect underlying structures. Like other synthetic substitutes, it puts the under lying Scalp vascularity in jeopardy.

Discussion

An ideal dural substitute must resemble the natural dura mater in all its properties. It should be immunologically inert, cause minimal or no inflammatory response in the host body, should be non-adherent to the underlying brain, be bio-degradable/ bio-resorb able, durable yet flexible, must aid in achieving watertight closure thereby forming a good protective barrier. From the operating surgeon's perspective, its use should be technically least demanding and must reduce operating time. From the patients point of view it should not cause additional pain or morbidity. Cost factor is a cause for concern in developing countries.

Watertight dural closure following any neurosurgical procedure seems to be an accepted norm worldwide. (Barth M Jonathan B, Neal, BS & Sameer A 2008). Animal studies have shown that use of Polyglactin (Vicryl) in suturing dural margins offers advantage over other suture materials like polyglycolic acid, polyester and silk. Bertil and colleagues through animal experiments showed that absorbable suture caused lesser foreign body reaction. Use of Polyglactin caused no subdural adhesions in reoperations. (Vallfros B, Hansson HA & Sevensson J 1981). Continuous interlocking sutures seem more effective in controlling CSF leak than interrupted sutures. Use of fibrin sealant as an adjunct helps in achieving better results irrespective of the suturing technique adopted (Sengupta S 2013).

Valsalva maneuver may serve as a useful confirmatory test of satisfactory water tight dural closure. However there is no scientific evidence validating this procedure.

Brian P. Walcott and colleagues studied the effects of synthetic graft for dural reconstruction in elective cranial surgeries and concluded that synthetic dural reconstruction material does not predispose to increased incidence of surgical site infection or CSF leak (Brian P, Jonathan B, Neal BS & Sameer A 2004).

Fibrin sealant seems to be a useful adjunct in preventing dural leaks. Pinar Akdemir Ozisik et al., through their rat experiments, have shown than, fibrin glue offers a better safety profile and watertight closure as compared to n-Butyl methacrylate and CO2 laser techniques. (Ozisik PA et al., 2006). Parizek and colleagues carried out detailed evaluation of 2959 connective tissue grafts. This included allogeneic and xenogeneic grafts from fascia lata, pericardium, and dura mater. These cases were followed up for 20 years. They found that irrespective of the dural graft material used, success rate of 96.9% can be achieved (Parízek J et al., 1997). Technology has transcended all aspects of neurosurgery. The search and research for an ideal dural substitute continues. Auto grafts, allografts, xenografts as well as synthetic materials have been used for dural repair so far. (Cobb M A, Badylak S F & Janas W 1999, Sabatino G, Della PGM & Bianchi F 2014, Flanagan KE, Tien LW & Elia R 2014).

In spite of rapid progress in fields of polymer science, immunology and biotechnology, biocompatibility remains a major challenge with biomaterials. (Williams DF 2008). Around 13 million biomaterial-based implants are used in US alone annually. (Wang X 2003). FDA (Food and Drug Administration) has currently approved many collagen-containing products. They find applications in diabetic ulcers management, spinal dural repair (duroplasty), and regeneration of bone graft substitute. (Narotam PK et al., 2004, Thornton JF & Rohrich RJ 2005). Current research and practices prove collagen to be ideally suited for dural reconstructive procedures. Since 1965 Collagen has been used for dural replacement. It offers large surface area for absorption of CSF. This promotes graft adherence to dura by way of surface tension. Collagen attracts fibroblasts by chemo taxis leading to rapid re-colonization. Collagen is relatively stiffer in comparison to other elastic proteins. It has a resilience of 90% making it capable of reversible deformation. Collagen is a natural substrate for promoting cellular activities. These properties make it an ideal material for tissue engineering (Gosline J et al., 2002).

Duragen (Integra Life sciences, Plainsboro, NJ, USA) serves as a suture less dural substitute graft. It is a bovine origin purified type I collagen taken from Achilles tendon. Host fibroblasts invade the collagen matrix thereby promoting fibrin clot formation. Within a period of 6 to 8 weeks, it is fully reabsorbed as the wound heals. This not only repairs the defect but, in due course of time, restores a normal dura. This prevents peri-dural fibrosis. (Heuer G et al., 2003) Pradeep and Colleagues studied the radiological findings in Cranial and spinal cases undergoing dural collagen matrix reconstruction. They concluded that it provides 100% CSF containment with a complication rate, less than 3.2%. Complications included radiologically evident pseudomeningocele and, sub dural or sub galeal collections. The same group also found similar results in posterior fossa surgeries. (Narotam PK et al., 2007). Jorn A Horaczek and colleague's evaluated collagen based dural graft in covering large dural defects in patients undergoing decompressive hemicraniectomies. They found that the operating time was considerably reduced and so were the complication rates and overall duration of treatment. However there was no change in the rehabilitative outcomes (Horaczek JA et al., 2008). This aspect needs further elucidation as, one needs to see, if the cost of using a large collagen based graft translates to reducing the cost of treatment.

Guidelines for Good Clinical Practice

Literary evidence and personal experience tell us that dural substitutes have become an important part of surgeon's armamentarium. The search for an ideal substitute continues because, a single substitute does not have all the desired qualities. As on date, Ultrapure Type I collagen matrix based dural substitutes fulfills all important issues relating to safe, fast and effective dural reconstruction. For complex dural reconstructive procedures, a hybrid/mixed technique seems to be a desirable approach. Experiences learnt from senior surgeons reaffirm the fact that, till date there is no substitute for a sound surgical closure technique which follows standard principles of neurosurgery. A Case to Case basis method of dural reconstruction seems reasonable in present scenario. The purpose of this study is to Keep our fellow neurosurgeons well informed about the options available for dural reconstruction because, Information bring you choices and choices bring you power. Educating oneself of the available options and choices ultimately transform to better outcomes.

Conflicts of Interest

None.

References

Barth M, Tuettenberg J, Thomé C, Weiss C, Vajkoczy P, Schmiedek P. Watertight dural closure: is it necessary? A prospective randomized trial in patients with supratentorial craniotomies. *Neurosurgery*. 2008 Oct; 63(4 Suppl 2):352-8; discussion 358.

Brian P W, Jonathan B Neal, B S, Sameer A, The incidence of complications in elective cranial neurosurgery associated with dural closure material. *J. Neurosurg*. 120:278–284, 2014.

Cobb M A, Badylak S F, Janas W, *Surgical Neurology*, 1999, 51(1), 99.

Flanagan K E, Tien L W, Elia R, *Journal of Biomedical Materials Research Part B Applied Biomaterials*, 2014, 103(3), 494.

Gosline J, Lillie M, Carrington E et al., (2002) Elastic proteins: biological roles and mechanical properties. *Philos. Trans. R. Soc. B. Biol. Sci*. 357(1418):121–132.

Heuer G Stiefel M, Maloney-Wilensky et al., Duragen is effective dural substitute: Clinical experience with 100 cases. *American Association of Neurological Surgeons Annual Meeting*, April 2003.

Horaczek J A, Jan Zeirski, Alexander Graewe, Collagen Matrix in Decompressive Hemicraniectomy. *Neurosurgery* 63[ONS Suppl 1]:ONS178–ONS183, 2008.

Narotam P K, Jose S, Nathoo N et al., (2004) Collagen matrix (Duragen) in dural repair: analysis of a new modified technique. *Spine* 29(24):2861–2867, discussion 2868-2869.

Narotam P K, Kesava Reddy, Derek Fewer et al., *J. Neurosurg.* 2007 Jan;106(1):45-51.

Ozisik P A, Servet T, Inci, Soylemezoglu F, Orhan Hilmi, Tuncalp Ozgen, Comparative dural closure techniques: a safety study in rats. *Surgical Neurology* 65 (2006) 42 – 4.

Parízek J, Měricka P, Husek Z, Suba P, Detailed evaluation of 2959 allogeneic and xenogeneic dense connective tissue grafts (fascia lata, pericardium, and dura mater) used in the course of 20 years for duraplasty in neurosurgery. *Acta Neurochir (Wien)*. 1997;139(9):827-3.

Sabatino G, Della P G M, Bianchi F, *Clinical Neurology & Neurosurgery*, 2014, 116(2), 23.

Sengupta S, Watertight dural closure! An in vitro study to explore the myth. *IJNS* 2013; 02(01): 077-080.

Thornton J F, Rohrich R J (2005) Dermal substitute (Integra) for open nasal wounds. *Plast. Reconstr. Surg.* 116(2):677.

Vallfros B, Hansson H A, Sevensson J, Absorbale or Nonabsorbable Suture Materials for Closure of the dural closure. *Neurosurgery* 9(4):407-413 • October 1981.

Wang X (2013) Overview on biocompatibilities of implantable biomaterials. *Adv. Biomater. Sci. Appl. Biomed.*

Williams D F (2008) On the mechanisms of biocompatibility. *Biomaterials* 29(20):2941–2953.

Chapter 20

Stem Cell Therapy in Spinal Cord Injury

Bhawan Nangarwal, Priyadarshi Dikshit,
Vikas Dwivedi and Ved Prakash Maurya
Department of Neurosurgery, Sanjay Gandhi Postgraduate Institute of Medical Sciences, Lucknow, India

Abstract

Spinal cord injury lead to significant functional impairment because severed nerves in the spinal cord lead to interruption in the upward and downward passage of signals across the level of injury. There are nearly 30 million people across the globe who are handicapped with motor dysfunction following SCI. In addition to motor disability, injury to the cord affects sensory and autonomic functions, which finally carries a substantial financial and psychological burden to the individual and society. With the advent of industrialization, road traffic accidents and falls from height are the leading cause of spinal cord injury leading to disability. The maximum mobility of the cervical spine contributes to most of the deaths occurring after SCI. Following trauma, the management of the spinal cord has been a colossal topic of neurological research for several decades. Pharmacological, cell therapy, various surgical interventions, and rehabilitative measures are the therapeutic strategies being employed for spinal cord injury at a broader spectrum. Advancements in the biology of stem cells have opened an enormous opportunity in applying stem cell therapy for pathologies such as spinal cord injury. This chapter addresses the basics of stem cell therapies, the essential characteristics, and the mode of action of the relevant cells involved in the management of SCI.

In: Neurosurgery Research
Editors: Amit Agrawal, Pradeep Chouksey, Adesh Shrivastava et al.
ISBN: 978-1-68507-837-9

Introduction

Spinal cord injury is a complex pathophysiological series of events initiated by injury to the spinal cord. These mechanical insults may be in the form of abrupt inflicting events or maybe the result of gradual compressive myelopathy due to a variety of pathology arising either from the cord (intramedullary) or from the structures adjacent (intradural extramedullary, extradural intraspinal) to the cord. The overall global incidence of acute spinal cord injury is estimated to be around 10 cases per 100,000 persons, resulting in over 700,000 new cases diagnosed per year worldwide (Kumar R et al.). A most common cause for SCI is road traffic accidents (38%), followed next in order by falls from height (>22%), violence (13.5%), sports-related injuries (9%), and other everyday traumatic events (McKinley et al.). Cancer, inflammation, infections, or spinal disc degeneration can also cause SCI (Sekhon LH et al.). Spinal cord injury is amongst the most severe and debilitating neurological ailments throughout the globe. SCI involves a high disability rate and a profound financial burden in managing these patients. This burden carries a significant impact on the health system of a country reported that in the United States of America, an average expenditure of 1.1 million to 4.6 million $ (USD) is being spent on each patient over their lifetime who sustained spinal cord injury (Ahuja CS et al.).

There has been a continuous effort in the medical and surgical management of these patients, but the results to date are not very encouraging. The advent of stem cell therapy in the management of spinal cord injury carries a great hope to the millions of patients who are suffering from this debilitating ailment. The influence of this therapy can be estimated from the fact that by the end of 2018, a total of 18 clinical trials had been completed while nine trials were ongoing. The stem cells carry an inherent tendency of asymmetrical division, resulting in a daughter cell and a progenitor cell. The stem cells can differentiate and mature into all the possible terminal cell populations. Recent advances have modulated the differentiation pathway, leading to the production of homogeneously differentiated cell populations. In experimental rodent models, the transplantation of multipotent cells has resulted in elongation in the length of axons and synapse formation despite a hostile environment following trauma (Lu P et al.). The clinical application of stem cell transplant in SCI patients had initiated a 2010 Geron Corporation Trial. This trial explores the possibilities and their clinical outcome regarding applying human ESC-derived Oligodendrocyte Progenitor Cells (OPCs) over the site of injury (Frantz S et al.). The cell-based therapies have found broad applicability following this trial, ranging from transplantable cells derivation from neural progenitor and establishment of methodology for optimized transplant delivery.

Pathophysiology of Spinal Cord Injury

Pathophysiology consists of two phases - primary and secondary. Primary injury occurs during the initial mechanical damage of the spinal cord tissue. Primary injury can cause haemorrhage, disruption of the cell membrane, and neurotransmitter imbalance resulting in immediate compromise of neuronal function. The secondary injury results from the inflammatory, ischemic, and apoptotic events after the initial insult to the cord. Even more than 23% of SCI patients who suffered secondary injuries within ten years have been reported by many studies (Krause JS et al.). SCI constitutes three phases: acute, subacute and chronic.

The first phase of the injury initiates an inflammatory response that causes the recruitment of inflammatory substances such as macrophages, T lymphocytes, neutrophils and microglia and release cytokines such as Tumor Necrosis Factor-alpha Interleukin 1-beta, and Interleukin-6 (Nakamura M et al.). The free radical formation also has a role in secondary SCI damage. Inadequate reduction of oxygen molecules at the mitochondrial level causes Reactive Oxygen Species (ROS) release, leading to lipid peroxidation, DNA damage, and cell death. The increase in ROS and Reactive Nitrogen Species further damage neuronal tissue (Ahuja CS et al.). All these cascades of events are collectively known as "secondary injury."

The subacute phase occurs after these events and may last for about one year in humans. This becomes a chronic disease after several days due to further expansion of the lesion. Meanwhile, astrocytes are activated along with neuronal damage from high levels of the extracellular matrix, which inhibit cell migration and repair of nerve growth. Stem cell therapies for SCI aim to decrease secondary injury, accelerate the function of remaining cell populations, and help regenerate neuronal and glial populations (Silva NA et al.). SCs are the cells that can proliferate and regenerate under certain circumstances and can differentiate into other functional cells.

Principle of Stem Cell Therapy in SCI

SC therapy involves multiple aspects, which recent studies have shown. Transplantation of SC can repair damaged nerve cells and tissues, including neurons and glial cells. Meanwhile, SCs also releases neurotrophic factors, changing the injured site's microenvironment and potentiating axonal growth. SCs can also differentiate into glial cells and help myelination and functional recovery (Ceci M et al.).

In recent years, there has been a steep surge in the medical conditions that have advocated SC therapy's role. There exists a broad spectrum of clinical conditions where the benefits of stem cell therapy can be advocated. Other than SCI, stem cell therapy has also been used in clinical conditions such as intracerebral haemorrhage, ischemic stroke, head injury and subarachnoid haemorrhage (Reis C et al.).

Classification of Stem Cells

There are two popular ways for the classification of stem cells.

a. The first classification is based on various developmental stages. SCs may be divided into embryonic stem cells (ESCs), and adult stem cells (ASCs); ASCs found in many adult tissues and divided into mesenchymal stem cells (MSCs), hematopoietic stem cells (HSCs), neural stem cells (NSCs) and induced pluripotent stem cells (iPSCs).
b. The second classification is based on differentiation potential and divided into totipotent stem cells (TSCs), pluripotent stem cells (PSCs), and unipotent stem cells (USCs) (Weissman IL et al.).

Stem Cells in SCI

The common SCs used to treat spinal cord injury are MSCs, NSCs, ESCs and iPSCs (Reis C et al., Weissman IL et al.).

Bone Marrow Mesenchymal Stem Cells

These are partially differentiated progenitor cells found in the adult bone marrow and have the potential for haematopoiesis and bone regeneration. When these cells are introduced at the site of injury, they cause a decrease in inflammatory reactions, astroglial scarring, and blood-spinal cord barrier (BSCB) disruption; modulated astrogliosis; decrease in pain; and help in the improvement of functional recovery of limb movement, which can be mediated by the matrix metalloproteinase (MMP) 2/STAT3 pathway (Charbord P et al.). The intradural injection of BM-MSC-based cells has been studied in cervical SCI patients' treatment. After six months of transplantation, there was an improvement in upper extremities function, and MRI images were seen in six out of ten candidates (Han D et al.).

Neural Stem Cells and Neural Progenitor Cells

These are types of pluripotent cells isolated from the subventricular region of the ventricles and hippocampus and the ependymal lining of the central canal of the spinal cord. These cells can differentiate into specific neuronal or glial cells, which helps in myelination and provide nutritional support, thus being used as cell transplantation therapy in spinal cord injury (Sankavaram SR et al.). NPCs can differentiate into oligodendrocytes, promotes myelination and enhance hindlimb function. NPCs inhibit the secretion of macrophages and T cells, and neuroprotective cytokines help in the modulation of inflammatory response. In a study done in 2018, they observed that perilesional intramedullary injections of NSCs were found safe, but the dose should be further investigated. NPCs have shown a substantial potential in spinal cord injury treatment, but functional recovery remains the main limiting factor (Levi AD et al.).

Embryonic Stem Cells

These cells are multipotent stem cells that can differentiate into neurons and glial cells. Embryonic Stem Cells (ESCs) are first fused with cell adhesion molecule L1, which helps in the survival of neurons and sprouting. Human embryonic stem cell-derived oligodendrocytes or oligodendrocyte progenitor cells and motor neuron progenitors bear the capability of astrogliosis and improve motor recovery (Cloutier F et al.). ESC-derived neural cells provide a network for axons to pass via chondroitin sulphate proteoglycan (CSPG), a significant barrier for regeneration. In 2014, a clinical study was done with human ESC-derived oligodendrocyte progenitor cell transplantation, demonstrating their safety in spinal cord injury patients (Shroff G et al.).

Induced Pluripotent Stem Cells

Because of the teratogenic potential of ESCs, the next viable option was to develop induced pluripotent stem cells, which have the same pluripotent capacity with the advantage of reduced side effects. These cells are obtained from somatic cells like autologous skin, thus avoiding ethical concerns. At the same time, it allows autologous cell transplantation and prevents rejection (Salewski RP et al.). IPSCs-derived neural stem/progenitor cells (iPSC-NS/PCs) prevent demyelination and accelerate the formation of synapse and secretion of neurotrophic factor that helps improve functional recovery in SCI (Cloutier F et al.). A study was done to compare iPSC-NPs and BM-MSCs and NPS from spinal fetal cell line (SPC-01), which demonstrated better effect due to their firm graft survival, inhibition of glial scar and axonal sprouting (Ruzicka J et al.).

Novel Biological Therapies for Spinal Cord Injury

There are various strategies developed to enhance Stem cell therapy, including SC secretory product-based therapy, scaffold-based and immunotherapy, which can be used simultaneously with MSC therapy. They can improve cell survival, migration, and proliferation (Stastna M et al.).

Stem Cell Secretome Therapy

The SCs purely do not rely on its differentiation capacity and regeneration but also needs paracrine and autocrine mechanisms by its secretome activity. Stem cells derived-secretome are the various factors secreted in extracellular space, including soluble proteins, nucleic acids, lipids, cytokines, neurotrophins, growth factors, and extracellular vesicles (EV) (Huang JH et al.). There is a gradual shift to adopt secretome therapy because of their low tumorigenicity, easy production, easily modifiable, and storage without toxic substances such as dimethyl sulfoxide (DMSO) (Ha D et al.). Several studies have shown their immunomodulatory neurotrophic/neuroprotective and angiogenetic effects in the treatment of SCI. There are various secretome components out of which EVs of microvesicles and exosomes are most effective and can be administered as intravenous or intranasally in animals and from there can reach injured neurons (Sarko DK et al.).

EVs also promote angiogenesis, inhibit inflammation, decrease the lesion size, prevent apoptosis, and support neuronal cell survival and regeneration. In a study done by Lu et al. recently, it was found that MSC-EV administration decreased the pericytes and helped improve the integrity of the BSCB via down-regulation of NF-κB p65 signalling (Lu Y et al.). EVs can also effectively nerve injury-induced pain, demonstrated in rat models. A previous study demonstrated that miR-133b has a vital role in neuron differentiation and neurite growth. So, MSCs were engineered to secrete miR-133brich EVs for the treatment of SCI and found to accelerate the recovery of hindlimb motor function, decrease in lesion size, protection of neurons, and axon regeneration (Ren ZW et al.). There are several hindrances in the clinically applying secretome/EVs, including biodistribution of secretome/EVs and unestablished regulatory requirements for the manufacturing and application of secretome/EVs (Liu S et al.) (Table 1).

Table 1. Summary of Stem Cells used in Spinal Cord Injury

Cell type	Action
BM-MSCs	Secrete neurotrophic factors Promote axonal regeneration Decrease astroglial scarring density Decrease inflammatory reactions Decrease BSCB leakage Reduce neuropathic pain Improve bladder compliance
NSCs and NPCs	Increase neuroprotective cytokines Improve cell proliferation Promote myelination Modulate the inflammatory response
ESCs	Promote astrogliosis Sustain nodal architecture Decrease neuropathic pain
iPSCs	Improve neurotrophic factor secretion Promote axonal sprouting Inhibit demyelination Promote synapse formation Inhibit glial scar Decrease lesion size Improve respiratory function
EVs derived from stem cells	Regulate axon regeneration Protect cells from apoptosis Inhibit inflammation Decrease injury size Protect the integrity of the BSCB

Immunotherapy

After trauma, there is a secretion of multiple growth-suppressive molecules that impairs healing and regeneration. Despite this, several types of research have been carried out to use Immunotherapy in acute spinal cord injury, which can modulate molecular signalling pathways and modify the injury site to favour regeneration (Bregman BS et al.). Rat models have demonstrated that antibodies to myelin-associated inhibitors can improve motor function (Lee JK et al.). Similarly, B-cell depleting antibodies have also been found to decrease inflammation, promote cell survival and reduce hindlimb dysfunction. Hence, Immunotherapy and MSC treatment are more effective in treating SCI due to a simultaneous decrease in inflammation and spinal cord regeneration (Liebscher T et al.). However, their safety must be demonstrated before humans use them, as these antibodies should not affect normal healthy myelin.

Scaffolds

Scaffolds and injectable hydrogels are used as a matrix to enhance cell engraftment and survival. They can be made up of natural, synthetic, or combined materials. In previous studies, it has been demonstrated that MSCs incorporated in fibrin scaffold showed viability up to 10 weeks. With time, new scaffolds have been developed that do not retain cells at the site of lesion, and they help in the survival of cells and, at the same time, modulation of the immune system and prevent fibrosis (Liu S et al.).

Yousefifard et al. demonstrated in their systematic review and meta-analysis that combined use of MSCs and scaffolds is more effective in SCI than MSCs and scaffolds alone (Yousefifard M et al.). A phase I clinical trial on 40 patients who had acute complete spinal cord injury was done and found that the patients who received collagen scaffold along with UC MSC had improvement in American Spinal Injury Association (ASIA) grade, bowel and bladder function, and MEP and the control group without UC-MSCs-loaded scaffold they showed no improvement even after 12 months (Mukhamedshina YO et al.). Even in MRI and diffusion tensor imaging, these patients showed nerve regeneration and electrophysiological activity was also recovered. A similar study done by Zhao et al. showed that treatment with NeuroRegen, a collagen scaffold used with umbilical cord blood-derived MSCs in eight patients with complete chronic SCI, successfully improved the sensation level and increased the MEP-responsive area without even change in ASIA grade (Zhao Y et al.). These studies showed that scaffolds facilitate regeneration of the spinal cord. However, several parameters, including biodegradation rate, biocompatibility, material safety and thickness of the matrix, need to be studied further before clinical translation.

Challenges and Conclusion

SCs have neuro-regenerative and neuroprotective effects in the treatment of SCI. Cell-based therapies act by mechanisms such as immunomodulation, cell replacement nutrition, and scaffold support and provide functional recovery. However, stem cell therapies have safety concerns, such as immunotoxicity, immunogenicity, and tumorigenicity, shown in preclinical studies (Sabino L et al.). Another concern is their short cell survival and low integration to ensure the genetic stability, generation consistency and storage safety of these stem cells. The clinical application requires first to ensure the quality and reciprocality of SC transplantation as even small changes in cell origin and growth conditions can significantly impact the outcomes (Zholudeva LV et al.). In clinical trials, it has been found that small sample size, limited supervision, and poor quality were the main limiting factors in the development of stem cell therapy (Nori S et al.). However, multiple ongoing trials will provide more information in the clinical application of stem cell therapy in SCI. Besides several experimental/animal-based trials, the clinical trials focussing on the SCI are still limited. Despite the encouraging results in the initial studies, the scope for establishing the most effective treatment strategy, which includes the type of cell therapy, route and dose, and the frequency of administration, is still there. To date, most of the clinical trials are restricted to a single centre and are investigator-oriented studies. Besides these challenges, there is always a significant patient safety issue, bringing ethical issues into the picture. These include the use of ESCs, high financial burden over the participant and the centre involved and lack of volunteers to participate in novel therapy in the absence of encouraging results or data. Despite all the developments in cell-based therapy for SCI management, there is a significant deficit of phase III trials that explore the therapeutic efficacy of stem cell transplantation. There should be a standardized regulatory system between international agencies such as the United States Food and Drug Administration and the European Medicines Agency (Yamazaki K et al., Jin MC et al.).

References

Ahuja CS, Nori S, Tetreault L, Wilson J, Kwon B, Harrop J et al., 2017. Traumatic spinal cord injury-repair and regeneration. *Neurosurgery.* Vol. 80, pg. S9-S22.

Bregman BS, Kunkel-Bagden E, Schnell L, Dai HN, Gao D, Schwab ME, 1995. Recovery from spinal cord injury mediated by antibodies to neurite growth inhibitors. *Nature.* Vol. 378(6556), pg. 498-501.

Ceci M, Mariano V, Romano N, 2018. Zebrafish as a translational regeneration model to study the activation of neural stem cells and role of their environment. *Rev. Neurosci.* Vol. 30, pg. 45-66.

Charbord P., 2010. Bone marrow mesenchymal stem cells: historical overview and concepts. *Hum. Gene. Ther.* Vol. 21(9), pg. 1045-56.

Cloutier F, Siegenthaler MM, Nistor G, Keirstead HS, 2006. Transplantation of human embryonic stem cell-derived oligodendrocyte progenitors into rat spinal cord injuries does not cause harm. *Regen. Med.* Vol. 1(4), pg. 469-79.

Frantz S: Embryonic stem cell pioneer Geron exits field, cuts losses, 2012. *Nat. Biotechnol.* Vol. 30, pg. 12-13.

Ha D, Yang N, Nadithe V, 2016. Exosomes as therapeutic drug carriers and delivery vehicles across biological membranes: current perspectives and future challenges. *Acta Pharm. Sinica B.* Vol. 6(4), pg. 287-96.

Han D, Wu C, Xiong Q, Zhou L, Tian Y, 2015. Anti-inflammatory mechanism of bone marrow mesenchymal stem cell transplantation in rat model of spinal cord injury. *Cell Biochem. Biophys.* Vol. 71(3), pg. 1341-7.

Huang JH, Yin XM, Xu Y, Xu CC, Lin X, Ye FB et al., 2017. Systemic administration of exosomes released from mesenchymal stromal cells attenuates apoptosis, inflammation, and promotes angiogenesis after spinal cord injury in rats. *J. Neurotrauma.* Vol. 34(24), pg. 3388-96.

Jin MC, Medress ZA, Azad TD, Doulames VM, Veeravagu A, 2019. Stem cell therapies for acute spinal cord injury in humans: a review. *Neurosurg. Focus.* Vol. 46(3), pg. E10. https://thejns.org/doi/abs/10.3171/2018.12.FOCUS18602.

Krause JS, 2010. "Risk for subsequent injuries after spinal cord injury: a 10-year longitudinal analysis," *Archives of Physical Medicine and Rehabilitation.* Vol. 91(11), pg. 1741-6.

Kumar R, Lim J, Mekary RA, Rattani A, Dewan MC, Sharif SY et al., 2018. Traumatic spinal injury: global epidemiology and worldwide volume. *World Neurosurg.* Vol. 113, pg. 345-363.

Lee JK, Zheng B, 2012. Role of myelin-associated inhibitors in axonal repair after spinal cord injury. *Exp Neurol.* Vol. 235(1), pg. 33-42.

Levi AD, Okonkwo DO, Park P, Jenkins AL 3rd, Kurpad SN, Parr AM et al., 2018. Emerging safety of intramedullary transplantation of human neural stem cells in chronic cervical and thoracic spinal cord injury. *Neurosurgery.* Vol. 82(4), pg. 562-75.

Liebscher T, Schnell L, Schnell D, Scholl J, Schneider R, Gullo M et al., 2005. Nogo-A antibody improves regeneration and locomotion of spinal cord-injured rats. *Ann. Neurol.* Vol. 58(5), pg. 706-19.

Liu S, Jia Y, Yuan M, Guo W, Huang J, Zhao B et al., 2017. Repair of osteochondral defects using human umbilical cord Wharton's jelly-derived mesenchymal stem cells in a rabbit model. *Biomed. Res. Int.* 2017:8760383.

Liu S, Xie YY, Wang B., 2019. Role and prospects of regenerative biomaterials in the repair of spinal cord injury. *Neural Regen. Res.* Vol. 14(8), pg. 1352-63.

Lu P, Wang Y, Graham L, McHale K, Gao M, Wu D et al., 2012. Long-distance growth and connectivity of neural stem cells after severe spinal cord injury. *Cell.* Vol. 150, pg. 1264-73.

Lu Y, Zhou Y, Zhang R, Wen L, Wu K, Li Y et al., 2019. Bone mesenchymal stem cell-derived extracellular vesicles promote recovery following spinal cord injury via improvement of the integrity of the blood-spinal cord barrier. *Front. Neurosci.* Vol. 13, pg. 209.

McKinley, WO, Seel RT, Hardman JT, 1999. Nontraumatic spinal cord injury: Incidence, epidemiology, and functional outcome. *Arch. Phys. Med. Rehab.* Vol. 80, pg. 619-23.

Mukhamedshina YO, Zakirova EY, Galieva LR, Kostennikov AA, Akhmetzyanova ER, Rizvanov AA, 2017. Distribution and survival of transplanted adipose derived mesenchymal stem cells in the spinal cord injury. *Bio Nanoscience.* Vol. 7(4), pg. 608-12.

Nakamura M, Houghtling RA, MacArthur L, Bayer BM, Bregman BS, 2003. Differences in cytokine gene expression profile between acute and secondary injury in adult rat spinal cord. *Exp. Neurol.* Vol. 184. pg. 313-25.

Nori S, Okada Y, Nishimura S, Sasaki T, Itakura G, Kobayashi Y et al., 2015. Long-term safety issues of iPSC-based cell therapy in a spinal cord injury model: oncogenic transformation with epithelial-mesenchymal transition. *Stem Cell Reports.* Vol. 4(3), pg. 360-73.

Reis C, Wilkinson M, Reis H, 2017. A look into stem cell therapy: exploring the options for treatment of ischemic stroke. *Stem Cells International.* Article ID 3267352:14.

Ren ZW, Zhou JG, Xiong ZK, Zhu FZ, Guo XD, 2019. Effect of exosomes derived from MiR-133b-modified ADSCs on the recovery of neurological function after SCI. *Eur. Rev. Med. Pharmacol. Sci.* Vol. 23(1), pg. 52-60.

Ruzicka J, Machova-Urdzikova L, Gillick J, Amemori T, Romanyuk N, Karova K, et al., 2017. A comparative study of three different types of stem cells for treatment of rat spinal cord injury. *Cell Transplant.* Vol. 26(4), pg. 585-603.

Sabino L, Maria CA, Luca L, Valerio V, Edda F, Giacomo R, et al., 2018. Engraftment, neuroglial trans differentiation and behavioral recovery after complete spinal cord transection in rats. *Surg. Neurol. Int.* Vol. 9, pg. 19.

Salewski RP, Buttigieg J, Mitchell RA, van der Kooy D, Nagy A, Fehlings MG, 2013. The generation of definitive neural stem cells from PiggyBac transposon-induced pluripotent stem cells can be enhanced by induction of the NOTCH signaling pathway. *Stem Cells Dev.* Vol. 22(3), pg. 383-96.

Sankavaram SR, Hakim R, Covacu R, Frostell A, Neumann S, Svensson M, et al., 2019. Adult neural progenitor cells transplanted into spinal cord injury differentiate into oligodendrocytes, enhance myelination, and contribute to recovery. *Stem Cell Reports.* Vol. 12(5), pg. 950-66.

Sarko DK, McKinney CE, 2017. Exosomes: origins and therapeutic potential for neurodegenerative disease. *Front. Neurosci.* Vol. 11, pg. 82.

Sekhon LH, Fehlings MG, 2001. Epidemiology, demographics, and pathophysiology of acute spinal cord injury. *Spine (Phila Pa 1976).* Vol. 26(24), pg. 2-12.

Shroff G, Dhanda Titus J, Shroff R, 2017. A review of the emerging potential therapy for neurological disorders: human embryonic stem cell therapy. *Am. J. Stem Cells.* Vol. 6(1), pg. 1-12.

Silva NA, Sousa N, Reis RL, Salgado AJ, 2014. From basics to clinical: A comprehensive review on spinal cord injury. *Progress Neurobiol.* Vol. 114, pg. 25-57.

Stastna M, Van Eyk JE, 2012. Investigating the secretome: lessons about the cells that comprise the heart. *Circ. Cardiovasc. Genet.* Vol. 5(1), pg. 08-18.

Weissman IL, Anderson DJ, Gage F, 2001. Stem and progenitor cells: origins, phenotypes, lineage commitments, and trans differentiations. *Annual Review of Cell and Developmental Biology.* Vol. 17(1), pg. 387-403.

Yamazaki K, Kawabori M, Seki T, Houkin K, 2020. Clinical Trials of Stem Cell Treatment for Spinal Cord Injury. *Int. J. Mol. Sci.* 2021:3994. doi:10.3390/ijms21113994.

Yousefifard M, Maleki SN, Askarian-Amiri S, Vaccaro AR, Chapman JR, Fehlings MG, et al., 2019. A combination of mesenchymal stem cells and scaffolds promotes motor functional recovery in spinal cord injury: a systematic review and meta-analysis. *J. Neurosurg. Spine.* Vol. 32(2), pg. 269-84.

Zhao Y, Tang F, Xiao Z, Han G, Wang N, Yin N et al., 2017. Clinical study of NeuroRegen scaffold combined with human mesenchymal stem cells for the repair of chronic complete spinal cord injury. *Cell Transplant.* Vol. 26(5), pg. 891-900.

Zholudeva LV, Lane MA, 2019. Transplanting cells for spinal cord repair: who, what, when, where and why? *Cell Transplant.* Vol. 28(4), pg. 388-99.

Chapter 21

Nanotechnology in Neurosurgery: A Prospective Shift Towards Extremely Minimally Invasive Surgery

Brig (Dr) S. Shashivadhanan[1]
and Shivangi Shashivadhanan[2]
[1]Professor Surgery and Neurosurgeon, Military Hospital Bathinda, India
[2]Biotechology RV College of Engineering Bangalore, India

Abstract

Introduction

Nanotechnology is that branch of engineering which deals with materials whose smallest functional unit is at least one billionth of a meter, in one dimension. The central nervous system poses challenges to newer therapeutic strategies incorporating nanotechnology. Each region of brain has a unique cytoarchitecture and molecular environment. There are multiple processing centers and the formidable "blood brain barrier," which needs due consideration. Studies done so far have demonstrated that, incorporation of nanotechnology into neurosurgical practice has the potential to transform practice of neurosurgery once for all.

Aim

Through this paper, authors have attempted to focus on research work being carried out in field of nanotechnology that have a potential to enhance the practice of neurosurgery. Promising research is going on in

In: Neurosurgery Research
Editors: Amit Agrawal, Pradeep Chouksey, Adesh Shrivastava et al.
ISBN: 978-1-68507-837-9

field of nano electromechanical systems to mimic the brain circuitry, neural regeneration using nano scaffolds, attempting neural continuity using suture less anastomosis, molecular imaging for functional neuro imaging, nano technology driven targeted drug delivery, and nano robots.

Observation

Nanotechniques are making contribution to neurosurgery in the following main fields (1) nanomanipulation or nano neurosurgery, (2) nano neuro imaging, (3) non-surgical neural nanorepair, and (4) nano neuromodulation, (5) nanobiotechnology (nanorobots).

Nanomanipulation or Nanoneurosurgery includes techniques for performing neurosurgery at cellular level. This is focused at level of neuron, neural processes or at intra cellular level. A nanoknife has been developed having a diameter of 40 nanometer for performing axonal surgery. Using these techniques, controlled axonal transection can be performed. Further, the cut ends can be aligned into position using dielectrophoresis. Fusion between the two cut ends can be effected by techniques which include electrofusion, chemical like polyethylene glycol or laser-induced cell fusion. Nanodevices provide a new dimension to neurosurgeon enabling extreme precision and control with nerves.

Cavalcanti et al. are working on an intravascular nanorobot. They work on the principle that aneurysms have increased levels of nitric oxide Synthetase. The nanorobots can detect aneurysm formation based on increase in levels of nitric oxide synthase protein. These nanorobots can also detect dynamic vascular changes and communicate the same to health care providers. This has the potential for reducing cost of screening through conventional imaging and frequent follow ups. Expanding the scope of this platform will find wider application in detection of tumor or ischemic changes.

Nano imaging aids viewing of the nervous system at the cellular or molecular level thereby throwing light on functionality. Quantum dots provide qualitative and quantitative data which allows visualizing neural physiology at molecular level.

Nano Surgical repair makes use of non-organic materials which help in axonal regeneration and halt neuronal degeneration and prevent damage. This translates to extended neuronal life span.

Neural Nano modulation refers to the monitoring and alteration of neuronal function by intervening on electrical and electrochemical function. This may work by stimulation or inhibition mechanisms.

Nano biotechnology Nanotechnology incorporated with robotics, gives rise to miniaturized robots called nanobots. They are capable of performing surgical interventions within the vascular system and other cavities. Empowered by programming functions, these surgical nano robots can function autonomously. They can detect, diagnose and remove disease process at cellular level. This revolutionary concept of having an onsite surgeon, changes the concept of neurosurgery, offering it a whole new dimension. They can be used to carry out neuro manipulation using an on board computer. Nano robots can perform extremely precise and refined intracellular surgery. This precision in neuro manipulation can never be achieved by the best trained human hand.

Conclusion

Nanotechnology is not an independent emerging scientific discipline. Rather it's an intelligent integration of traditional science with the latest that science and engineering has to offer. In order to derive tangible benefits, three things must occur concurrently for nanotechnology applications. This includes, 1. advances in chemistry and materials science leading to synthesis of sophisticated nano neuro materials 2. advancement in the neuro pathophysiology and molecular biology. 3. Design and integration of engineering and biology to produce specific Nano engineered applications for the nervous system. It is a convergence of biology with nano engineering and electronics.

Keywords: nano neurosurgery, nano imaging, nanoneuromodulation, nano biotechnology nano robots

Introduction

Richard Feynman is considered as the "Father of Nanotechnology." The term nanotechnology was first coined by Norio Taniguchi in 1974. He concluded that materials can be manipulated very precisely at dimensions of nanometer. In terms of SI unit, Nano represents one-billionth of a unit meter (1.0 × 10-9). "Nanotechnology is the science of design, synthesis, characterization and application of materials and extremely small devices." Nano materials, by virtue of their size, acquire unique physical and chemical properties. They possess certain surface characteristics which prove advantageous over their original size. (Mariappan N 2014).

Neurosurgery began as a specialty where the surgeon was primarily focused on excision of tumors, removal of ruptured discs or fixing unstable spines. Subsequently, came the neuroendoscope, interventional neuroradiology and later stereotactic surgery. Neurosurgeon, who so far have relied on tactile and visual feedback are being pushed by newer technologies which rely less on primitive feedback mechanisms.

The association of nanotechnology with neurosurgery has grown in the recent past. It holds promise for a wide range of neurological conditions. These include newer treatment options for Glioblastoma Multiforme, diagnosis of Alzheimer's disease, newer neuro protective strategies against oxidative stress, Nano nerve repair, Nano neuro imaging using nanoparticles and quantum dots, use of Nanofibres and nanowires for nano neuromodulation with surgical nanobots. (Khawaja AM 2011).

The Nano neurosurgeon will have to rely on optical spectroscopy and electron microscopy. There is a paradigm shift from macro excision and implantation, to surgery at axonal level with manipulation and functional neuromodulation. Research is directed towards restoring structural and functional normalcy of diseased nervous system. Palliative care will gradually become obsolete from dictionary. More neurological conditions like, neurodegenerative diseases, neuropsychiatric conditions and mood disorder will come into the realm of neurosurgery. There is a speculation that neurosurgery which is considered an art might transform into a technology-intensive specialty where outcomes can be made more precise, predicable and less labor intensive. (Russell J 2009).

Although the integration of nanotechnologies with nervous system, in vivo, seems slow and challenging, it is poised to disrupt future of applied Neurosciences of which neurosurgery is an integral part.

Nano Manipulation and Nano Neurosurgery

We have already gathered principal proof of core technologies which can accomplish axonal repair. This methodology utilizes combination of micro technology, electro kinetic axon manipulation, and biological principles of cell fusion. Nano surgery is an integrated multidisciplinary approach which will change the concept of neurosurgery. It focuses on surgical intervention at axonal level and concurrently attempts to restore functionality. (David W 2005)

Following neuronal injury there is up regulation of inhibitory proteoglycans with concurrent down regulation of growth factors. Current research is directed towards up regulation of growth factors and down regulation of inhibitory factors. It aims to complete the repair process before degeneration and apoptosis takes place. The strategy for regeneration includes promoting regeneration at site of injury, providing tension mediated axonal bridging so as to establish normal neural circuitry which results in restoration of function. Work has been done more on peripheral nerve injury. Focus is now shifting to central nervous system.

Proposed Mechanism

Stretavan et al., have done experimental work on this high technology surgery and come out with useful insights. Their work suggests, that what we so far thought was fiction, is soon going to become reality.

The single cell axonal repair is done in three principal steps. In the first stage damaged regions of axons are excised so as to have healthy ends. Next, donor axon is placed to bridge the gap. This requires precise alignment. The final stage consists of fusion of the two segments. The final step would be to confirm functionality of the repaired axon.

Stage 1

Small Nano scale needles/ cutting devices have been developed which can precisely cut the axon in a repeatable manner. They have a radius of curvature of 20 nm. (Locish H et al. 2004. Kandel E et al. 2000). Silicon nitride knife with an ultra-sharp knife edge is used. The mechanical compliance of the suspension can be modulated to give the necessary force for cutting a single axon. It can also harvest required cells from a histological specimen. The Nano cutting knife uses the Micro Electro Mechanical System (MEMS) (Petersen KE et al., 2000). This eliminates the need for manual manipulation. The process can be initiated following which on board sensing devices takeover the function in a semiautonomous manner.

Stage 2

Next step consists of aligning the cut ends in a precise manner. This can be achieved through contact or non-contact methods. The challenge lies in manipulation without altering function. Non-contact alignment is achieved by

Di electrophoresis (DEP) which utilizes the principle of creating a net charge on axonal elements leading to movement in one direction within a stationary electrical field. (Gascoyne P 1997, Wang X 2004).

Computer-controlled activation triggers the optimal stimulus under human command. It does not affect the axonal physiology. (Heida T et al. 2001, Heida T et al., 2002)

Stage 3

Fusion of cut ends can be achieved by polyethylene glycol, laser-induced fusion, or electro fusion (Hui SW et al., 1993). Electro fusion causes breakdown of cell membranes with pore formation which finally seals. (Bates G, 1987) Pairing of DEP with electro fusion simplifies the two stages of axonal surgery wherein the same electrodes can be used to align and fuse axons operating in MEMS. Checking functionality of fusion can be ascertained by incorporating green fluorescent protein into axoinc cytoplasm. Flow of fluorescent material across the fused ends confirms axonal continuity. (Okabe M et al. 1997).

Challenges

Setting up a micro device surgical chamber incorporating all the core technologies, so as to make it of practical use in repair of CNS, is the current challenge. An axon surgery platform needs to carry out repair in a coordinated and sequential manner. Control of microfluidic environment requires putting in, growth factors. All this also requires optical monitoring. (Rafuse VF, 1996. Schucht P 2002, You SW 2003).

Repair needs to be undertaken before Wallerian degeneration can set in. Repair of multiple axons needs to be carried out in a time bound manner. A cell replacement strategy is under research which can effect re myelination of repaired axons. After axon repair, the seeded cells and growth factors require a three dimensional bio scaffold which supports all stages of regeneration. It must assist revascularization, in addition to providing mechanical support. And finally, to offer tangible benefits, each stage of surgical repair and regeneration must follow a favorable sequence. This will require constant monitoring and intervention. (Liu CY et al., 2003, Huang JH et al. 2004, Huang JH et al. 2004).

Nano Neuro Imaging

Nanotechnology is an exciting field that will greatly impact neurosciences in diagnostics and therapeutics. It will herald personalized and targeted medicine. It impact will be seen in fields of stem cell therapy, immunotherapy, immunoimaging, pre- and intraoperative brain tumor characterization, and targeted payload delivery to the CNS.

Gold Nanocages are used in Photoacoustic tomography. Photoacoustic tomography imaging is a hybrid technique that combines optical and sonographic imaging modalities and detects absorbed photons sonographically. It provides accurate 3Dimensional imaging of tumors. (Sun Y et al, 2002, Li W 2011) Evaluation and Validation of Antiangiogenic Therapy can be accomplished using super paramagnetic iron oxide (SPIO) nanoparticle (Lu M et al., 2011). These agents remained confined to the vascular compartment for hours after administration and will not extravasate in the presence of a compromised blood-brain barrier. This can help to distinguish pseudo progression from true tumor progression in patients suffering from Glioblastoma Multiforme. (Peer DK et al., 2001, Gerstner ER et al., 2010).

Detection of Nitric Oxide (NO): NOs have a number of physiologic functions related to neurotransmission and neovascularization. It may contribute to neurotoxicity associated with tissue injury, apoptosis, and ischemia. (Calabrese V et al., 2007, Garthwaite J &, Boulton CL 1995).

Multidimensional in vivo NO monitoring has been achieved by using amperometric trimethylsilane conjugated platinum nanodisks.

Nanotechnology is also being used in Stem Cell Tracking with MR Imaging, Noninvasive Detection of Neural Progenitor Cells in Living Brains by MR Imaging, enhanced delivery of Blood-Brain Barrier Impermeable Probes, offers definite advantage over conventional Imaging. Role of Nano bodies are being studied in cancer therapy. Quantum Dots are finding application in biological imaging. The future neuroradiologist is poised to make forays into diagnosing, monitoring and treating a host of pathologies which have so far been falling into realm of Neurosurgeon or Neurophysician. (Suffredini G. East JE and Levy LM 2014)

Nano Robots and Nano Biotechnology

Endoscopes & Micro devices have enhanced many neurosurgical procedures in recent years. Advances in bio molecular science and manufacturing techniques, is helping in miniaturization of devices from microelectronics to Nano electronics. Development of Nano robots with embedded Nano biosensors and actuators is opening up vistas for early detection of brain aneurysms.

Cavalcanti and team developed a Nano robot prototype which can detect cerebral aneurysm. It has embedded Nano biosensors for detection of Nitric Oxide Synthetase overexpression with telemetric control and data transmission capability. This Nano machine platform design is based on clinical data, proteomic signals, cell morphology and numerical analysis. The Nano robots can recognize the chemical gradient in blood stream. This can find application in wide varieties of vascular pathologies in addition to aneurysm detection. (Cavalcanti, Shirinzadeh, Fukuda, and Ikeda 2021).

Nano robots are bound to change practice of modern medicine. It will herald shift from a treatment model to a prevention model making extensive use of in-body sensors. They will check for abnormalities, kill pathogens, repair and correct structural and functional abnormalities even before the patient manifests with symptoms. (Kroeker K 2009).

Nanoneuromodulation

The conventional electroencephalogram (EEG) and the electrocorticogram (ECoG) allow continuous electrical monitoring on a macro scale, Nano electrodes offer us electrode size, which is roughly that of the molecules, to be detected. This improves the order of magnitude and helps monitoring at neuronal level. The Carbon nanotubes (CNTs) can be used for neuron-level electrical and chemical monitoring and modulation. In addition they can be 'grown' and modified to support growth of neural network. The CNT array can offer a 10-fold improvement in dopamine detection level and response time over carbon fiber microelectrodes, which is the current gold standard. Nano neuromodulation is set to make Procedures of deep brain stimulation more precise and effective (Russell J & Andrews 2009).

Nano Scaffolds

Nano fiber scaffolds for tissue engineering is a rapidly growing field. These structures provide support to neural tissue in addition to promoting growth and differentiation. Self-assembling peptide nanofiber scaffolds (SAPNS), are composed of positively and negatively charged L-amino acids which self-assemble into interwoven nanofibres. When substituted with desired molecules they enhance neural stem cell survival in 3-D cultures, enhance osteoblast proliferation, differentiation, and 3-D migration. They possess hemostatic properties. They metabolize slowly without causing toxicity to native tissue. These properties make them ideal, for use in neurotrauma, especially spinal cord injury. (Vasita R and D.S. Katti 2006, Gelain F, Lomander A, Vescove AL, and Zhang C 2007).

Conclusion

As nanotechnology forays into field of neurosurgery, demarcation between science and fiction is getting progressively blurred. The neurosurgeons of future need to be tech savvy. They have to understand and accept newer technologies which are changing the very philosophy of neurosurgical practice. There is a transformation from macro excision to Nano excision, mechanical to functional repair, clinical diagnosis to molecular diagnosis by in vivo Nano robots. Medicine seems to be transforming from prevention, to cure, to interventional prevention at cellular level. This field of transformational medicine will involve coming together of multiple stake holders from diverse fields. The focus is to make humanity disease free and probably immortal in near future.

References

Bates G, Saunders J, Sowers A: *Electrofusion: Principles and applications*, in Sowers A (ed): *Cell Fusion.* New York, Plenum Press, 1987, pp 376–395.

Cavalcanti, Shirinzadeh, Fukuda, and Ikeda / *Nano robot for Brain Aneurysm.* Downloaded from ijr.sagepub.com at University of Otago Library on 28 May 2021).

Calabrese V, Mancuso C, Calvani M, et al. Nitric oxide in the central nervous system: neuroprotection versus neurotoxicity. *Nat. Rev. Neurosci.* 2007;8:766–75.

David W. Stretavan, Wesley Chang, Elizabeth Hawkes, Christopher Keller et al. Microscale surgery on single axons. *Neurosurgery* 57:635-646, 2005.

Garthwaite J, Boulton C L. Nitric oxide signaling in the central nervous system. *Annu. Rev. Physiol.* 1995; 57:683–706.

Gascoyne P, Pethig R, Satayavivad J, Becker F F, Ruchirawat M: Dielectrophoretic detection of changes in erythrocyte membranes following malarial infection. *Biochim. Biophys. Acta* 1323:240–252, 1997).

Gelain F, Lomander A, Vescove A L, and Zhang C, Systematic studies of a self-assembling peptide nanofiber scaffold with other scaffolds. *J. Nanosci. Nanotechnol.* 7, 424 (2007).

Gerstner E R, Batchelor T T. Antiangiogenic therapy for Glioblastoma. *Cancer J.* 2012; 18:45–50.

Heida T, Rutten W L, Marani E: Dielectrophoretic trapping of dissociated fetal cortical rat neurons. *IEEE Trans Biomed. Eng.* 48:921–930, 2001.

Heida T, Rutten W L, Marani E: Experimental investigation on neural cell survival after dielectrophoretic trapping. *Arch. Physiol. Biochem.* 110:373–382, 2002.

Huang J H, Groff R F, Zhang J, Pfister B J, Zager E L, and Smith D H: Living Nerve Constructs Bridging Peripheral Nerve Lesions Demonstrate Long-term Survival and Restoration of Function. *Platform Presentation (373.7) at the 34th Annual Meeting of the Society for Neuroscience*, San Diego, California, October 2004.

Huang J H, Zager E L, and Pfister B J, Smith D H: *Human Dorsal Root Ganglia Neurons as Live Nerve Constructs: Implications for Transplantation*. Presented at the AANS Annual Meeting, Orlando, Florida, May 2004.

Hui S W, Stenger D A: Electrofusion of cells: Hybridoma production by electrofusion and polyethylene glycol. *Methods Enzymol*. 220:212–227, 1993.

Kandel E, Schwartz J, Jessell T (ed): *Principles of Neural Science*. New York, McGraw-Hill, 2000.

Khawaja A M. The legacy of nanotechnology: Revolution and prospects in neurosurgery. *International Journal of Surgery* 9 (2011) 608-614).

Kroeker K. Medical nanobots. *Commun. ACM.* 2009; 52(9):18–19.

Li W, Brown P K, Wang L V, et al. Gold Nanocages as contrast agents for Photoacoustic imaging. *Contrast Media Mol. Imaging* 2011; 6:370–77.

Liu C Y, Spicer M, Apuzzo M L: The genesis of neurosurgery and the evolution of the neurosurgical operative environment: Part II—concepts for future development, 2003 and beyond. *Neurosurgery* 52:20–33, 2003.

Lodish H, Berk A, Matsudaira P, Kaiser C A, Krieger M, Scott M P, Zipursky L, Darnell J: *Molecular Cell Biology*, 5th ed, W.H. Freeman, 2004).

Lu M, Cohen M H, Rieves D, et al. FDA report: ferumoxytol for intravenous iron therapy in adult patients with chronic kidney disease. *Am. J. Hematol.* 2010; 85:315–19.

Mariappan N. Recent Trends in Nanotechnology Applications in Surgical Specialties and Orthopedic Surgery. *Biomedical & Pharmacology Journal*, September 2019. Vol. 12(3), p. 1095-1127.

Okabe M, Ikawa M, Kominami K, Nakanishi T, Nishimune Y: 'Green mice' as a source of ubiquitous green cells. *FEBS Lett*. 407:313–319, 1997).

Peer D K, Hong S, Farokhzad O C, et al. Nano carriers as an emerging platform for cancer therapy. *Nat. Nanotechnology* 2007; 2: 751–60.

Petersen K E: Silicon as a mechanical material. *Proc. IEEE* 70:420–457, 1982.

Rafuse V F, Gordon T: Self-reinnervated cat medial gastrocnemius muscles. I. Comparisons of the capacity for regenerating nerves to form enlarged motor units after extensive peripheral nerve injuries. *J. Neurophysiol.* 75: 268–281, 1996.

Russell J. Andrews, Nanotechnology and Neurosurgery. *Journal of Nano science and Nanotechnology Vol.9*, 5008–5013, 2009).

Schucht P, Raineteau O, Schwab M E, Fouad K: Anatomical correlates of locomotor recovery following dorsal and ventral lesions of the rat spinal cord. *Exp. Neurol.* 176:143–153, 2002.

Suffredini G, J. E. East and L. M. Levy. New Applications of Nanotechnology for Neuroimaging. *American Journal of Neuroradiology* July 2014, 35 (7) 1246-1253).

Sun Y, Xia Y. Shape-controlled synthesis of gold and silver nanoparticles. *Science* 2002; 298: 2176–79Abstract/FREE Full Text 2.

Vasita R and D. S. Katti, Nanofibers and their applications in tissue engineering. *Int. J. Nano medicine* 1, 15 (2006).

Wang X, Becker F F, and Gascoyne P R: Membrane dielectric changes indicate induced apoptosis in HL-60 cells more sensitively than surface phosphatidylserine expression or DNA fragmentation. *Biochim. Biophys. Acta* 1564:412–420, 2002.

You S W, Chen B Y, Liu H L, Lang B, Xia J L, Jiao X Y, Ju G: Spontaneous recovery of locomotion induced by remaining fibers after spinal cord transection in adult rats. *Restor. Neurol. Neurosci.* 21:39–45, 2003.

Chapter 22

Adult Brachial Plexus Injuries

Balachandar D*, Abhishek Kumar, Priyadarshi Dikshit and Kuntal Kanti Das
Sanjay Gandhi Postgraduate Institute of Medical Sciences, Lucknow, India

Abstract

Brachial plexus injuries (BPI) are one of the most devastating injuries by dint of the population affected and the extent of the resulting functional impairment. Not only the victims but also the entire family suffers indirectly from the functional loss to the victim of such injuries. Recent decades have seen many advances in the understanding, diagnosis, surgical techniques, and outcomes of these injuries. From a therapeutic nihilism in the initial years to the well-proven efficacy of modern-day nerve transfer surgeries, the management of BPI has travelled a long road. This chapter provides an updated review on this condition, focusing on surgical treatment and outcome assessment with a brief perspective of the future in this field.

Keywords: brachial plexus, partial, complete, surgery, neurotization

Introduction

BPIs are rare (appx 1% of all injuries) but one of the most devastating injuries [1–4]. 5% of motorcycle accident victims have BPIs in addition to other injuries [5]. The affected individual may suffer from excruciating peripheral

*Corresponding Author's Email: drkuntalkantidas@gmail.com.

In: Neurosurgery Research
Editors: Amit Agrawal, Pradeep Chouksey, Adesh Shrivastava et al.
ISBN: 978-1-68507-837-9

or central deafferentation pain for the rest of their lives, which adds to the overall misery of such patients. In addition to the sensory-motor deficits, and pain, functional limitations can be massive. Even the best surgical outcomes can be associated with highly unsatisfied and functionally limited patient outcomes due to pain and loss of dexterity [7, 8]. Choi et al. showed that 3-50% of patients with BPIs remain out of employment [9].

Surgical management of BPIs started early in the 20th century, but it was not widely practised because of frequently reported unsatisfactory and poor results [3]. Recent decades have seen many advances like the use of operating microscopes, better micro suture techniques for nerve graft and nerve or tendon transfer repair, and advanced perioperative electrophysiological techniques. Millesi and Narakas first reported good results which encouraged others to be more aggressive in managing these cases [10, 11, 12].

This chapter discusses the management options focusing on the surgical techniques, outcomes, and future perspectives of brachial plexus injuries.

Surgical Anatomy

Brachial plexus has 5 roots [C5-T1], 3 trunks [upper, middle, and lower], 6 divisions [each trunk has 2 divisions one is anterior and the other is posterior], 3 cords [lateral, posterior, and medial] [named in relationship to axillary artery] and 5 main terminal branches [musculocutaneous, radial, axillary, median and ulnar]. Figure 1 shows the various components of the brachial plexus.

The brachial plexus is situated in the posterior triangle of the neck. The upper and middle trunks with their divisions are situated in the omotrapezial triangle. The lower trunk is situated in omoclavicular triangle. To be more specific, the trunks of the brachial plexus emerge out from the interscalene triangle [between anterior and middle scalene muscles]. The subclavian artery travels within the triangle, with the subclavian vein being anterior to the scalenus anterior. The anterior rami of the spinal nerve are situated posterior to the vertebral artery. The nerve roots C8 and T1 are more retroclavicular [in the lower part of the scalene triangle], 1st and 2nd rib lie posterior to it, and inferiorly it is related to pleura. Figure 2 shows these anatomical details in an artistic illustration.

The spinal nerves on their exit through the neural foramina distal to dorsal root ganglion (DRG) receive inputs from the cervical sympathetic chain. C5 and C6 roots receive contributions from the middle cervical ganglion while the C7 and C8 receive contributions from the inferior cervical ganglion.

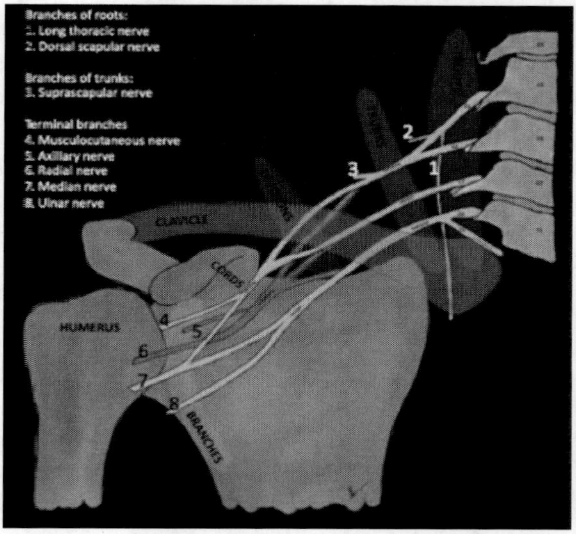

Figure 1. Schematic illustration of a right-sided brachial plexus showing roots, trunks, divisions, cords and branches with its relationship to clavicle, scapula and head of humerus.

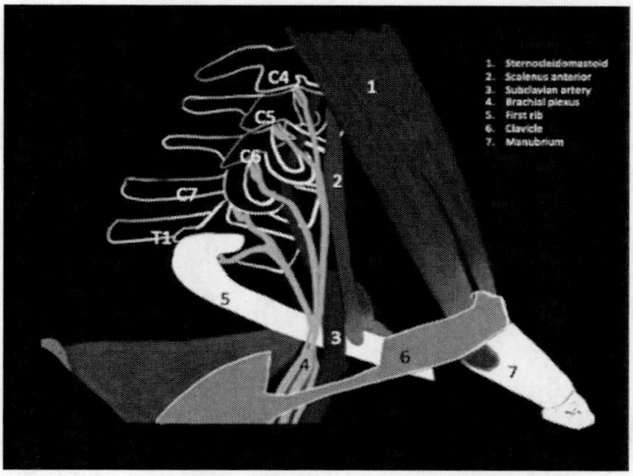

Figure 2. Schematic illustration of a Right-sided brachial plexus showing its relationship to neural foramen, vertebral artery, scalene muscles, subclavian artery, first rib and clavicle.

Anatomic Variations

Pre-fixed plexus is one that receives a contribution from C4, with minimal contribution from T1 and T2. Whereas, a post-fixed plexus receives contributions from T2, with no contribution from C4. Other variations commonly noted are: (a) ulnar nerve receives contributions from the lateral cord (relatively common 15-75%). (b) median nerve receives contributions from the lateral cord (less common), this variation most of the times accompanied by musculocutaneous nerve giving contributions to median neve. (c) entirely independent origins of radial and axillary nerves (20%) [12].

The important nerves arising from the brachial plexus and having significance in BPI evaluation and management include:

- *Musculocutaneous nerve:* It is a terminal branch of the lateral cord of the brachial plexus with a root value of C5, C6, C7. It is a mixed nerve. Its motor fibres innervate muscles of the anterior arm [biceps brachii, brachialis, coracobrachialis] while sensory fibres innervate skin on the lateral surface of the forearm through the lateral cutaneous nerve of the forearm.
- *Axillary nerve:* It is one of the terminal branches of the posterior cord. It carries fibres from C5 and C7. It is also a mixed nerve, having motor supply to the deltoid and teres minor muscles and carrying sensations over the deltoid.
- *Radial nerve:* It is the second terminal branch of the posterior cord, containing fibres from C5-T1. It is a mixed nerve. The motor supply involves all muscles of the posterior compartment of the arm and forearm. The sensory innervation territory includes the skin of the posterior surface of the arm, central posterior surface of the forearm, skin of lateral part of the dorsum of the hand including lateral 2 ½ fingers.
- *Median nerve:* It is formed by the joining of two roots, one each from the lateral and the medial cord. It is a mixed nerve with the following functions:

Motor supply to:

1) Flexor compartment of forearm except for flexor carpi ulnaris (FCU) and the medial ½ of the flexor digitorum profundus.

2) Thenar muscles [abductor pollicis brevis, flexor pollicis brevis, and opponens pollicis] except for adductor pollicis.
3) 2 lateral lumbricals.

Sensory supply to the skin of lateral ½ of palm, anterior aspect of lateral 3 ½ fingers, and posterior aspect of lateral 2 ½ fingers.

Ulnar Nerve

It is a terminal branch of the medial cord of the brachial plexus that contains fibres of C8-T1. It is a mixed nerve with a motor supply to flexor carpi ulnaris and medial ½ of flexor digitorum profundus of the forearm. It supplies all intrinsic muscles of the hand except for LOAF muscles [lateral 2 lumbricals, opponens pollicis, abductor pollicis brevis, flexor pollicis brevis].

Anatomy of Spinal Accessory Nerve

After giving cranial root to vagus nerve ganglion, the spinal root of the spinal accessory nerve (SAN) passes down anterior to the transverse process of the atlas. From there, it descends down posterior to the sternocleidomastoid muscle, innervating it. Approximately 9 cm above the clavicle, posterior to sternocleidomastoid, SAN takes a posterior inferior and lateral turn to enter the anterior border of the trapezius. On its way, it lies 1cm above the Erb's point and courses superficial to levator scapulae separated from it by the prevertebral layer of the deep cervical fascia.

The Pattern of Injury and Clinical Findings

Clinical examination is mandatory to identify:

i. the nerves injured,
ii. the level of injury: i.e., pre or post-ganglionic injuries. Pre-ganglionic injuries affect the roots alone while post-ganglionic injuries affect the trunk, division, cord, etc.

iii. the severity of the injury—incomplete or complete. It is important to identify whether the injury is a pan-brachial plexus injury or a partial injury of the upper (most common) or the lower brachial plexus.

Pre-ganglionic injuries have a poor prognosis and mandate earlier surgical management as they do not recover spontaneously. Thus, it is paramount to diagnose these injuries using certain features like i) Horner's syndrome, ii) injury to proximal nerves such as long thoracic, phrenic, and dorsal scapular nerve, iii) denervation of cervical paraspinal musculature on EMG, iv) absence of Tinel's sign in the supraclavicular fossa, and v) severe deafferentation pain.

Motor Function Evaluation

Table 1 shows the myotomes innervated by the roots of the brachial plexus. Many times, triceps function may be preserved even with avulsion of C7 root as it also receives contributions from C6 and C8. Severe deafferentation pain is seen in C8–T1 root avulsion. C5–C7 root avulsions also have deafferentation pain but it is usually less severe in nature. Worst deafferentation pain is seen in pan plexus injuries with multiple root avulsions.

Table 1. Nerve root injuries and their involved myotomes

C5	Shoulder abduction
C6	Elbow flexion
C7	Elbow extension
C8-T1	Intrinsic hand muscles

Sensory Function

Sensations of the affected limb are compared with the uninvolved limb. A relative decrease in response to touch and pinprick is looked for. Damage to the axon causes degeneration in the distal segment through a process known as Wallerian degeneration. Tinel's sign will be absent in the neck in case of total plexal avulsion. Whereas an elicitable but static Tinel's sign indicates poor recovery. The absence of Tinel's sign distal to the injury even after 4-6 weeks of injury indicates total neural interruption and poor axonal growth, making a spontaneous recovery impossible. Generally, the expected rate of progression of ingrowing neurons and hence the Tinel's sign is 1 mm/day.

Autonomic Function

The postganglionic lesion is associated with dry skin in the anaesthetic region. Whereas the anaesthetic region with sweating suggests a preganglionic lesion. The denervated skin has the least resistance on moving examiner's fingers, causing gliding of the palpating fingers. Return of sweating in the denervated skin may precede motor or sensory recovery by weeks or months.

Role of Preoperative, Intraoperative, and Postoperative Electrophysiology

Nerves respond to injuries by a process called Wallerian degeneration (WD). Depending on the grade and site of injury, such reparative processes may lead to regenerating nerves (provided cell body, here the dorsal root ganglion) to reach the distal nerve tube and eventually the target muscle. The muscle, on the other hand, undergoes denervation changes and eventually degenerative changes unless a timely re-innervation takes place. Therefore, it is understandable that electrophysiology can display, at a physiological level, the dynamics of post-injury or post-surgical changes supplementing our clinical assessment.

For the ease of understanding, this section is divided into:

1) Pre and postoperative electrophysiology.
2) Intraoperative physiology.

Preoperative Electrophysiology

It is useful during the initial patient workup in localizing the site of the lesion; and, also in documenting recovery in a patient with BPI, while awaiting surgical intervention.

Postoperative electrophysiology, similarly determines whether the surgical procedure is providing the expected degree of nerve regeneration and eventual muscle re-innervation. Thus, it can help prognostication and help therapeutic decision-making vis-à-vis secondary brachial plexus procedures.

Electromyography (EMG)

As nerves respond to injuries by WD, there is a period of denervation which is followed by re-innervation of the muscle. These changes are reflected in the EMG studies differently. So, the affected muscle will show electrical changes suggestive of denervation approximately by 2–3 weeks. The baseline EMG is therefore planned at 3 weeks after injury, and this is repeated every 1–2 months for lesions showing serial improvements on clinical examination [6].

There are three phases of activity noted during an EMG study [13]. This is depicted in Figure 3.

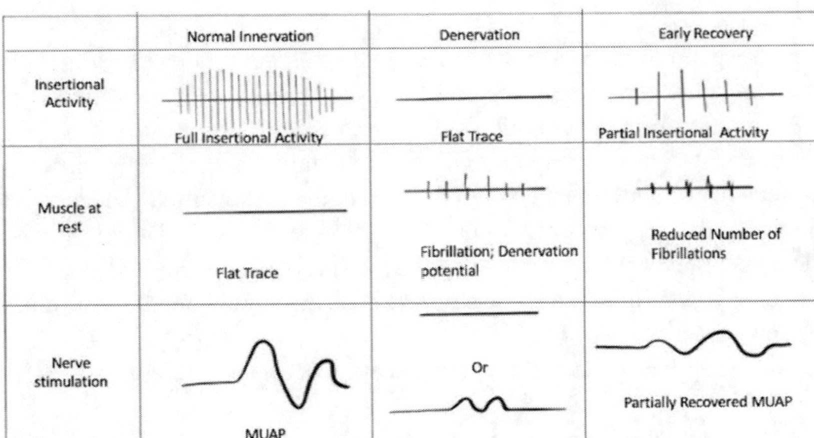

Figure 3. Showing EMG findings in various stages of a nerve injury.

1) The first phase – The insertional phase (assesses insertional activity) It is the burst of muscle fibre discharges due to needle electrode insertion through the normal muscle tissue (the needle electrode mechanically depolarizes the muscle fibres in its path). Its presence indicates muscle tissue viability.
2) The second phase – The resting phase (assesses spontaneous activity)

Spontaneous activity, which may be physiological (endplate activity) or pathological (e.g., fibrillation potentials), is sought using a screen sensitivity setting of 50 μV/division. Unlike the transient nature of the insertional activity, most forms of spontaneous activity are sustained.

3) Third phase – The activation phase (assesses voluntary activity)
Normal muscle – patient slightly contracts the muscle so that 2 to 4 MUAPs appear on the screen, the sensitivity of which is set at 200 μV/division.
The presence of spontaneous fibrillation in a muscle on electromyography is an indication of denervated yet vital muscle.

Nerve Conduction Studies

Motor NCS is performed for motor nerves and compound muscle action potential (CMAP) is recorded at the distal target muscle [14]. Similarly, a sensory nerve conduction study reveals sensory nerve action potential (SNAP).

The action potentials are analyzed for (i) amplitude (milli- or microvolts) and (ii) latency (time between the stimulus and the potential, in milliseconds). The conduction velocities can then be measured by dividing the distance from the latency. The velocities should be more than 50 m/s in the upper limbs and more than 40 m/s in the lower limbs [15]. Table 2 shows the findings on NCS in various grades of nerve injury.

Table 2. NCS findings in different types of injury

Type of injury	Amplitude	Conduction Velocity
Axonal disruption	Reduced	Near normal
Conduction block	CMAP amplitude normal for distal stimulation	Normal CMAP observed in weak muscle is considered as conduction block
	50% reduction in CMAP amplitude for stimulation proximal to the lesion [this is not possible in brachial plexus injuries]	

The main role of the preoperative SNAP is to differentiate preganglionic from postganglionic injuries. A distal sensory loss, but a preserved sensory conduction and hence a normal SNAP indicates a preganglionic injury.

However, if both pre-and postganglionic injuries co-exist, there will be a flat trace or negative SNAP.

The same tests are conducted serially after a surgical repair. Regeneration potential in the muscle, improvements in the NCV (amplitude as well as latency) are observed. Many a time though, these electrophysiological improvements do not concur with clinical improvements.

Intraoperative Electrophysiological Monitoring (IOEPM)

Intraoperative electrophysiological monitoring (IOEPM) helps the surgeon to

i. judge the function of nerves and to
ii. assess the severity of the injury in real-time and its potential for neural recovery [16].

Without IOEPM, it is difficult to assess the nerve roots completely and distinguish between pre and postganglionic injuries during surgery. The accuracy of CT myelography and MRI (85% and 52% respectively) in diagnosing pre and postganglionic injuries are much less when compared with an intradural exploration [17]. According to Oberlin et al. [18], intraoperative evoked potential recording is 100% sensitive for ventral as well as dorsal root avulsion. Generally, it is advised that a combination of SEPs, MEPs and NAP for IOEPM is utilized to most accurately verify the type of injury [19].

Kline and Happel, (1993) maintain that NAP is the most useful intraoperative test in adult brachial plexus injuries [20]. The presence of a NAP has clinical significance. The operative series by Kline and Hudson (1995) showed better functional results in 92% of neuromas in continuity where NAP is present [19]. If NAP is present in nerves with less favourable outcomes (supplying distal muscles), then also recovery is possible. In this scenario, neuroma resection is not advised. Rather neurolysis is performed. Moreover, the proximal ends of the severed nerve roots like C5/C6 may be utilised as intraplexal nerve donors, NAP is documented. Thus IOEPM helps in intraoperative decision making.

Role of Imaging

Neuroimaging has a supportive role in the evaluation of BPIs, unlike many other neurosurgical ailments.

Plain Skiagram

Plain skiagram is a very useful investigation that helps to localise the region of brachial plexus and peripheral nerve injuries. Table 3 shows the different kinds of fractures associated with BPIs.

Also, shoulder dislocation or fractures can be associated with nerve injury. C3–C5 spinal nerve injury usually shows elevated diaphragm, owing to ipsilateral phrenic nerve palsy. Also, the presence of rib fractures may indicate that harvesting the intercostal nerves may be difficult during surgery owing to their damage or extensive local fibrosis.

Table 3. Various fractures and their associated nerve injuries

Neck of humerus fracture	Axillary nerve injury
Mid shaft of humerus fracture	Radial Nerve injury
Radius and Ulanar fracture	Median and Ulnar nerve injury
Cervical spine Transverse process fracture	Root of brachial plexus injury

CT Myelography

CT myelography helps in identifying traumatic pseudo meningoceles [17], a characteristic finding in root avulsions. Tearing of arachnoid sleeves around the root with seepage of CSF into the adjacent area explains this radiological finding. Traumatic pseudo meningoceles extending outside the neural foramen is highly suggestive of root avulsion [21]. CT myelogram has better visualisation of traumatic pseudo meningocele if it is done at least a month after the injury by which time the adjoining hematomas generally resolve.

MRI

MRI has become the imaging modality of choice for greater resolution and overall characterization of lesions within the brachial plexus [17]. An injured peripheral nerve due to endoneurial or perineural oedema shows increased T2WI and STIR increased signal intensity changes. Atrophied muscles will show high-intensity signals compared with normal muscles on T1WI [22]. Table 4 shows the MRI signal patterns in different types of nerve injuries. Figure 4 shows a pseudomeningocele on MRI in a case of BPI.

Table 4. Different types of nerve injuries and their pattern of signal changes

Neuropraxia	Focal increase in signal intensity
Axonotmesis	Transient increase in nerve signal intensity distal to injury, followed by normalization
Neurotmesis	Increased signal intensity which is disappearing very late

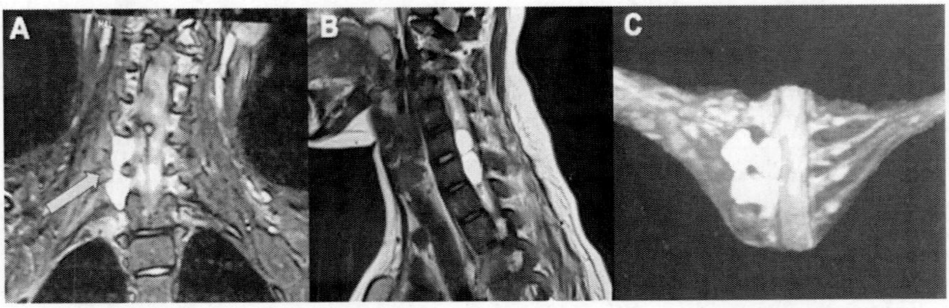

Figure 4. MRI of the cervical spine and brachial plexus shows hyperintensity similar to cerebrospinal fluid, indicating a pseudomeningocele on coronal (A, yellow arrow) and sagittal (B) sections. MR myelogram (C) shows more clearly depicts this finding.

MR Myelography

MR myelography is quick, non-invasive and provides multiplanar imaging having a diagnostic accuracy comparable with the conventional and CT myelograms [23]. CT Myelography and MR myelography have the same sensitivity (92.9%) for detecting root avulsions [21].

Management

Spontaneous Recovery

Given that injuries with nerves in continuity can show spontaneous recovery, the patient is usually given a trial for 3-4 months for potential recovery. However, documented preganglionic injuries, sharp injuries with possible nerve discontinuity etc. are contraindications for a wait and watch strategy [24]. Kline [1] from his personal experience reported that lesions with C5-C6 involvement had 40% spontaneous recovery rates while the results were far inferior when C7 root was also involved (15%-16%). In the complete plexus involvement, there was only a 4%-5% chance of spontaneous recovery.

Timing of Surgery

For most postganglionic injuries, 3-4 months waiting time is generally a standard. The first 3 months after injury is the time for best recovery [1, 5, 25, 26] followed by the next 3 months. Surgery is indicated for patients who do not show improvement beyond the first three months [24]. Neuromuscular junction becomes increasingly incapable of receiving reinnervation after 20-24 months [24] and hence many surgeons discourage any delays beyond 5-6 months of injury [25, 27].

Poor results after a delayed surgical intervention can be explained by:

1) chronically axotomized proximal stump that has reduced regenerating capacity,
2) the distal stump loses its capacity to support regenerating axons from the proximal stump, and
3) atrophied muscle has less chance to recover from a re-nervation.

Martin et al. [27] mention that surgery performed on or before 3 months for stretch and blunt injuries showed better recovery regardless of the level of injury. Waiting for three months causes most of the neuropraxic injuries to recover, also the regenerating nerves can be assessed [28] by an intra op NAP. Nerve axons regenerate at a speed of only 1-2.5 mm per day, hence the timing is important. Hems et al. [29] noted that postoperative inflammation was highest between 2 and 8 weeks, so it seems reasonable to operate after 2-3 months in such injuries. For preganglionic injuries with root avulsion, surgery [nerve transfer] is performed as early as possible.

Table 5 shows the indications of an immediate or an early brachial plexus repair. In early surgery, the surgical field is clean and anatomy is clear and postoperative rehabilitation can be started early. But a neuroma with regenerating fascicles can sometimes be mistakenly resected and grafted, this is because a direct perioperative recording cannot reliably exclude regeneration in the first few weeks after injury.

Table 5. Indications for immediate/early surgery and repair (< 3-4 weeks) – Indications

1)	Lacerated sharp, open injuries
2)	Associated vascular injuries
3)	Flail limb with severe de-afferentiation pain
4)	Pseudo meningoceles

Surgical Options

The anterior approach consists of supraclavicular and infraclavicular exposures. Depending on the extent of injury, either or in the majority of cases, a combined approach is taken.

The surgical techniques commonly performed in brachial plexus injuries are [24]:

1) *Direct end-to-end repair:* Done in a clean nerve transection injury where the cut ends of two nerves can be brought together without tension.
2) *Neurolysis:* It is the release of a nerve or neuroma from the surrounding scar tissue. It can be freeing the nerve from encircling scar (external neurolysis) or from scars within (internal neurolysis).
3) *Nerve grafting:* It is used after resection of a nonconducting neuroma, or in postganglionic injuries where the proximal and distal nerve stumps are separated by a large distance. The sural nerve is commonly used for grafting. It is believed that there is a loss of 30% axons at one anastomosis site and hence using a nerve graft has the risk of losing a significant number of ingrowing axons.
4) *Nerve transfer (neurotization):* A functionally less important nerve is transferred to a distal but more important nerve when a significant

segment of the nerve is lost or damaged proximally. The prerequisites for neurotization include: a functioning muscle recipient whose nerve is denervated due to a proximal injury and EMG of the recipient's muscle shows spontaneous fibrillation (indicates denervated yet a vital muscle).

Priorities of Nerve Repair

Restoring Shoulder Function

For upper plexus injury (absent shoulder abduction, external rotation and elbow flexion), the standard choice of reconstruction includes triple nerve transfer which is – (i) SAN to suprascapular nerve, SSN (causes restoration of shoulder stability) (ii) motor nerve of triceps to axillary nerve, Somsak's procedure (causes abduction > 90° and deltoid strength ≥M4) and (iii) ulnar nerve fascicle to biceps motor nerve, Oberlin's procedure [30, 31]. Figures 5 and 6 show intraoperative steps of Somsak's and Oberlin's procedures.

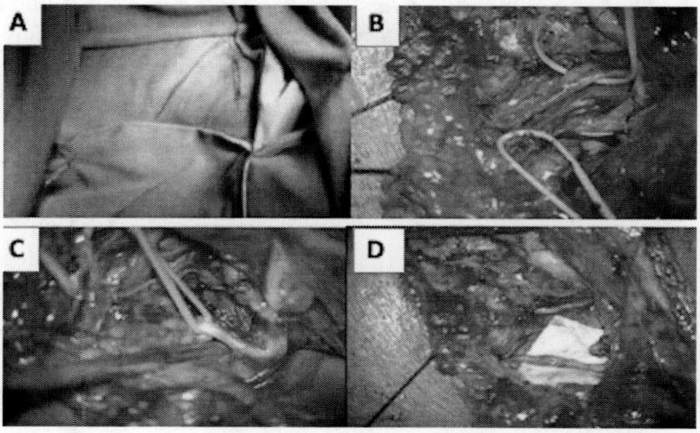

Figure 5. Left supraclavicular brachial plexus exploration is seen, with an incision marked along the lower end of the posterior border of SCM and upper border of clavicle (A). The upper trunk is identified and both C5 and C6 roots are taken in a loop and suprascapular nerve is isolated (B) and dissected for a segment. The SAN is found on the anterior border of trapezius and dissected distally, preserving innervation of medial part of the muscle (C). The SAN is cut sharply at right angles as distally as possible (donor distal) while the SAN is similarly cut close to the Erb's point (recipient proximal). The two cut ends are co-apted using 2-4 interrupted sutures (8-0 nylon) and reinforced with fibrin glue (D).

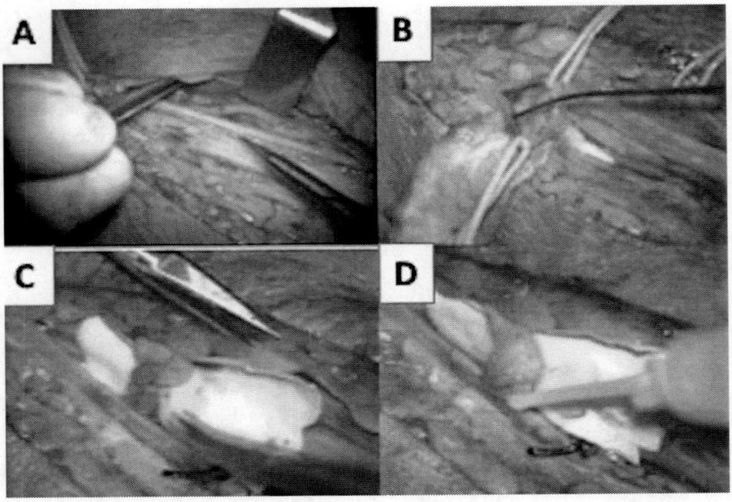

Figure 6. Through a longitudinal incision over the medial part of the arm, along the inter-mascular septum, the ulnar nerve and musculocutaneous nerves are exposed. MCN is found beneath the biceps brachii muscle (A). It is traced till some branches entering the biceps brachii are defined and retrogradely dissected on the MCN to obtain a good length. The ulnar nerve is dissected and fascicle supplying flexor carpi ulnaris (FCU) is identified and dissected for a length (B). Then the donor (FCU fascicle of ulnar nerve) is divided as distal as possible while the branch entering the biceps brachii is divided as proximal to the muscle as possible and co-apted using 2-4 interrupted sutures (8-0 nylon) and reinforced with fibrin glue (C, D).

Elbow Flexion and Extension

Oberlin Transfer

Done in upper plexus injury which involves the transfer of an ulnar nerve fascicle to biceps motor nerve (MRC grade $\geq$ M4 achieved in most of the patients [32, 33]).

Median to Biceps Motor Never Transfer

Non-essential branches of the median nerve (usually those that innervate the muscle causing radial deviation of the wrist joint) to wrist and finger flexors used to neurotize biceps of brachialis motor nerve [34].

Double fascicular transfer (Oberlin transfer + median nerve fascicle transfer) remains a topic of controversy as studies show it is not superior to single fascicle transfer [35].

Hand and Wrist Reanimation

Done in lower plexus injuries where anterior interosseous nerve branch to pronator quadratus is transferred to the distal ulnar motor branches [36]. This helps in the restoration of functions of the median nerve. The nerve transfers for reinnervation of the radial nerve include nerve to brachioradialis or supinator to posterior interosseous nerve.

Flail Arm Reconstruction

The flail arm generally results from extensive pan-brachial avulsions and remain a difficult problem to treat. Generally, multistage and multi-disciplinary teamwork is needed to optimise outcomes in these patients. Extra plexal donors like SAN, contralateral spinal accessory nerve, hypoglossal nerve, intercostal nerves, phrenic nerve, contralateral C7 [37] are used as donors for nerve transfers for shoulder and elbow function restoration. The primary aim of reconstruction of a flail arm is shoulder stability, abduction and elbow flexion. The secondary aim is to achieve elbow extension with wrist and hand function [38].

Contralateral C7 Nerve as a Donor in Brachial Plexus Injuries

The first case of contralateral C7 nerve transfer was done in 1986 [39]. This concept came in due a limited availability of donor nerves for neurotisation in cases of high-velocity injury in more extensive trauma.

Why Choose the C7 Nerve Root?

This is because C7 forms the middle trunk and there is no single muscle in the upper limb which is supplied only by C7. So, dividing it is not going to cause permanent sensory or motor deficits. It should never be sectioned below infraclavicular level as the other adjoining trunks from the upper and lower trunk might get injured which can cause permanent motor and sensory deficits.

Which Fascicle to Use for Neurotization? – (Anterior Division, Posterior Division or Whole C7 Root?)

It is to be noted that the diameter of the selected C7 fascicle should match the diameter of the donor ulnar nerve from the contralateral side. Partial neurotization of C7 can also be done. Generally, the posterior division of the C7 nerve root has more motor fibres than the anterior division [40]. So, the posterior division is used to restore motor power and the anterior division is used to restore desired sensory function.

Procedure

Under general anaesthesia, the patient is positioned supine, and the C7 is exposed on the healthy side. Either the trunk or the anterior or posterior division is selected according to the calibre of the ulnar nerve from the affected side. The ulnar nerve is cut at wrist level and it is subcutaneously tunnelled up to the level of mid-arm and tunnelled across the chest in the subcutaneous plane and brought near the cut end of C7 for a tension-free suturing. Care should be taken to preserve the superior ulnar collateral vessels which provide blood supply to the graft. Subsequently, as the nerve regeneration from the contralateral C7 reaches the ipsilateral axilla (confirmed by positive Tinel's sign and electrophysiological studies), the ulnar nerve is divided in the affected arm side and transferred to the desired recipient nerve [41, 42].

In a case series published by Zang and Gu, motor recovery rate i.e., >=M3 was 50-80% and the sensory recovery rate (>=S3) was above 60% [43]. Waikakul et al. in a case series of 96 patients showed that only 52% of patients had >=M3 recovery with contralateral C7 to musculocutaneous nerve transfer [44]. Hierner et al. reported 100% M3 biceps recovery and 25% recovery for median nerve [45]. The two most important factors for improved surgical outcome include (i) choosing the right fascicle of C7 for neurotization and (ii) maintaining the vascularity of the graft used.

Sensory Neurotization

Secondary injuries are more prone to occur in an anaesthetic hand in the event of complete brachial plexus injuries or in lower trunk injuries [46]. Thus, sensory reconstruction should be one of the goals of BPI repair, whenever feasible.

Due to its wider sensory cutaneous distribution in the hand, the median nerve, which is called the "eye of the hand," is usually chosen as the recipient for sensory neurotization. The lateral cord, being primarily sensory, is usually chosen as a recipient [24]. Ulnar nerve has also been used as a recipient because its diameter matches the intercostal nerves (a frequently used donor). Different donor nerves reported in the literature are intercostal nerves, intercostobrachial nerves (ICBN), contralateral C7 nerve and supraclavicular nerves.

Foroni et al. [47] showed good recovery using ICBN in 11 patients. They described a close anatomical proximity of the cortical area of ICBN and the upper limbs leading to a more complete cortical plasticity and better results in their study. Although the sensory recovery is only marginal (S2 or S2 plus), it was still good enough in a completely insensate hand. Table 6 shows the sensory examination gradings for outcome assessment in BPIs.

Hattori et al. [49] used ICBN as a donor for sensory neurotization for the hand. He said that it had better results in comparison with previously used intercostal nerves. He even noted the capability of heat and cold following the nerve transfer.

Table 6. Sensory recovery according to Highet's scale

S0: No recovery of sensitivity in the autonomous zone of the nerve
S1: Recovery of deep cutaneous pain sensation within the autonomous zone of the nerve
S1+: Recovery of superficial pain sensitivity
S2: Recovery of superficial pain and some touch sensitivity
S2+: As in S2, but with overresponse
S3: Recovery of pain and touch sensitivity with disappearance of the overresponse
S3+: As in S3, but localization of the stimulus is good and there is imperfect recovery of two-point discrimination
S4: Complete recovery

Factors Affecting Outcome

As surgical results in BPI are not always good and uniform, it is important to understand the factors that affect the postoperative outcomes. These factors are helpful in the case of selection as well as in prognostication.

i. *Age* – Multiple case series have demonstrated that worse motor outcomes are associated with older age [50–52]. The higher cortical plasticity in young patients could be a factor contributing to their better recovery [53].
ii. *Level of brachial plexus injury* – Upper plexus (C5-C7) have improved outcomes when compared to lower plexus injuries (C8-T1). Complete plexus injuries have the worst outcomes.
iii. *Donors used* – The motor outcome depends on the donor nerve used, whether it is intra or extra-plexal. Due to the need for cortical plasticity, extra-plexal donors have usually inferior outcomes than the intra-plexal donors.
iv. *Technique* – Nerve transfer (neurotization) has better recovery in comparison with nerve grafting, this was reported by Ali et al. [54] in a systemic review. Also, minimising suture material, use of glue cast etc. have been shown to have better results.
v. *Length of the graft* – outcome worsens with the increasing length of the graft. Terzis and Kostas [55] say that 7cm is the cut-off point. Graft below and equal to 7cm were found to have improved outcomes. Grafts more than 10 cm were found to have the worst outcome [56].

Post-Operative Care and Assessment of Improvement

Postoperative rehabilitation plays an important role in the extent of functional improvement after surgery [57, 58]. Socolowski et al. [58] used a 4-point scale to assess the quality of rehabilitation programs for their patients and showed a statistically better motor recovery in patients who receive good rehabilitation.

Every patient should receive a tailored rehabilitative programme depending on the type of injury. But all patients with BPIs, irrespective of the type of injury should receive these general aspects of rehabilitation considerations [59].

i. maintaining range of motion of the extremity,
ii. providing support to the extremity,
iii. preserving or improving strength in weak muscles,
iv. preventing oedema in the weak or paralysed extremity,

v. educating proper use of contralateral healthy extremity to prevent musculoskeletal symptoms of overuse,
vi. pain management.

Pain Management

Pain with plexopathy (weakness) gives rise to neuropathic pain. This pain is not due to inflammatory mediators but actually due to tissue damage (a stretch of damaged nerve endings). Absence of sensation with pain is the most common finding here. Damage to the somatosensory system causes sensitization of peripheral nerves by ectopic or spontaneous hyperexcitability in the modulatory pathway. Possible mechanisms for this neuropathic pain can be excitatory neurotransmission through N-methyl-D-aspartate (NMDA) receptors. This plays a major role in neuropathic pain, leads to tolerance to opioids and other analgesics. So, drugs that block NMDA receptors block the excitatory neurotransmission pathway, stabilize neuron excitability and suppress central sensitization.

Diagnosis of neuropathic pain is mostly by patients' verbal description. Bedside screening tools like Leeds assessment of neuropathic symptoms and signs (LANSS), pain scale can be used or the pain DETECT questionnaire which shows approximately 80% accuracy in diagnosing neuropathic pain [61]. For neuropathic pain, combination therapy works better [59]. Amitriptyline or duloxetine with gabapentin or pregabalin is started and continued for 2 – 8 weeks. Also, the physical and emotional aspect of the illness is treated along with pain. Patients should be encouraged to engage in physical activities. Poor sleep, anxiety and depression have to be addressed at the same time.

Non-Pharmacological Treatment of Pain

Neuromuscular Electrostimulation (NMES)

Here a stimulator that uses pulsating alternate current for stimulating nerve and innervated muscle is used [62]. This causes an increasing range of motion around the joints, increases muscle contraction and tone, reduces the chance of shoulder subluxation, reduction of pain. This also helps in motor relearning, muscle strengthening and prevents muscle atrophy.

Techniques

1) TENS (Transcutaneous electrical nerve stimulation)
   Functions based on gate control theory mechanism of pain. And it has no adverse effects.
2) Dorsal column stimulation
   It inhibits nociceptive transmission by stimulating large afferent fibres. Evidence is there for using dorsal column stimulation in refractory neuropathic pain involving the back and leg [63].
3) Deep brain stimulation
   Done for refractory neuropathic pain, but it takes months to years for desired benefits (pain reduction)
4) DREZotomy
   Done disrupt the signals generated in the dorsal root entry zone (DREZ) of the dorsal columns. This is reserved for long-standing pain [59].

Acupuncture and hypnosis have also been tried in addition to drug treatment [64, 65].

Amputation and Prosthesis

Patients who are not candidates for nerve repair, who do not gain significant recovery or improvement and who have complete flail arm are left with an extremity which has little or no useful function. In this scenario, the options available for patients are (i) hand dominance retraining, (ii) functional arm arthrosis, or (iii) more aggressive limb amputation with prosthetic restoration.

Amputation is done for patients with complete flail arm with no further chance of neurological recovery. It is done at mid humeral level with shoulder fusion. Prosthetic restoration is either passive or cosmetic-only or functional. Functional prosthetic restoration is body-powered (cable operated) or externally powered or hybrid.

Functional Outcomes Other Than Muscle Power

Surgical outcome assessment in BPI predominantly focuses on motor and sensory outcomes. What remains neglected but very important for the patient is pain and loss of dexterity. It is understood that motor and sensory functions can be examined by the physician while pain and quality of life are best assessed by the patient himself/herself. Thus, it has been suggested that patient-reported outcomes be given equal importance during follow-up examination. Different authors have used validated questionnaires like Short form-36 (SF 36) [66, 67], Disability of the arm, shoulder and hand (DASH) score [68–70] and pain visual analogue scale (PVAS) [71]. Ahmed Labib et al. [5] showed that the mean DASH score, as well as SF-36 scores, were significantly worse in these patients than the normal population. They also noted that DASH score and SF-36 scores were better in patients who underwent surgery within 6 months of injury. Moreover, they noted that those who were operated on within 5 months had significantly better PVAS scores. As far as the type of injury was concerned, pre-ganglionic injuries had more severe PVAS scores and consistently low DASH and SF 36 scores.

Rasulic et al. [72] reported their 20-year-old experience with BPIs in 2017. They used ULM scoring in addition to the DASH questionnaire in their patients. The mean DASH score of their patients was 58.7. They noted that DASH scores were lower in higher injuries i.e., spinal nerve avulsion and root level injuries. Similarly, DASH scores were higher in those who underwent delayed surgeries. They also noted that nearly 76% of patients reported pain in the follow-up period and 18.8% of patients suffered from depression, primarily from feeling discriminated against in society. They noted that the DASH questionnaire was particularly suited for QOL evaluation as it was a quick method and because of the calculation involved, patients are not able to influence the final score. They also noted that despite nearly 95% of their patients improving in motor functions, only 82% of patients were eventually satisfied with surgery, implying that QOL was more than just motor functions!

Secondary Brachial Plexus Procedures

For patients in whom initial nerve reconstruction does not give promising results and in patients with a delayed presentation where primary nerve reconstruction is not recommended, a set of secondary procedures can still be considered [73]. These include free muscle transplantation, pedicled muscle and tendon transfers, rotational osteotomies of humerus and radius, and joint fusion techniques. Table 7 shows the various free muscle transfer options in BPIs.

Table 7. Showing various free muscle transfer options in BPIs

<table>
<tr><td>Restoration of function</td><td>Muscle transplantation needed</td><td>Nerves used for neurotizing these muscles</td></tr>
<tr><td>Elbow flexion or extension</td><td>Latissimus dorsi or rectus femoris</td><td rowspan="2">Accessory nerve or intercostal nerves, or contralateral anterior (for the flexors) or posterior (for the extensors) divisions of the C7 root</td></tr>
<tr><td>Finger flexion or extension</td><td>Gracilis transferred to forearm</td></tr>
</table>

Pedicled Muscle and Tendon Transfer

Here one muscle function is sacrificed to replace another function. The muscle to be transferred has to be adequately innervated and should have at least M4 strength [73].

Rotational Osteotomies of Humerus and Radius

Rotational osteotomies of the humerus help improve external rotation by 30 degrees and rotational osteotomies of humerus and radius can correct supination or pronation deformities [73].

Joint Fusion Techniques

Many surgeons prefer to stabilize the wrist when free muscle transfer is planned for hand reanimation. It allows the tension of the free muscle to be adjusted better if crossing a stable joint. Although many authors have recommended humeroscapular arthrodesis, this is helpful only if active scapulothoracic motion is preserved [73].

Future Perspectives

The next revolutionary step is already been witnessed in work done by Aszmann et al. [74] where they have deliberately performed amputation for patients with paralyzed and flail arms due to non-recovering severe brachial plexus injury. These patients are given intense systemic training for the amputated arm and reliable myoelectric signals from the forearm are used to create movements in a prosthetic hand (movements between thumb and other fingers). Patients were able to do bimanual tasks with this prosthesis. Apart from functional recovery with a bionic limb, there was a significant reduction in neuropathic pain.

The advancement in robotic technology with an improved conception of the brain-machine interface will lead to further evolution of peripheral rewiring procedures along with central re-education.

Conclusion

BPIs are rare but functionally disabling, causing not only loss of function but also severe pain and psychological issues. A sound anatomical knowledge, proper and accurate determination of injury site, type and operability are essential. A number of surgical options are available now and distal nerve transfers have changed surgical management drastically in recent years. That said, management of BPIs is a long drawn battle.

References

Ahmed-Labib M, Golan JD, Jacques L (2007) Functional Outcome of Brachial Plexus Reconstruction after Trauma. *Neurosurgery* 61:1016–1023.

Ali ZS, Heuer GG, Faught RW, Kaneriya SH, Sheikh UA, Syed IS, Stein SC, Zager EL (2015) Upper brachial plexus injury in adults: comparative effectiveness of different repair techniques. *Journal of neurosurgery* 122:195–201.

Andreisek G, Crook DW, Burg D, Marincek B, Weishaupt D (2006) Peripheral neuropathies of the median, radial, and ulnar nerves: MR imaging features. *Radiographics* 26:1267–1287.

Aszmann OC, Roche AD, Salminger S, Paternostro-Sluga T, Herceg M, Sturma A, Hofer C, Farina D (2015) Bionic reconstruction to restore hand function after brachial plexus injury: a case series of three patients. *The Lancet* 385:2183–2189.

Beaton DE, Schemitsch E (2003) Measures of health-related quality of life and physical function. *Clinical Orthopaedics and Related Research®* 413:90–105.

Bertelli JA, Ghizoni MF (2007) Transfer of the accessory nerve to the suprascapular nerve in brachial plexus reconstruction. *The Journal of hand surgery* 32:989–998.

Birch R (2009) Brachial plexus injury: the London experience with supraclavicular traction lesions. *Neurosurgery Clinics of North America* 20:15–23.

Bowen BC, Pattany PM, Saraf-Lavi E, Maravilla KR (2004) The brachial plexus: normal anatomy, pathology, and MR imaging. *Neuroimaging Clinics* 14:59–85.

Brucker PU, Gruen GS, Kaufmann RA (2005) Scapulothoracic dissociation: evaluation and management. *Injury* 36:1147–1155.

Bruxelle J, Travers V, Thiebaut JB (1988) Occurrence and treatment of pain after brachial plexus injury. *Clin Orthop Relat Res* 87–95.

Carvalho GA, Nikkhah G, Matthies C, Penkert G, Samii M (1997) Diagnosis of root avulsions in traumatic brachial plexus injuries: value of computerized tomography myelography and magnetic resonance imaging. *Journal of neurosurgery* 86:69–76.

Chen N, Yang LJS, Chung KC (2011) Anatomy of the brachial plexus. *Practical Management of Pediatric and Adult Brachial Plexus Palsies* E-Book 0.

Choi PD, Novak CB, Mackinnon SE, Kline DG (1997) Quality of life and functional outcome following brachial plexus injury. *The Journal of Hand Surgery* 22:605–612.

Chuang DC, Lee GW, Hashem F, Wei F-C (1995) Restoration of shoulder abduction by nerve transfer in avulsed brachial plexus injury: evaluation of 99 patients with various nerve transfers. *Plastic and reconstructive surgery* 96:122–128.

Coulet B, Boretto JG, Lazerges C, Chammas M (2010) A comparison of intercostal and partial ulnar nerve transfers in restoring elbow flexion following upper brachial plexus injury (C5-C6±C7). *The Journal of hand surgery* 35:1297–1303.

Dubuisson AS, Kline DG (2002) Brachial plexus injury: a survey of 100 consecutive cases from a single service. *Neurosurgery* 51:673–683.

El-Gammal TA, Fathi NA (2002) Outcomes of surgical treatment of brachial plexus injuries using nerve grafting and nerve transfers. *Journal of reconstructive microsurgery* 18:007–016.

Ferrante MA (2021) *The Needle EMG Examination.* Springer Publishing Company.

Flores LP (2006) [Epidemiological study of the traumatic brachial plexus injuries in adults]. *Arq Neuropsiquiatr* 64:88–94.

Foroni L, Siqueira MG, Martins RS, Heise CO, Sterman Neto H, Imamura AY (2017) Good sensory recovery of the hand in brachial plexus surgery using the intercostobrachial nerve as the donor. *Arq Neuro-Psiquiatr* 75:796–800.

Freynhagen R, Baron R, Gockel U, Tölle TR (2006) Pain DETECT: a new screening questionnaire to identify neuropathic components in patients with back pain. *Current medical research and opinion* 22:1911–1920.

Garg R, Merrell GA, Hillstrom HJ, Wolfe SW (2011) Comparison of nerve transfers and nerve grafting for traumatic upper plexus palsy: a systematic review and analysis. *JBJS* 93:819–829.

Garratt A, Schmidt L, Mackintosh A, Fitzpatrick R (2002) Quality of life measurement: bibliographic study of patient assessed health outcome measures. *Bmj* 324:1417.

Gu Y, Chen D, Zhang G, Cheng X, Xu J, Zhang L, Cai P, Chen L (1998) Long-term functional results of contralateral C7 transfer. *Journal of reconstructive microsurgery* 14:57–59.

Gu Y, Xu J, Chen L, Wang H, Hu S (2002) Long term outcome of contralateral C7 transfer: a report of 32 cases. *Chinese medical journal* 115:866–868.

Gu Y, Zhang G, Chen D, Yan J, Cheng X, Chen L (1992) Seventh cervical nerve root transfer from the contralateral healthy side for treatment of brachial plexus root avulsion. *The Journal of Hand Surgery: British & European Volume* 17:518–521.

Hattori Y, Doi K, Sakamoto S, Yukata K (2009) Sensory recovery of the hand with intercostal nerve transfer following complete avulsion of the brachial plexus. *Plastic and reconstructive surgery* 123:276–283.

Hems T (2015) Timing of surgical reconstruction for closed traumatic injury to the supraclavicular brachial plexus. *Journal of Hand Surgery (European Volume)* 40:568–572.

Hierner R, Berger A (2007) Did the partial contralateral C7-transfer fulfil our expectations? Results after 5 year experience. In: *How to Improve the Results of Peripheral Nerve Surgery.* Springer, pp 33–35.

Hudak PL, Amadio PC, Bombardier C, Beaton D, Cole D, Davis A, Hawker G, Katz JN, Makela M, Marx RG (1996) Development of an upper extremity outcome measure: the DASH (disabilities of the arm, shoulder, and head). *American journal of industrial medicine* 29:602–608.

Huskisson EC (1974) Measurement of pain. *The lancet* 304:1127–1131.

Kelly BM, Leonard Jr JA (2011) Rehabilitation concepts for adult brachial plexus injuries. *Practical Management of Pediatric and Adult Brachial Plexus Palsies E-Book* 301.

Kim DH, Cho Y-J, Tiel RL, Kline DG (2003) Outcomes of surgery in 1019 brachial plexus lesions treated at Louisiana State University Health Sciences Center. *Journal of Neurosurgery* 98:1005–1016.

Kim DH, Midha R, Murovic JA, Spinner RJ, Teil R (2007) Kline and Hudson's nerve injuries: operative results for major nerve injuries, entrapments and tumors. Elsevier Health Sciences.

Kitajima I, Doi K, Hattori Y, Takka S, Estrella E (2006) Evaluation of quality of life in brachial plexus injury patients after reconstructive surgery. *Hand Surg* 11:103–107.

Kline D (2009) Timing for brachial plexus injury: a personal experience.

Kline DG (1982) Timing for exploration of nerve lesions and evaluation of the neuroma-in-continuity. *Clinical orthopaedics and related research* 42–49.

Kline DG, Happel LT (1993) A quarter century's experience with intraoperative nerve action potential recording. *Canadian journal of neurological sciences* 20:3–10.

Leechavengvongs S, Witoonchart K, Uerpairojkit C, Thuvasethakul P, Ketmalasiri W (1998) Nerve transfer to biceps muscle using a part of the ulnar nerve in brachial plexus injury (upper arm type): a report of 32 cases. *The Journal of hand surgery* 23:711–716.

Mackinnon SE (1988) Surgery of the peripheral nerve. *Carpal tunnel syndrome* 146–169.

Mallik A, Weir A (2005) Nerve conduction studies: essentials and pitfalls in practice. *J Neurol Neurosurg Psychiatry* 76:ii23–ii31.

Martin E, Senders JT, DiRisio AC, Smith TR, Broekman MLD (2019) Timing of surgery in traumatic brachial plexus injury: a systematic review. *Journal of Neurosurgery* 130:1333–1345.

Martins RS, Siqueira MG, Heise CO, Foroni L, Teixeira MJ (2013) A prospective study comparing single and double fascicular transfer to restore elbow flexion after brachial plexus injury. *Neurosurgery* 72:709–715.

McHorney CA, Ware Jr JE, Raczek AE (1993) The MOS 36-Item Short-Form Health Survey (SF-36): II. Psychometric and clinical tests of validity in measuring physical and mental health constructs. *Medical care* 247–263.

Midha R (1997) Epidemiology of brachial plexus injuries in a multitrauma population. *Neurosurgery* 40:1182–1189.

Nakamura T, Yabe Y, Horiuchi Y, Takayama S (1997) Magnetic resonance myelography in brachial plexus injury. The Journal of bone and joint surgery *British volume* 79:764–769.

Narakas AO (1985) The treatment of brachial plexus injuries. *International Orthopaedics* 9:29–36.

Narakas AO, Hentz VR (1988) Neurotization in brachial plexus injuries. Indication and results. *Clin Orthop Relat* Res 43–56.

Novak CB, Mackinnon SE (2002) Distal anterior interosseous nerve transfer to the deep motor branch of the ulnar nerve for reconstruction of high ulnar nerve injuries. *Journal of reconstructive microsurgery* 18:459–464.

Oberle J, Antoniadis G, Kast E, Richter H-P (2002) Evaluation of traumatic cervical nerve root injuries by intraoperative evoked potentials. *Neurosurgery* 51:1182–1190a.

Oberlin C, Beal D, Leechavengvongs S, Salon A, Dauge M, Sarcy J (1994) Nerve transfer to biceps muscle using a part of ulnar nerve for C5–C6 avulsion of the brachial plexus: anatomical study and report of four cases. *The Journal of hand surgery* 19:232–237.

Ochiai N, Nagano A, Sugioka H, Hara T (1996) Nerve grafting in brachial plexus injuries: results of free grafts in 90 patients. *The Journal of bone and joint surgery British volume* 78:754–758.

Pittler MH, Ernst E (2008) Complementary therapies for neuropathic and neuralgic pain: systematic review. *The Clinical journal of pain* 24:731–733.

Rasulić L, Savić A, Živković B, et al. (2017) Outcome after brachial plexus injury surgery and impact on quality of life. *Acta Neurochir* 159:1257–1264.

Ruchelsman DE, Price AE, Valencia H, Ramos LE, Grossman JA (2010) Sensory restoration by lateral antebrachial cutaneous to ulnar nerve transfer in children with global brachial plexus injuries. *Hand* 5:370–373.

Saitoh Y, Yoshimine T (2007) Stimulation of primary motor cortex for intractable deafferentation pain. *Operative neuromodulation* 51–56.

Sheffler LR, Chae J (2007) Neuromuscular electrical stimulation in neurorehabilitation. *Muscle & Nerve: Official Journal of the American Association of Electrodiagnostic Medicine* 35:562–590.

Shin AY, Spinner RJ, Steinmann SP, Bishop AT (2005) Adult traumatic brachial plexus injuries. *J Am Acad Orthop Surg* 13:382–396.

Sinha S, Khani M, Mansoori N, Midha R (2016) Adult brachial plexus injuries: Surgical strategies and approaches. *Neurology India* 64:289.

Sinha S, Pemmaiah D, Midha R (2015) Management of brachial plexus injuries in adults: Clinical evaluation and diagnosis. *Neurol India* 63:918.

Socolovsky M, Di Masi G, Battaglia D (2011) Use of long autologous nerve grafts in brachial plexus reconstruction: factors that affect the outcome. *Acta neurochirurgica* 153:2231–2240.

Socolovsky M, Malessy M, Lopez D, Guedes F, Flores L (2017) Current concepts in plasticity and nerve transfers: relationship between surgical techniques and outcomes. *Neurosurgical focus* 42:E13.

Sungpet A, Suphachatwong C, Kawinwonggowit V (2003) One-fascicle median nerve transfer to biceps muscle in C5 and C6 root avulsions of brachial plexus injury. *Microsurgery: Official Journal of the International Microsurgical Society and the European Federation of Societies for Microsurgery* 23:10–13.

Terzis JK, Barbitsioti A (2012) Primary restoration of elbow flexion in adult post-traumatic plexopathy patients. *Journal of Plastic, Reconstructive & Aesthetic Surgery* 65:72–84.

Terzis JK, Kostas I (2006) Suprascapular nerve reconstruction in 118 cases of adult posttraumatic brachial plexus. *Plastic and reconstructive surgery* 117:613–629.

Terzis JK, Kostopoulos VK (2007) The Surgical Treatment of Brachial Plexus Injuries in Adults. *Plastic and Reconstructive Surgery* 119:73[e].

Vissers K (2006) The clinical challenge of chronic neuropathic pain. *Disability and rehabilitation* 28:343–349.

Waikakul S, Orapin S, Vanadurongwan V (1999) Clinical results of contralateral C7 root neurotization to the median nerve in brachial plexus injuries with total root avulsions. *The Journal of Hand Surgery: British & European Volume* 24:556–560.

Wang H, Bishop AT, Shin AY, Spinner RJ (2008) Intraoperative testing and monitoring during brachial plexus surgery. In: *Handbook of Clinical Neurophysiology*. Elsevier, pp 720–730.

Wang S, Li P, Xue Y, Yiu H, Li YC, Wang H (2013) Contralateral C7 nerve transfer with direct coaptation to restore lower trunk function after traumatic brachial plexus avulsion. *JBJS* 95:821–827.

Ware Jr JE, Sherbourne CD (1992) The MOS 36-item short-form health survey (SF-36): I. Conceptual framework and item selection. *Medical care* 473–483.

Wilbourn AJ (2002) Nerve conduction studies: Types, components, abnormalities, and value in localization. *Neurologic Clinics* 20:305–338.

Xu J, Wang H, Hu S, Gu Y (2004) Selective transfer of the C7 nerve root: an experimental study. *Journal of reconstructive microsurgery* 20:463–470.

Zhang CG, Gu YD (2014) Contralateral C7 nerve transfer - Our experiences over past 25 years. *J Brachial Plex Peripher Nerve Inj* 06:e62–e65.

Chapter 23

Management of Cerebral Metastasis

Mohan Raj Sharma[1] and Sagar Koirala[2]
[1]Department of Neurosurgery, Tribhuvan University Teaching Hospital, Institute of Medicine, Kathmandu, Nepal
[2]Upendra Devkota Memorial National Institute of Neurological and Allied Sciences Kathmandu, Kathmandu, Nepal

Abstract

Brain metastases are a common neurological problem encountered by neurosurgeons and are the most common type of brain tumor. The five most common primary sources are lungs, breasts, kidneys, colorectal, and melanomas. The primary source may be unidentifiable in 10% to 30% at the time of diagnosis. Common presenting features include features of raised intracranial pressure, hydrocephalus, or focal deficits based on the location of the tumor. The imaging investigation of choice is magnetic resonance imaging. They represent some of the challenging cases in neurosurgery in terms of treatment. The mainstay of treatment is surgical excision for an accessible solitary lesion with radio and chemotherapy. For multiple lesions, multiple factors need to be considered before recommending treatment to the patient and family. In this chapter, we review the current literature regarding the epidemiology, clinical features, diagnostic workup, and treatment recommendations for cerebral metastasis.

Introduction

With the increasing availability of advanced diagnostic modalities and the increased life expectancy, both the incidence and prevalence of brain

In: Neurosurgery Research
Editors: Amit Agrawal, Pradeep Chouksey, Adesh Shrivastava et al.
ISBN: 978-1-68507-837-9

metastasis are on the rise. The systemic treatment given for extracranial primary malignancies may not penetrate the blood-brain barrier creating a 'safe heaven' [1]. The metastases are broadly classified as synchronous when diagnosed along with primary source or metachronous if diagnosed at a later date. The five most common primary sources are lungs, breasts, kidneys, colon and rectum, and melanomas in descending order [2]. 15 to 30% of patients with cancer elsewhere in the body eventually end up developing cerebral metastasis [3]. The primary source may be unidentifiable in 10 to 30% at the time of diagnosis [3].

Epidemiology

Brain metastases are regarded as the most common intracranial tumors in adults. Brain metastases are identified even before the primary tumor in 15% of cases. Multiple metastases are noted in up to 30-50% of the cases [3, 4]. Metastasis to the brain stem is rare. In children, metastases to the brain are mostly from Ewing's sarcoma, neuroblastoma and rhabdomyosarcomas [5].

Clinical Features

The majority of patients present with features of raised intracranial pressure, hydrocephalus, or focal deficits based on the location of the tumor. Seizure and mental status changes may also occur. Based on the site of the primary lesion other clinical features are not uncommon. Sometimes, the metastasis mimics a hemorrhagic stroke especially those from renal cell carcinomas, choriocarcinomas, and melanomas.

Investigation

A computed tomography (CT) scan shows contrast-enhancing lesion(s) typically at the grey-white junction often with extensive fingerlike vasogenic edema. Edema is strikingly more pronounced than in primary tumors. However, a magnetic resonance imaging (MRI) is the gold standard because of its superiority in picking up multiple lesions compared to CT and in detecting posterior fossa metastasis [6]. Usually, the lesions are located in the anterior circulations, more toward middle cerebral artery distribution [7]. Magnetic resonance spectroscopy can help in distinguishing metastasis from gliomas [8]. The intratumoral metabolic parameters like high choline with low N-acetylaspartate are similar in both metastases and high-grade glioma but peritumoral areas are significantly different. The peritumoral choline levels are high with low N-acetylaspartate in gliomas whereas both these parameters are normal in metastases [9].

Positron emission tomography (PET) scan can also be obtained to diagnose the occult primary, systemic metastasis elsewhere in the body using fluoro-2-deoxy-D-glucose as a tracer. The metastases are mostly hypermetabolic but in a small proportion of cases can be hypometabolic or normal [10].

Common mimickers of brain metastases are high-grade gliomas, brain abscesses, lymphomas, tuberculomas, and neurocysticercoses [6]. Rarely multifocal tumefactive demyelination and cardioembolic multifocal strokes can also be considered in the differential diagnosis [11].

Metastasis Work-up

Once metastasis is suspected or confirmed, a thorough search for primary is necessary to determine the line of further management. A CT scan of the chest and abdomen is better than X-rays and ultrasound of the abdomen. Mammogram for suspected breast source and ultrasound-guided fine-needle aspiration biopsy (FNAB) may be required if lumps are present. Similarly, other tests like PET scan for the search of tumors causing bone metastasis, prostate-specific antigen (PSA) for prostate, a genetic workup for genetic/familial cancer syndromes may be required.

Considerations before Treatment

Metastasis to the brain means it is stage IV disease for any primary tumor thereby indicating a generally poor prognosis. Treatment planning also depends on whether the primary is under control, its responsiveness to adjuvant therapies, and the overall biological behavior of primary cancer.

The treatment protocol is also governed by the aim of treatment. If our goal is histological confirmation of the lesion, easier accessible sites may be the first choice to take a biopsy. However, if the primary tumor is under control and the patient is fit for a major surgery, a complete resection of the metastasis may be contemplated.

Table 1. RPA classification with prognosis

RPA Class	Description	Median survival in months
1	KPS > 70 Age < 60 years Controlled (stable over 3 months)/absent primary with brain only site of metastasis	7
2	All others	4
3	KPS < 70	2

RPA = Radiation Therapy Oncology Group recursive partition analysis
KPS = Karnofsky Performance Scale.

The Radiation Therapy Oncology Group recursive partition analysis (RPA) classification uses Karnofsky Performance Scale (KPS), age, and nature of primary tumor to prognosticate these patients (Table 1) [12]. This classification is extremely useful to formulate the management plan.

Patients in RPA class three will not benefit from any modalities of treatment as opposed to class 1 [12].

Different management options include surgery (biopsy, partial or subtotal resection, gross total surgical excision), radiotherapy, chemotherapy, and immunotherapies either singly or in combination depending on the number of brain lesions as well as responsiveness to these therapies. It is important to involve the patient and family in the decision-making process to formulate the choice of treatment as the overall prognosis is poor.

Pretreatment with steroids is required for most of these patients to control the presenting symptoms due to the lesion and its surrounding edema [13].

Treatment Options for a Single Metastasis

Studies done in the 1990s by Patchell, Vecht, and Mintz all pointed towards the benefit of surgery followed by whole-brain radiotherapy (WBRT) in such patients [14-16]. When compared with the needle biopsy followed by radiotherapy, the surgery group had a decreased local recurrence rate (20% vs 50%), an improved overall survival (40 weeks vs 15 weeks), and prolonged functional independence (38 weeks vs 8 weeks) [14].

Indications of surgery in a patient with controlled primary and good KPS include accessible dominant lesions with a mass effect. Also, in cases where the primary is unknown or tissue diagnosis is needed, surgery is required. Patients with lesions presenting as life-threatening tumoral bleed or mass effect may also be the candidates for surgery [17].

In deep-seated lesions less than three cm in diameter, stereotactic radiosurgery (SRS) alone or in combination with whole-brain radiation can be considered [18]. One randomized controlled trial and two retrospective studies have compared the SRS against surgery followed by WBRT showing an equivalent survival [18]. However, a retrospective study done by Bindal et al., in 1996 showed a significantly longer median survival time in the surgery followed by the WBRT group when compared to SRS followed by the WBRT group (16.4 months vs 7.5 months) [19]. A recent systematic review failed to add any new information on this topic [20].

Treatment Options for up to Three Metastasis

A retrospective study by Schackert in 2002 found some benefit of surgery in patients with a limited number of metastases [21]. Surgery may be offered to patients with good preoperative health whose primary disease is under control or to those whose disease is radio-resistant. At times the dominant large lesion may have to be operated on leaving the rest of the lesion for radiotherapy in an effort to decrease the need for prolonged steroids use.

Treatment Options for Multiple Metastases

When the primary site is unknown, a biopsy may be required for diagnosis. The role of surgery is very limited otherwise. An SRS is increasingly being used for such lesions. Yamamoto and colleagues compared the effectiveness of SRS in one, two to four, and four to 10 lesions with an overall volume less than 15 ml or the largest lesion <three cm size in newly diagnosed patients

with a KPS >70. They found that the results of SRS for five to 10 lesions are not inferior to SRS for two to four lesions [22].

Recent Advances

Laser interstitial thermal therapy is an upcoming treatment modality for radioresistant metastasis and cases with recurrence after treatment. Image guidance is used to navigate the laser probe within the tumor where it is thermally ablated. It is also being used in cases failing to respond to SRS [23-24].

Studies in various phases are ongoing to evaluate the safety and efficacy of immunotherapy in brain metastasis. Of them, melanomas and non-small cell lung carcinomas seem to respond better to Ipilimumab and Pembrolizumab respectively [25-26].

Photodynamic therapy and sonodynamic therapy are other areas where research is in the preliminary stages in animal models [27]. Tumor treatment fields device that delivers alternating electric fields targeting tumor cells is also in the trial phase for various brain metastases [28].

Palliative Care

One of the most important and often neglected factors in treating these patients to consider is the quality of life of these patients as survival in most cases is limited to months. Clinicians should consider palliative care or end-of-life care to ease suffering. Hospice services are therefore equally important.

Prognosis

The median survival of the untreated patients is about one month [14]. Steroids alone might double the survival [14]. With the addition of WBRT to steroids, it has been found that the survival increases to three to six months. Surgery along with WBRT as compared to WBRT alone increases survival to 9-10 months and a better quality of life for solitary metastasis [29].

Conclusion

Brain metastasis is one of the most complex problems in neurosurgery. There is still a lot of uncertainty regarding treatment and prognosis. Though some patients may be obviously untreatable due to a delayed presentation and presence of widespread disease at diagnosis, the majority can achieve a variable increase in survival with a combined treatment with surgery, radiotherapy and chemotherapy. Further research is needed to define the optimal treatment strategy in this area.

References

Bastos D. C. A., Rao G., Oliva I. C. G., Loree J. M., Fuentes D. T., Stafford R. J., Beechar V. B., Weinberg J. S., Shah K., Kumar V. A., Prabhu S. S. Predictors of Local Control of Brain Metastasis Treated With Laser Interstitial Thermal Therapy. *Neurosurgery*. 2020 Jul 1;87(1):112-122. doi: https://10.1093/neuros/nyz357. PMID: 31539421.

Bindal A. K., Bindal R. K., Hess K. R., Shiu A., Hassenbusch S. J., Shi W. M., Sawaya R. Surgery versus radiosurgery in the treatment of brain metastasis. *J Neurosurg*. 1996 May;84(5):748-54. doi: https://10.3171/jns.1996.84.5.0748. PMID: 8622147.

Borah B. M., Cacaccio J., Durrani F. A., Bshara W., Turowski S. G., Spernyak J. A., Pandey R. K. Sonodynamic therapy in combination with photodynamic therapy shows enhanced long-term cure of brain tumor. *Sci Rep*. 2020 Dec 11;10(1):21791. doi: https://10.1038/s41598-020-78153-0. PMID: 33311561; PMCID: PMC7732989.

Delattre J. Y., Krol G., Thaler H. T., Posner J. B. Distribution of brain metastases. *Arch Neurol*. 1988 Jul;45(7):741-4. doi: https://10.1001/archneur.1988.00520310047016. PMID: 3390029.

Fares J., Kanojia D., Rashidi A., Ulasov I., Lesniak M. S. Genes that Mediate Metastasis across the Blood-Brain Barrier. *Trends Cancer*. 2020 Aug;6(8):660-676. doi: https://10.1016/j.trecan.2020.04.007. Epub 2020 May 13. PMID: 32417182; PMCID: PMC7392815.

Galldiks N., Langen K. J., Albert N. L., Chamberlain M., Soffietti R., Kim M. M., Law I., Le Rhun E., Chang S., Schwarting J., Combs S. E., Preusser M., Forsyth P., Pope W., Weller M., Tonn J. C. PET imaging in patients with brain metastasis-report of the RANO/PET group. *Neuro Oncol*. 2019 May 6;21(5):585-595. doi: https://10.1093/neuonc/noz003. PMID: 30615138; PMCID: PMC6502495.

Garsa A., Jang J. K., Baxi S., Chen C., Akinniranye O., Hall O., Larkin J., Motala A., Hempel S. Radiation Therapy for Brain Metastases: A Systematic Review. *Pract Radiat Oncol*. 2021 Sep-Oct;11(5):354-365. doi: https://10.1016/j.prro.2021.04.002. Epub 2021 Jun 9. PMID: 34119447.

Gaspar L., Scott C., Rotman M., Asbell S., Phillips T., Wasserman T., McKenna W. G., Byhardt R. Recursive partitioning analysis (RPA) of prognostic factors in three Radiation Therapy Oncology Group (RTOG) brain metastases trials. *Int J Radiat Oncol Biol Phys.* 1997 Mar 1;37(4):745-51. doi: https://10.1016/s0360-3016(96)00619-0. PMID: 9128946.

George T., Cicilet S., Hoisala R., Rout P. Multifocal Tumefactive Demyelination Mimicking Intracranial Neoplasm. *J Clin Diagn Res.* 2016 Mar;10(3):TD10-1. doi: https://10.7860/JCDR/2016/15589.7465. Epub 2016 Mar 1. PMID: 27134967; PMCID: PMC4843352.

Ghiaseddin A. P., Shin D., Melnick K., Tran D. D. Tumor Treating Fields in the Management of Patients with Malignant Gliomas. *Curr Treat Options Oncol.* 2020 Jul 30;21(9):76. doi: https://10.1007/s11864-020-00773-5. PMID: 32734509; PMCID: PMC7391234.

Hayakawa T., Yoshimine T., Arita N., Mogami H., Nakagawa H. [Metastases to the brain-prognosis and surgical indications]. *Gan To Kagaku Ryoho.* 1990 Apr;17(4 Pt 2):761-7. Japanese. PMID: 2344191.

Kaye J., Patel N. V., Danish S. F. Laser interstitial thermal therapy for in-field recurrence of brain metastasis after stereotactic radiosurgery: does treatment with LITT prevent a neurologic death? *Clin Exp Metastasis.* 2020 Jun;37(3):435-444. doi: https://10.1007/s10585-020-10035-1. Epub 2020 May 6. PMID: 32377943.

Linskey M. E., Andrews D. W., Asher A. L., Burri S. H., Kondziolka D., Robinson P. D., Ammirati M., Cobbs C. S., Gaspar L. E., Loeffler J. S., McDermott M., Mehta M. P., Mikkelsen T., Olson J. J., Paleologos N. A., Patchell R. A., Ryken T. C., Kalkanis S. N. The role of stereotactic radiosurgery in the management of patients with newly diagnosed brain metastases: a systematic review and evidence-based clinical practice guideline. *J Neurooncol.* 2010 Jan;96(1):45-68. doi: https://10.1007/s11060-009-0073-4. Epub 2009 Dec 4. Erratum in: J Neurooncol. 2010 Jan;96(1):69-70. PMID: 19960227; PMCID: PMC2808519.

Mintz A. P., Cairncross J. G. Treatment of a Single Brain Metastasis: The Role of Radiation Following Surgical Resection. *JAMA.* 1998;280(17):1527-1529. doi: https://10.1001/jama.280.17.1527.

Mintz A. P., Cairncross J. G. Treatment of a single brain metastasis: the role of radiation following surgical resection. *JAMA.* 1998 Nov 4;280(17):1527-9. doi: https://10.1001/jama.280.17.1527. PMID: 9809735.

Ostrom Q. T., Wright C. H., Barnholtz-Sloan J. S. Brain metastases: epidemiology. *Handb Clin Neurol.* 2018;149:27-42. doi: https://10.1016/B978-0-12-811161-1.00002-5. PMID: 29307358.

Patchell R. A., Tibbs P. A., Regine W. F., Dempsey R. J., Mohiuddin M., Kryscio R. J., Markesbery W. R., Foon K. A., Young B. Postoperative radiotherapy in the treatment of single metastases to the brain: a randomized trial. *JAMA.* 1998 Nov 4;280(17):1485-9. doi: https://10.1001/jama.280.17.1485. PMID: 9809728.

Pope W. B. Brain metastases: neuroimaging. *Handb Clin Neurol.* 2018;149:89-112. doi: https://10.1016/B978-0-12-811161-1.00007-4. PMID: 29307364; PMCID: PMC6118134.

Ryken T. C., McDermott M., Robinson P. D., Ammirati M., Andrews D. W., Asher A. L., Burri S. H., Cobbs C. S., Gaspar L. E., Kondziolka D., Linskey M. E., Loeffler J. S., Mehta M. P., Mikkelsen T., Olson J. J., Paleologos N. A., Patchell R. A., Kalkanis S. N. The role of steroids in the management of brain metastases: a systematic review and evidence-based clinical practice guideline. *J Neurooncol.* 2010 Jan;96(1):103-14. doi: https://10.1007/s11060-009-0057-4. Epub 2009 Dec 3. PMID: 19957014; PMCID: PMC2808527.

Schackert G. Surgery of brain metastases - pro and contra. *Onkologie.* 2002 Oct;25(5):480-1. doi: https://10.1159/000067444. PMID: 12415204.

Server A., Josefsen R., Kulle B., Maehlen J., Schellhorn T., Gadmar Ø., Kumar T., Haakonsen M., Langberg C. W., Nakstad P. H. Proton magnetic resonance spectroscopy in the distinction of high-grade cerebral gliomas from single metastatic brain tumors. *Acta Radiol.* 2010 Apr;51(3):316-25. doi: https://10.3109/02841850903482901. PMID: 20092374.

Soffietti R., Ahluwalia M., Lin N., Rudà R. Management of brain metastases according to molecular subtypes. *Nat Rev Neurol.* 2020 Oct;16(10):557-574. doi: https://10.1038/s41582-020-0391-x. Epub 2020 Sep 1. PMID: 32873927.

Stelzer K. J. Epidemiology and prognosis of brain metastases. *Surg Neurol Int.* 2013 May 2;4(Suppl 4):S192-202. doi: https://10.4103/2152-7806.111296. PMID: 23717790; PMCID: PMC3656565.

Suki D., Khoury Abdulla R., Ding M., Khatua S., Sawaya R. Brain metastases in patients diagnosed with a solid primary cancer during childhood: experience from a single referral cancer center. *J Neurosurg Pediatr*. 2014 Oct;14(4):372-85. doi: https://10.3171/2014.7.PEDS13318. Epub 2014 Aug 15. PMID: 25127097.

Tabouret E., Chinot O., Metellus P., Tallet A., Viens P., Gonçalves A. Recent trends in epidemiology of brain metastases: an overview. *Anticancer Res*. 2012 Nov;32(11):4655-62. PMID: 23155227.

Trinh A., Wintermark M., Iv M. Clinical Review of Computed Tomography and MR Perfusion Imaging in Neuro-Oncology. *Radiol Clin North Am.* 2021 May;59(3):323-334. doi: https://10.1016/j.rcl.2021.01.002. Epub 2021 Mar 23. PMID: 33926680.

Valiente M., Ahluwalia M. S., Boire A., Brastianos P. K., Goldberg S. B., Lee E. Q., Le Rhun E., Preusser M., Winkler F., Soffietti R. The Evolving Landscape of Brain Metastasis. *Trends Cancer.* 2018 Mar;4(3):176-196. doi: https://10.1016/j.trecan.2018.01.003. Epub 2018 Feb 21. PMID: 29506669; PMCID: PMC6602095.

Vecht C. J., Haaxma-Reiche H., Noordijk E. M., Padberg G. W., Voormolen J. H., Hoekstra F. H., Tans J. T., Lambooij N., Metsaars J. A., Wattendorff A. R., et al., Treatment of single brain metastasis: radiotherapy alone or combined with neurosurgery? *Ann Neurol.* 1993 Jun;33(6):583-90. doi: https://10.1002/ana.410330605. PMID: 8498838.

Yamamoto M., Serizawa T., Shuto T., Akabane A., Higuchi Y., Kawagishi J., Yamanaka K., Sato Y., Jokura H., Yomo S., Nagano O., Kenai H., Moriki A., Suzuki S., Kida Y., Iwai Y., Hayashi M., Onishi H., Gondo M., Sato M., Akimitsu T., Kubo K., Kikuchi Y., Shibasaki T., Goto T., Takanashi M., Mori Y., Takakura K., Saeki N., Kunieda E., Aoyama H., Momoshima S., Tsuchiya K. Stereotactic radiosurgery for patients with multiple brain metastases (JLGK0901): a multi-institutional prospective observational study. *Lancet Oncol.* 2014 Apr;15(4):387-95. doi: https://10.1016/S1470-2045(14)70061-0. Epub 2014 Mar 10. PMID: 24621620.

Chapter 24

Initiating, Developing and Structuring a Pediatric Neurosurgery Healthcare System: A Quality Improvement Venue

Hector E. James*, **MD, FAANS, FAAP, FCCM**

Department of Neurosurgery, University of Florida College of Medicineand Pediatric Neurosurgery Consultant, Wolfson Children's Hospital/Baptist Health of Northeast Florida, Jacksonville, Florida, USA

Abstract

Family-centered care has been identified as a major advance in the quality of care. This is a report on the initiation, development and structuring of a child/family-centered pediatric neurosurgery healthcare system. The organizational matrix for the development of a pediatric neurosurgery healthcare system was structured through a multi-institutional and multidisciplinary effort, centered at a tertiary care children's hospital. The Division of Pediatric Neurosurgery was created in September 2003 at the University of Florida College of Medicine Jacksonville and Wolfson Children's Hospital/Baptist Health of Northeast Florida. The pediatric neurosurgery service was developed with a medical matrix (pediatric neurosurgeon and physician assistant), and administrative matrix (two medical secretaries) and a hospital matrix (pre-operative, operative and post-operative patient care). The second phase consisted of a staged development of a pediatric neurosurgery healthcare system consisting of multidisciplinary and multi-institutional supporting matrices for a care continuum: Fetal Diagnosis and Therapy

*Correspondence to: Hector E. James, MD, 400 E. Bay Street, Suite 507, Jacksonville, FL 32202. Email: hector.james@jax.ufl.edu.

In: Neurosurgery Research
Editors: Amit Agrawal, Pradeep Chouksey, Adesh Shrivastava et al.
ISBN: 978-1-68507-837-9

Center, Spinal Defects Clinic, Pediatric Neurosciences Clinic, Spasticity Program and Clinic, Brachial Plexus Program and Clinic, Craniofacial Program and Clinic, Epilepsy Surgery Program, Neuro-Oncology Clinic, and Telemedicine Clinics. Neurosurgeons can and should take the lead in creating venues for child/family-centered care by co-opting with physicians and allied healthcare professionals from other specialties, healthcare authorities and hospital administrations, in organizing the framework for comprehensive programs and clinics.

Introduction

Major advances have taken place in the neurosurgical care of infants, children, and adolescents. Clinical outcome measures are being documented and reported and are subject of ongoing research. The neurosurgical care of infants, children and adolescents requires a dedicated team with neurological surgeons, allied health, and administrative personnel. This team is necessary for the preoperative evaluation and diagnosis, planning and execution of neurosurgical interventions, operative procedures, postoperative care, recovery and initiating rehabilitation. For this manuscript we will call this team the pediatric neurosurgery service (PNS) and its primary purpose is the care of the *child's neurosurgical condition.*

Many infants, children and adolescents with neurosurgical conditions require ongoing and long-term care to provide best clinical outcomes. The parents/caregivers of the child with a neurosurgical condition are faced with a child who has *chronic healthcare needs* (CCHN). Comprehensive and coordinated care models in pediatrics have been shown to lower healthcare and social costs by reducing hospitalization and fewer days lost from work by the parents. [1-6] The PNS is not designed to meet chronic healthcare needs, and consequently the child ultimately may not attain the best outcome. To facilitate care of neurosurgical conditions as well as the chronic healthcare needs of the child and family, it is necessary to have access to a healthcare system. For this manuscript this will be called a *pediatric neurosurgery healthcare system* (PNHCS).

Many pediatric neurosurgery services provide comprehensive healthcare to their patients. The purpose of this report is to describe the initiation, structuring and development of a PNS and a PNHCS (Table 1), with the ultimate intent to provide information that may help those considering developing or improving healthcare services for the child/family with a neurosurgical condition and chronic healthcare needs.

Materials and Methods

Initiation and Development of the Pediatric Neurosurgery Service (PNS)

The PNS was initiated with the creation of the Division of Pediatric Neurosurgery in the Department of Neurosurgery at the University of Florida (UF) College of Medicine Jacksonville and Wolfson Children's Hospital (WCH)/Baptist Health of Northeast Florida in September 2003. At that time, the team consisted of one pediatric neurosurgeon, one physician assistant (PA) and two administrative personnel. The primary office of the PNS was located within WCH, the only pediatric tertiary care center for Northeast Florida and Southeast Georgia, with a multi-institutional medical faculty from the UF Health Jacksonville and Nemours Children's Health (NCH) Jacksonville, along with pediatricians and subspecialty pediatricians from within the community. Supporting services already established included, but were not limited to neonatology, perinatology, pediatric anesthesia, pediatric critical care, pediatric endocrinology, pediatric general surgery, pediatric hematology/oncology, pediatric hospitalists, pediatric neurology, pediatric pulmonary medicine, pediatric radiology, pediatric urology, radiation therapy and radiosurgery (Figure 1). The pediatric neurosurgery outpatient and inpatient services were initiated in October 2003 (Figure 2). Operative interventions were performed by the neurosurgeon and assisted by the PA (Figure 3). In 2006 a second pediatric neurosurgeon joined the faculty, as well as an advance practice registered nurse (APRN). The clinical roles of the PA and the APRN were interchangeable, and previously reported by the author [7]. In 2010 a second APRN joined the team, followed by two additional pediatric neurosurgeons in 2012, and a third APRN in 2013. Multidisciplinary outpatient clinics and services were progressively developed (Figure 4).

Initiation and Development of the Pediatric Neurosurgery Healthcare System (PNHS)

A series of organizational steps were taken with the hospital administration, interested parties and medical personnel. Some of these developed more rapidly than others and are listed in the chronological order in which they occurred (Table 1).

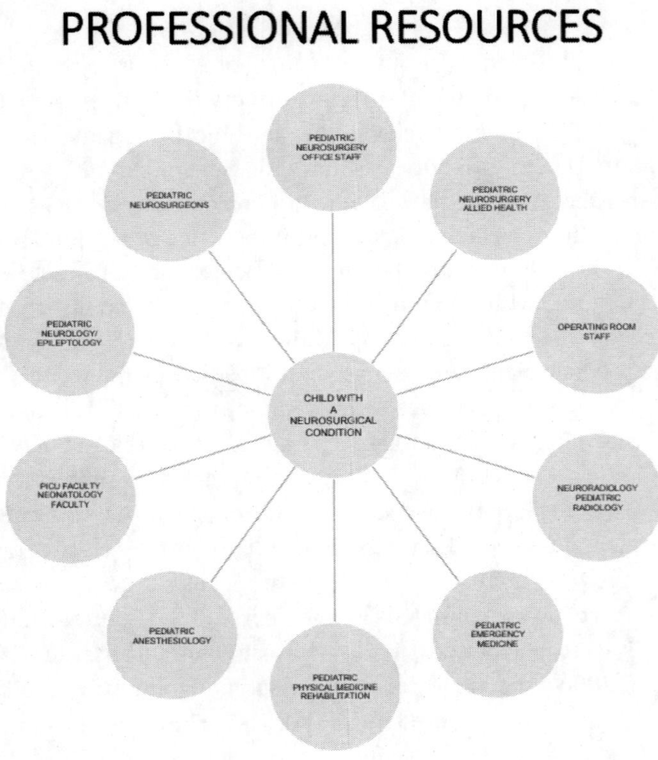

Figure 1. Professional Resources for a Child with a Neurosurgical Condition.

Fetal Diagnosis and Therapy Center

Preliminary communication between perinatology, neonatology and neurosurgery started in September 2003 for the purpose of initiating a forum to discuss pregnancies of a fetus with a clinically significant condition. This led to an organizational team meeting in March 2004. Subsequently, clinical genetics, pediatric cardiology and radiology were requested to participate in the monthly sessions. Over the ensuing months, other disciplines were invited, and membership was expanded, followed by the establishment of a meeting format. Meetings have since been held monthly. During the sessions, ongoing pregnancies with a fetus with a significant clinical condition are presented, imaging is reviewed, and management decisions are made. By creating a collaborative venue, lines of communication were established within the team, permitting prompt availability for urgent interdisciplinary consultations. A detailed description of the creation and development of the Fetal Diagnosis and Therapy Center has previously been published by the author [8].

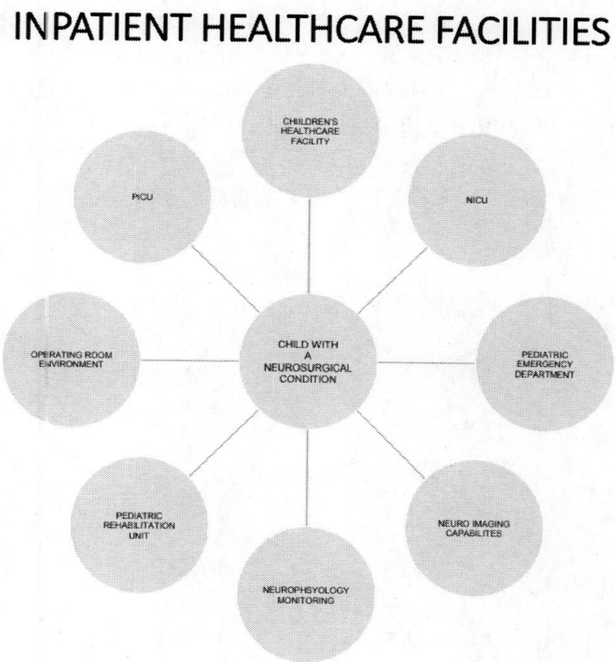

Figure 2. Inpatient Health Care Facilities for a Child with a Neurosurgical Condition.

Spinal Defects Clinic

In December 2003 communications between pediatric neurosurgery, WCH administration and the WCH Department of Rehabilitation led to establishing a location as well as administrative support for a multidisciplinary clinic for children with spina bifida. The purpose was to provide ongoing comprehensive long-term care for the child/family with spina bifida and other forms of spinal disorders. Additional members that were subsequently added were: pediatrician, pediatric urology, pediatric orthopedics, physical therapy, and social services. Subsequently, developmental medicine and physical medicine/rehabilitation physicians joined the team. The first clinic was held in June 2004. Half day monthly clinics have been held since. The patient and family are evaluated by the team, and upon completion of the examinations, a clinic management conference is held. The clinic Medical Director (the developmental medicine pediatrician) presides the conference, during which time medical and social needs are discussed, care decisions and return to clinic appointments are made. A clinic report is generated and distributed to the patient's primary care physician, parents, and medical personnel of interest. Further details on the initiation, development and structuring of the Spinal Defects Clinic are published elsewhere [9].

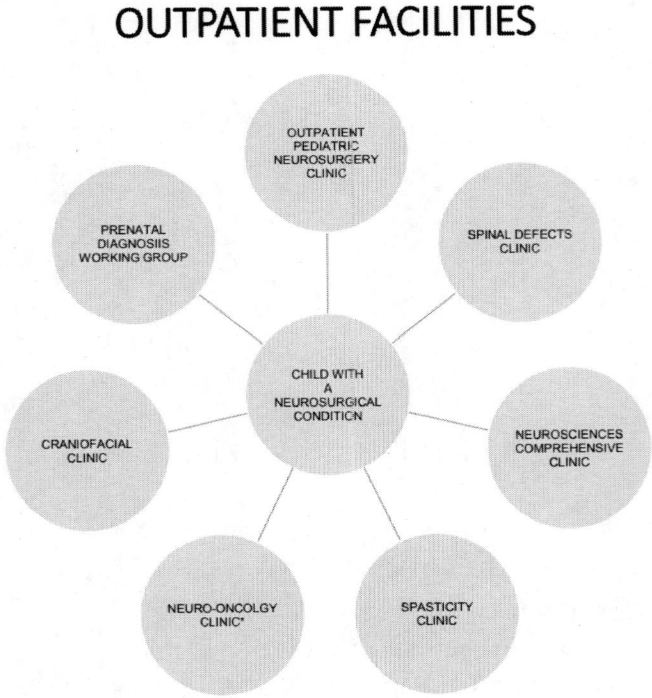

Figure 3. Schematic Representation of the Inpatient Care Sequence for a Child with a Neurosurgical Condition.

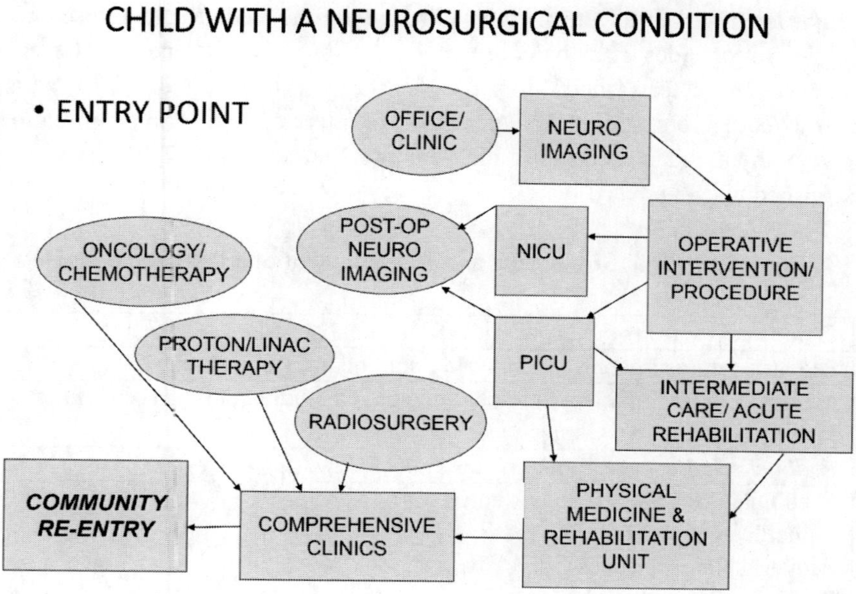

Figure 4. Key Outpatient Care Facilities for a Pediatric Healthcare System.

Pediatric Neurosciences Clinic

In early 2006 discussions were initiated between pediatric neurosurgery, WCH administration, the director of the UF Division of Developmental Medicine, and the administrative director of WCH Rehabilitation, as to establishing ongoing outpatient care for children with a neurosurgical condition with chronic healthcare needs, *other than spina bifida.* The neurosurgical conditions were to be, but not limited to hydrocephalus, moderate or severe head injury, encephaloceles and others. Meeting location, format and team members were discussed. The clinic was titled "Pediatric Neurosciences Clinic" and team members included, but were not limited to pediatric neurosurgery, developmental medicine, pediatric physical/occupational therapy, and social services. Pediatric physical medicine and rehabilitation subsequently became part of the consulting team. The first clinic was held in April 2007, and the monthly half-day clinics have been ongoing. At each clinic, the patient and family are evaluated by the team members and a clinic conference is held at completion of the evaluations. At the conference, medical and social issues are addressed, management issues discussed and priorities in care and return clinic visits, are determined. The developmental medicine pediatrician serves as the medical director of the Pediatric Neurosciences Clinic and presides over the conference. A team report is generated for each patient and forwarded to the child's primary care physician, parents/caregivers, and medical personnel of interest. Details on the initiation, development and structuring of the Pediatric Neurosciences Clinic have been published elsewhere [10].

Table 1. Initiation, Structuring and Development of a PNS and a PNHCS

Pediatric Neurosurgery Service (PNS)
Pediatric neurosurgeons, allied health, administrative personnel.
Medical Center: Inpatient Service, Imaging, Operating and Interventional Facilities, Outpatient Clinics.
Pediatric Neurosurgery Healthcare System (PNHCS)
Fetal Diagnosis and Therapy Center Spinal Defects Clinic Pediatric Neurosciences Clinic Spasticity Program and Clinic Brachial Plexus Program and Clinic Craniosynostosis/Craniofacial Program and Clinic Epilepsy Surgery Program Neuro-Oncology Clinic Telemedicine Clinics

Spasticity Program and Clinic

In the period of 2007 through 2009 conversations were established between pediatric neurosurgery, WCH administration, and the chairman of the UF Department of Pediatrics, as to the need to recruit a pediatric physical medicine physician. The purpose was to develop a comprehensive program for the evaluation, diagnostic work up, management strategies and long-term care of the child/family with spasticity.

In July 2009, a pediatric physical medicine (PPM) physician was recruited and following organizational discussions with WCH administration, the administrative director of the WCH Department of Rehabilitation, a clinic site was selected, and clinic staffing was determined. The first Spasticity Clinic was held in December 2009. In the clinic, patient and parents are jointly evaluated by the PPM physician and physical therapist. Pediatric neurosurgery is available for consultations. One APRN was recruited in 2011 to assist with the PPM program and spasticity clinics. Subsequently, WCH administration assigned a social services worker to the clinic team. At each clinic visit, the parents are informed as to the clinical findings and management recommendations, consultations, potential procedures, and interventions. Return to the clinic for reassessment following ongoing therapy, as well as interventions and further therapeutic decisions are outlined. Patients who are candidates for baclofen pumps or rhizotomies are referred to pediatric neurosurgery for evaluation and consultation. Monthly interdisciplinary management conferences were initiated in January 2010 for patients who are considered candidates for operative interventions. Conference participants include, but are not limited to pediatric neurosurgery, pediatric orthopedics, physical therapy, occupational therapy, social services, and the PPM physicians (who serve as the meeting coordinators). Both medical and social needs of the patient/family are discussed, and the care plan is determined. Physical medicine then communicates meeting results to parents/caregivers.

In 2010 the clinics were held once per week, but the demand led to increasing the days to twice per week in 2011, followed by three days per week in 2013. A second PPM physician was recruited in 2012, followed by a third in 2013. A second APRN was recruited in 2014. A detailed report on the initiation, development and structuring of the spasticity program has been previously published [11].

Brachial Plexus Program and Clinic

In 2010 communication commenced between WCH Administration, WCH Rehabilitation and the UF Division of Pediatric Physical Medicine to establish a clinic for the evaluation, diagnostic tests, procedures, interventions, and long-term management of the child/family with a brachial plexus injury. A monthly half-day "Brachial Plexus Clinic" was initiated in 2011.

In this clinic, the children are jointly evaluated by pediatric physical medicine and pediatric occupational therapy. In addition, a pediatric neurosurgeon and an orthopedic hand surgeon are readily available for consultation. Diagnostic tests, therapy recommendations and follow up appointments are made during the clinic visit. A report is completed by a PPM physician and sent to the patient's primary care provider, and when necessary, to consultants. Patients are re-evaluated following an appropriate pediatric occupational therapy treatment course and treatment adjustments made. For those patients in whom surgical correction may be necessary, referrals are made to pediatric neurosurgery and orthopedic/hand surgery. The parents/caregivers are informed as to the team discussion of the proposed surgical alternatives. If the decision for surgery is made, interventions are performed by the pediatric neurosurgery and hand surgery orthopedic team. Long term follow-up and therapy recommendations are provided by PPM and pediatric occupational therapy. Due to an increase in patient volume, the Brachial Plexus Clinic was increased from monthly to weekly sessions.

Craniosynostosis/Craniofacial Program and Clinic

In 2003 communications were established between pediatric neurosurgery and the UF Department of Maxillofacial Surgery with the purpose of evaluating and caring for children with craniofacial disorders, which lead to establishing a monthly joint craniofacial clinic at UF Health Jacksonville. Team members include, but are not limited to plastic surgery, pediatrics, dentistry, clinical nursing, speech therapy, and social services. Clinical genetics provides consulting services. The clinic meets monthly and team members evaluate the medical and social needs of the child and family. A team meeting is held following patient evaluation during which clinical findings are discussed, management decisions made, return visits determined, and a clinic visit report generated. This report is forwarded to the patient's primary care physician and team members. Referrals to other disciplines, including healthcare and or state agencies, medical insurance companies and/or schools, are followed-up by the nurse coordinator and/or social worker. Craniofacial reconstructions are performed by a surgical team consisting of a pediatric neurosurgeon and a maxillofacial surgeon. Postoperative continuity of care is performed in the craniofacial clinic visits. In 2011 the clinic relocated to the State of Florida Children's Medical Services Clinic in downtown Jacksonville, with expansion of the team to include other specialties and resources.

Epilepsy Surgery Program

In 2009 communications were initiated between pediatric neurosurgery, NCH Division of Pediatric Neurology and WCH Administration, as to the initiation of a pediatric surgical epilepsy program. Following a series of administrative steps, the program structure was defined and initiated in 2010, with further development of phases in the pre-operative care sequence through 2015. The NCH Division of Pediatric Neurology has had a longstanding presence in Jacksonville and serves the region of Northern Florida and Southern Georgia in the caring of children with epilepsy. Inpatient continuous EEG monitoring was established for the pediatric critical care unit, and inpatient EEG/video monitoring unit was built into the Neurosciences Floor at WCH. Recruitment of EEG technologists was completed and training on continuous monitoring in an inpatient and outpatient setting provided. Protocols were established and defined for the preoperative work up sequence of neurology evaluation, patient selection, and continuous video EEG inpatient monitoring (length of monitoring was determined by the patient's clinical status, video, and MRI findings). Results are then presented in a multidisciplinary epilepsy conference. If indicated, the patient is referred to a pediatric neurology epileptologist. Preoperative work-up is then pursued when indicated with, but not limited to positron emission tomography (PET), scintillating positron emission computed tomography (SPECT), clinical neuropsychology and preoperative video EEG continuous monitoring. The results are then presented at a second epilepsy multidisciplinary conference. If it is then decided that surgical intervention is warranted, the patient and family are scheduled to meet with pediatric neurosurgery. The reason for the planned interventions, objectives, potential risks, and complications are discussed with the parents/caregivers. Interventions discussed include but are not limited to placement of cortical grids/ depth electrodes, postoperative monitoring in the neurosciences ward or pediatric intensive care unit, subsequent definitive surgery, recovery, and rehabilitation therapy.

In 2010 the National Association of Epilepsy Centers certified WCH as a Pediatric Epilepsy Center. At that time, the Jacksonville center was only one of two Pediatric Epilepsy Centers in the entire State of Florida.

Neuro-Oncology Clinic

In 2012 and 2013 communications were established between UF Division of Pediatric Neurosurgery and the NCH Division of Hematology/Oncology for providing continuity and longitudinal long-term care to children with tumors of the nervous system. The first multidisciplinary Neuro-Oncology Clinic was held in October 2013.

Patients and parents/caregivers are evaluated by the team members in the UF Department of Pediatrics Multispecialty Clinic, located next to WCH. Team members include, but are not limited to pediatric neurosurgery, pediatric oncology, pediatric neurology, radiation oncology, clinical neuropsychology, and social work. Each specialty prepares a clinic report which is then forwarded to the primary care physician and team members. The NCH Division of Hematology/Oncology informs the parents/caregivers as to the recommendations made from the team.

In the early stages, the clinic met quarterly, but due to the clinical volume it was changed to every other month. A total of 45 patients were seen in the clinic during the period October 2014 through March 2015.

Telemedicine Clinics

In 2009 the State of Georgia Department of Health/Children's Medical Services (CMS) communicated to UF Division of Pediatric Neurosurgery the need for a pediatric neurosurgery telemedicine clinic for patients residing in southern Georgia, which would provide healthcare services across geographical, social, and cultural barriers. The patients included those who had an established neurosurgical diagnosis and required follow-up assessments, and/or new patients identified by CMS medical staff. The region is comprised of 16 counties located in southeast Georgia (Area 9-2) and served by the CMS office centered in the town of Waycross. The office has a regional medical director, six nurses and an administrative staff. The organizational matrix established for the purpose of medical quality had three basic components: administrative, electronic connectivity and patient care.

The *administrative* matrix provides identification of the patient referral source and parent/legal guardian information, written authorization from the healthcare insurance, and completion of documentation of healthcare information. The *electronic connectivity* matrix provides full audiovisual point-to-point communications with the patient, parents, and nurse, in a private setting. The *patient care* matrix provides nurses knowledgeable of telemedicine patient care, face-to-face encounters with the pediatric neurosurgeon, documentation of the encounters, and generation of a medical report to the primary referral physician/nurse and local clinic(s). Following completion of the organizational steps, the first clinic was held in February 2011 and subsequent clinic sessions scheduled. A total of 40 clinic sessions have been held through January 2016, with a total of 43 patient evaluated. If urgent clinical situations arise in between clinics, consultations are placed to pediatric neurosurgery by telephone or by email. Patients requiring neurosurgical interventions are hospitalized at WCH.

Preliminary Outcomes

Studies on outcomes of the clinics/programs are ongoing. We here report some preliminary results.

In the Spinal Defects Clinic, program questionnaires were provided to patients seen during the period of June 2004 through February 2009. There was a response rate of 54%. Of these, 62% indicated because of the clinic visits they had acquired more knowledge of their child's condition and medical needs. Additionally, the 62% indicated they had more information on their child's condition than they had received prior to clinic participation. Fifty-two percent (52%) stated that the care of their child was better coordinated than it had been prior to clinic initiation. Twenty-six percent (26%) stated that the clinic had reduced their travel time between medical appointments, as compared to before clinic participation [9]. A survey tool was developed addressing access to healthcare and quality of life based on an established survey for those patients with spina bifida that were transitioned from the Spinal Defects Clinic at WCH to adult services through the Jacksonville Health and Transition Services (JaxHATS) Clinic located within UF Health Jacksonville. Ten of 12 patients responded to the survey. The mean age was 25.1 years. All reported regular medical home visits, and ready access to medical care with no delays. Seven respondents reported very good to excellent quality of life [12].

In the Pediatric Neurosciences Clinic, a follow-up assessment of 71 patients seen in the clinic, documentation was received from parents/caregivers in the subsequent clinic visits, as to whether they had followed the recommendations for educational placement and/or pediatric occupational assessments and therapy. Eighty percent (80%) of the patients whose parents/caregivers had private insurance followed up on the recommendations for changes in school placement to better meet their child's neurocognitive needs, and 20% did not. In those with parents with government sponsored insurance, only 45% of the parents/caregivers followed up on the recommendations for changes in school placement [13]. The impact of this discrepancy related to the socioeconomic status of the families and is still under investigation.

In the Fetal Diagnosis and Therapy Center, the team members were surveyed as to how the FDTC had impacted their day-to-day activities. The vast majority indicated they had found the lines of communication between team members and departments that were previously poor or nonexistent had now been established, which facilitated for more timely and efficient patient care. They indicated team members were able to have a cohesive and timely approach in providing information to parents, thereby facilitating better education for medical decision making. They found the delivery, timing and immediate postnatal management was more efficient. Palliative/hospice care personnel found they were able to establish timely prenatal contact with parents with a fetus with a significant condition and build a relationship for addressing postnatal management issues. The pediatric neurosurgery team members were able to perform a timely and coordinated postnatal management plan for the newborn because they had the opportunity to inform and educate the parents, in the prenatal consultations.

In the Telemedicine Clinic, the CMS nurses reported parent/caregiver satisfaction from their TMC visits. They indicated they had acquired the necessary medical information to understand their child's medical condition, as well as future management needs. The CMS nurses also expressed that each session was a form of medical education that they would not have been otherwise exposed to, without telemedicine participation. Other venues for outcome/documentation are continuously being addressed.

Discussion

It has been recommended that new models of healthcare delivery and care coordination be entertained to address behavioral, social and environmental determinants of healthcare [14]. Comprehensive and coordinated patient care models have shown to lower healthcare and social costs through reduced hospitalizations and fewer days lost from work by the parents [1-6]. Parents/caregivers of children with chronic healthcare needs (CCHN) need to navigate not only medical issues and insurance, but also educational and social needs. It has been recently documented that a "patient-centered medical home" decreased the use of unnecessary or avoidable medical services, improved access to healthcare, improved preventive services and reduced healthcare costs [15]. Toomey and colleagues reported that 91% of parents of CCHN with some form of brain insult, stated they had unmet care coordination [16]. Children with some form of brain insult may provide a spectrum of various neurocognitive and mental health disorders, which then becomes a chronic learning disability and healthcare problem into adulthood [17-18].

The pediatric neurosurgery healthcare *system* was created in a stepwise fashion over time to help the pediatric neurosurgery *service* best provide continuity and long-term care for the CCHN and his or her parents/caregivers. Like any healthcare system, it is constantly being refined, and quality improvement needs are being addressed to meet new strategies and determinants of child/family health (Figure 5).

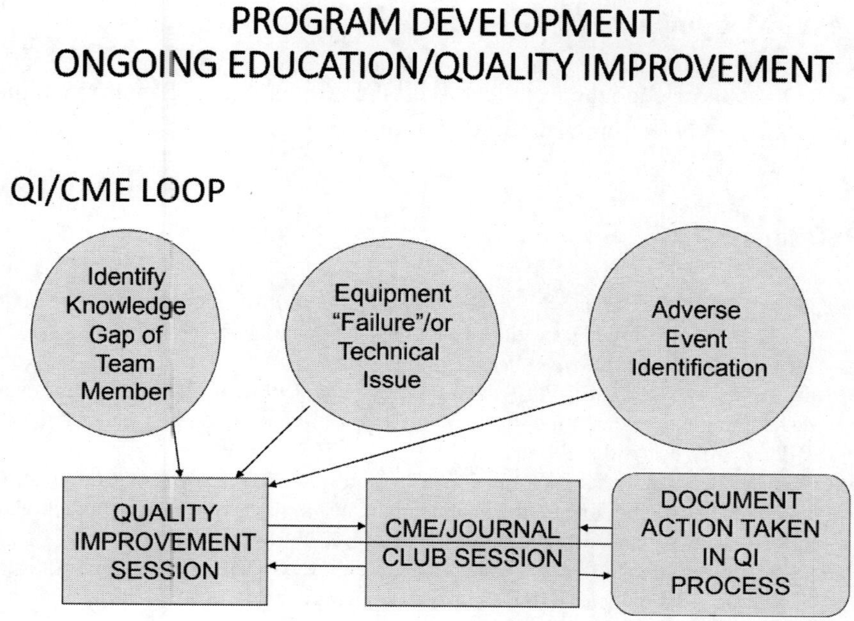

Figure 5. Schematic Representation of Ongoing Education and Quality Improvement Loop for Development and Maintenance of a Pediatric Neurosurgery Healthcare System.

Conclusion

Neurosurgeons can and should take the lead in creating systems that best provide continuity and long-term care for the child/family with a neurosurgical condition and chronic healthcare needs, which should provide a venue for best clinical outcomes for the child and his/her family. Neurosurgeons should strive by creating the necessary enthusiasm with their colleagues, allied health personnel, healthcare authorities and hospital administration for interdisciplinary communication and collaboration to enhance healthcare delivery to their patients and families.

Acknowledgments

I wish to acknowledge the excellent assistance from Jennifer Santarone in the preparation and electronic submission of this report.

References

Aguilera, A. M., Wood, D. L., Keely, C., James, H. E., and Aldana, P. R. (2016) Young adults with spina bifida transitioned to a medical home: a survey of medical care in Jacksonville, Florida. *J. Neurosurg. Pediatr.* 17:203-207.

Aldana, P. R., Wood, D. L., Postlethwait, R. A., and James, H. E. (2010) Initiating, developing and evaluating a comprehensive spinal defects clinic: a clinical report. *Pediatr. Neurosurg.* 46:329-334.

American Academy of Pediatrics Council on Children with Disabilities: Care Coordination in the medical home: integrating health and related systems of care for children with special health care needs. (2005) *Pediatrics* 116:1238-1244.

Barbaresi, W. J., Colligan, R. C., Weaver, A. L., Voigt, R. G., Killian, J. M., and Katusic, S. K. (2013) Mortality, ADHD, and psychological adversity in adults with childhood ADHD: a prospective study. *Pediatrics* 131:637-644.

Bilenker, J. H., Weller, W. E., Shaffer, T. J., Dover, G. J., and Anderson, G. F. (1998) The costs of children with sickle cell anemia: preparing for managed care. *J. Pediatr. Hematol. Oncol.* 20:528-533.

Farmer, J. E., Clark, M. K., Sherman, A., Marien, W. E., and Selva, T. J. (2005) Comprehensive primary care for children with special health care needs in rural areas. *Pediatrics* 116:649-656.

Hussey, P. S., Eibner, C., Ridgely, S., and McGlynn, E. A. (2009) Controlling US Health care spending – separate promising from unpromising approaches. *N. Engl. J. Med.* 361:2109-2111.

James, H. E., Hofrichter, P. B., Spierre, L. Z., and Aldana, P. R. (2013) Initiating a pediatric spasticity program with multi-specialty and multi-institutional support: a preliminary report. *Pediatr. Neurosurg.* 49:11-15.

James, H. E., MacGregor, T. L., Aldana, P. R. (2011) Creating a working group for prenatal diagnosis and management as a venue to facilitate neurosurgery health care delivery. *Pediatr. Neurosurg.* 47:176-179.

James, H. E., MacGregor, T. L., Childers, D. O. Jr, La Corte, E., and Aldana, P. R. (2014) Pediatric neurosurgery patients need more than a pediatric neurosurgeon: a clinical experience. *Pediatr. Neurosurg.* 49:63-68.

James, H. E., MacGregor, T. L., Postlethwait, R. A., Hofrichter, P. B., and Aldana, P. R. (2011) Advanced registered nurse practitioners and physician assistants in the practice of pediatric neurosurgery: a clinical report. *Pediatr. Neurosurg.* 47:359-363.

MacGregor, T. L., James, H. E., Everett, L., and Childers, D. O. Jr. (2016) Pediatric neurosurgery patients need more than a pediatric neurosurgeon. Part II. A clinical report: in the USA lack of parent/caregiver compliance interferes with the patient care sequence. *Pediatr. Neurosurg.* 51:229-235.

Nielsen, M., Olayiwola, J. N., Grundy, P., and Grumbach, K. (2014) *The patient-centered medical home's impact on cost and quality: an annual update of evidence 2012-2013.* Available via: https://www.pcpcc.org/resource/medical-homes-impact-cost-quality Accessed 16 Mar 2021.

Palfrey, J. S., Sofis, L. A., Davidson, E. J., Liu, J., Freeman, L., and Ganz, M. L. (2004) The pediatric alliance for coordinated care: evaluation of a medical home model. *Pediatrics* 113:1507-1516.

Starfield, B., and Shi, L. (2004) The medical home, access to care, and insurance: a review of the evidence. *Pediatrics* 113:1493-1498.

Toomey, S. L., Chien, A. T., Elliott, M. N., Ratner, J., and Schuster, M. A. (2013) Disparities in unmet need for care coordination. *National Survey of Children's Health* 131:217-224.

Van Lieshout, R. J., Boyle, M. H., Saigal, S., Morrison, K., and Schmidt, L. A. (2015) Mental health of extremely low birth weight survivors in their 30s. *Pediatrics* 135(3):452-459.

Wood, D. L., and Goldhagen, J. L. (2013) Promoting child health equity: family-centered care coordination is just one piece of the puzzle. *Pediatrics* 131:336-337.

Chapter 25

A Working Group for Prenatal Diagnosis and Management as a Venue to Facilitate Neurosurgery Health Care Delivery: A Report on a 14-Year Experience

Hector E. James[1,*], MD and Alexandra D. Beier[2], DO

[1]Department of Neurosurgery, University of Florida College of Medicine and Pediatric Neurosurgery Consultant, Wolfson Children's Hospital/Baptist Health of Northeast Florida, Jacksonville, Florida, USA

[2]Department of Neurosurgery, University of Florida College of Medicine Jacksonville and Lucy Gooding Pediatric Neurosurgery Center at Wolfson Children's Hospital/Baptist Health of Northeast Florida, Jacksonville, Florida, USA

Abstract

To improve communication with the parents of a fetus with a neurosurgical condition, as well as care of the newborn, a working group was created in 2004. The University of Florida Division of Pediatric Neurosurgery created a staged process for the development of a prenatal working group. This addresses the activities of the group for the period of March 2004 to December 2018. This report provides results for a total of 1144 pregnancies discussed in the monthly sessions of the working group, 139 of which generated neurosurgical consultations based on prenatal imaging. Those requiring postnatal surgery were able to receive scheduled delivery and neurosurgical procedures. The interdisciplinary

*Correspondence to Hector E. James, MD, 400 E. Bay Street, Suite 507, Jacksonville, FL 32202. Email: hector.james@jax.ufl.edu.

In: Neurosurgery Research
Editors: Amit Agrawal, Pradeep Chouksey, Adesh Shrivastava et al.
ISBN: 978-1-68507-837-9

activity facilitated better communication with parents/families, coordination of delivery, and timely postnatal management.

Introduction

Progress in obstetrics, perinatology, prenatal imaging of the fetus with ultrasonography (US), and magnetic resonance imaging (MRI) has created improved venues of identifying fetal neurosurgical conditions. The consequence has been early referral of parents with a fetus who may need alternative delivery methods, possible intrauterine intervention, and/or postnatal surgery. Timely and effective communication with neurosurgeons, perinatologists and other healthcare personnel enables an efficient and caring venue. Early informed engagement between the parents and neurosurgeon provides education as to the care and timing of the neurosurgical condition. Sharing of information permits decisions related to mode of delivery and postnatal management.

Initiation, structuring and development of the prenatal diagnosis and management working group has previously been reported [1]. This report provides the experience of activities, sequence of patient care and administrative functions and healthcare delivery during the period of March 2004 to December 2018. We wish to share this experience with the hope that other neurosurgeons with restricted or no access to a team approach may develop a similar working group in their location.

Materials and Methods

In a previous report we address the process of initiation, formation, and structure of the Fetal Diagnosis & Therapy Center [1]. This provided initial exploratory lines of communication with interested parties (Phase I), organizational and initial meetings with a limited number of team members (Phase II), and expansion of team member participation with other specialists of interest as well as monthly clinical meetings (Phase III) [1].

Monthly Center Meetings

The multidisciplinary team has structured monthly clinical sessions. The initial meeting participation was limited to perinatology, neonatology, and neurosurgery. When format, style, and structure of the meetings was finalized, other specialties were invited to participate. The current working group includes pediatric cardiology, pediatric general surgery, genetics, neonatology, pediatric neurosurgery, perinatology, radiology, and pediatric urology. The team is constituted by members from the University of Florida College of Medicine Jacksonville (UFCOMJ), Wolfson Children's Hospital (WCH)/Baptist Health of Northeast Florida, Nemours Children's Specialty Care Jacksonville (NCSCJ), private practicing perinatologists from Regional Obstetric Consultants (ROC)/Mednex, palliative care from a regional hospice care organization (Community PedsCare). Current team members are listed on Table 1. Other services are listed as consultants and are contacted for specific clinical needs.

Table 1. Center team members

Clinical Genetics
Neonatology
Obstetrics
Palliative Care
Pediatric Cardiology
Pediatric Cardiac Surgery
Pediatric Neurosurgery
Pediatric Radiology
Pediatric Surgery
Pediatric Urology
Perinatology (presides and documents monthly meetings)

Results

The period of this report is from March 2004 to December 2018. Of the 1144 patients discussed in clinic sessions, 139 (12.2%) generated a pediatric neurosurgery consultation. Listed in Table 2 are the clinical diagnoses that initiated the consultation. Nonspecific cerebral anomalies such as dysgenesis, schizencephaly, and nondiagnostic anatomical variations were the most common intrauterine anomalies (43). Ventriculomegaly/hydrocephalus was the second most frequent condition (34). Myelomeningocele was detected in 19 and confirmed in 11. Other prenatally diagnosed anomalies are listed in Table 2.

Table 2. Nervous system anomalies

Brain Developmental Anomalies (non-surgical)	43
Hydrocephalus/Ventriculomegaly	34
Myelomeningocele	19
Dandy Walker Malformation/Variant	11
Encephalocele/Meningocele Complex	11
Sacral Teratoma	6
Brain Parenchymal Cyst	5
Intracranial Hemorrhage	3
Terminal Myelocystocele	2
Spine Anomaly, unspecified	2
Brain Tumor	1
Brain AVM	1
Mega Cisterna Magna	1

Patients with a suspected neurosurgical condition discussed in the prenatal conference were referred for consultation in the pediatric neurosurgery office. Exceptions to this were those requiring urgent consultation because of late diagnosis, and/or impending delivery. Pertinent postnatal studies and/or interventions were scheduled based on estimated delivery dates. Perinatology discussed with obstetrics the mechanism for delivery and preferable dates. The neurosurgeon met with and educated the parents prenatally and initiated postnatal care process with informed consents for procedures. For the high risk and potentially poor outcome patient population, prenatal referrals to palliative care were requested.

Prenatal Imaging Sequences

Obstetricians routinely perform prenatal ultrasounds for evaluation of the fetus and pelvic structure of the mother. A perinatology referral is initiated when the fetus with a clinical condition is identified and/or pathology of the maternal pelvis raises concern. Perinatology consultation and examination with 3D ultrasonography follows. The consulting of perinatology decides if clinical and imaging findings indicate the need for MRI for further evaluation of the pelvic structures and/or fetus. Request for authorization is initiated with the insurance industry and scheduling of prenatal imaging is performed at WCH. A pediatric radiologist supervises the study to ensure pertinent imaging is obtained. The report is sent to the referring perinatologist and obstetrician. Imaging findings are discussed in the subsequent monthly center meeting.

Aspects of Care Coordination

Perinatology communicates to the obstetrician the team report and studies. A decision is then made as to timing and location of delivery. When indicated, deliveries are performed at Baptist Medical Center Downtown, adjacent to WCH, for prompt access to neonatology, pediatric anesthesia, and pediatric subspecialists. For those with less perinatal needs, deliveries are performed at the institution preferred by the obstetrician, and subsequent outpatient or inpatient consultations are performed with pertinent pediatric subspecialists. The perinatologist informs the team members and specialists as to the management decisions.

Patient Outcomes and Quality Improvement

As part of the monthly center meeting, updates of ongoing pregnancies, outcomes, and patient management, are presented. Neonatology and pediatric subspecialists provide a summary of post-delivery management and outcomes. Quality improvement aspects of patient care are addressed. Patient care outcomes are documented in the meeting minutes.

Virtual Consultations for Acute Diagnostic and Management Decisions

Between each monthly meeting, perinatology, neonatology, and pediatric subspecialists have created pathways for prompt virtual consultations. These consultations are summarized and presented at the subsequent monthly meeting.

Pediatric Neurosurgery Care Sequence

Establishment of lines of communication between perinatology and pediatric neurosurgery has facilitated timely pediatric neurosurgery consultations. Communication between perinatology, pediatric neurosurgery, and pediatric radiology has created an efficient venue of discussing prenatal imaging and/or diagnostic studies. Sharing of healthcare information between perinatology, obstetricians, pediatric neurosurgery, and neonatology has simplified coordination of delivery, timing, and immediate postnatal diagnostic studies, and care in the neonatal intensive care unit. Communication between palliative care, perinatology, and pediatric neurosurgery is readily available for timely prenatal contact. Pediatric neurosurgery personnel provide a coordinated care plan for immediate postnatal management, diagnostic studies, consultations, and interventions.

Discussion

Models of postnatal comprehensive and coordinated care are effective at reducing barriers to unmet healthcare needs for disabled children and their families [2]. These models also have shown to lower healthcare and social costs through reduced hospital stays and fewer days lost from work by the parents/caregivers [3-5]. As well as with the stressors of childbirth as above, having discussed postnatal management of the infant provides parental education and comfort.

Prenatal diagnosis and management working groups are not new entities and other institutions have recommended team care [6-8]. Quality improvement aspects of the team approach have been previously documented

[6-8]. Most publications are in the area of fetal cardiology. Emphasis has been placed on the comprehensive imaging for screening fetal heart development and early fetal studies [8]. Discussions on the timing and mode of delivery in prenatally diagnosed congenital heart disease have been published [9-11]. The team approach to the management of prenatally diagnosed myelomeningocele has been reported [12]. Emphasis has been placed on prenatal surgery [12]. Reports of prenatal team management for neurosurgical conditions are scant. It is our desire to provide this information to neurosurgeons and other healthcare providers the experience of the Fetal Diagnosis & Therapy Center in Jacksonville. This may enable others to develop a similar prenatal healthcare system.

Issues Identified in the Patient Care Sequence

Diagnostic studies such as MRI, and subspecialty consultations are constantly burdened by need for authorization from the insurance industry. At times, medical directors or authorizing insurance personnel must be verbally contacted for approval, creating a delay in the care sequence. The increased patient volume has created an administrative burden to the perinatology service because of demands for authorizations for prenatal MRI, and referrals to neonatology and pediatric subspecialists. We are attempting to obtain institutional support for care coordinators/navigators. A medical social worker is the person most indicated to deal with assisting the parents, navigate the private insurance industry and/or government insurance. A nurse may facilitate the medical aspects of care coordination with healthcare providers and subspecialists.

Conclusion

The prenatal diagnosis and management center provides a venue for coordinated and timely pediatric neurosurgery consultations. The working group is continuing to develop methodology and quality improvement aspects. We hope this report will assist other pediatric neurosurgeons who do not have a structured prenatal team for patient care to facilitate the development of such a service in their location.

Acknowledgments

We wish to acknowledge the assistance of Mrs. Jennifer Santarone in the preparation of this manuscript.

References

Adzick, N. S., Thom, E. A., Spong, C. Y., Brock, J.W. 3rd, Burrows, P. K., Johnson, M. P. Howell, L. J., Farrell, J. A., Dabrowiak, M.E., Sutton, L. N., Gupta, N., Tulipan, N. B., D'Alton, M. E., Farmer, D. L.; and MOMS Investigators. (2011) A Randomized Trial of Prenatal Versus Postnatal Repair of Myelomeningocele. *N. Engl. J. Med.* 364(11):993-1004. doi: 10.1056/NEJMoa1014379.

Donofrio, M. T., Moon-Grady, A. J., Hornberger, L. K., Copel, J. A., Sklansky, M. S., Abuhamad, A., Cuneo, B. F., Huhta, J. C., Jonas, R.A., Krishnan, A., Lacey, S., Lee, W., Michelfelder, E. C. Sr., Rempel, G.R., Silverman, N. H., Spray, T. L., Strasburger, J. F., Tworetzky, W., Rychik, J.; American Heart Association Adults With Congenital Heart Disease Joint Committee of the Council on Cardiovascular Disease in the Young and Council on Clinical Cardiology, Council on Cardiovascular Surgery and Anesthesia, and Council on Cardiovascular and Stroke Nursing. (2014) Diagnosis and treatment of fetal cardiac disease: a scientific statement from the American Heart Association. *Circulation.* 129(21):2183-2242. doi: 10.1161/01.cir.0000437597.44550.5d.

Farmer, J. E., Clark, M.J., Sherman, A., Marien, W.E., and Selva, T.J. (2005) Comprehensive primary care for children with special health care needs in rural areas. *Pediatrics* 116(3):649-656. doi: 10.1542/ peds.2004-0647.

James, H. E., MacGregor, T. L., and Aldana, P. R. (2011) Creating a working group for prenatal diagnosis and management as a venue to facilitate neurosurgery health care delivery. *Pediatr. Neurosurg.* 47(3):176-179. doi: 10.1159/000331567.

Li, Y. F., Zhou, K. Y., Fang, J., Wang, C., Hua, Y.M., and Mu, D. Z. (2016) Efficacy of Prenatal Diagnosis of Major Congenital Heart Disease on Perinatal Management and Perioperative Mortality: A Meta-Analysis. *World J. Pediatr*. 12(3):298-307. doi: 10.1007/s12519-016-0016-2.

Palfrey, J.S., Solis, L.A., Davidson, E.J., Jihong, L., Freeman, L., Ganz, M.L., and Pediatric Alliance for Coordinated Care. (2004) The Pediatric Alliance for Coordinated Care: Evaluation of a medical home model. *Pediatrics* 113(5 Suppl):1507-1516.

Perry, L.A. (1994) A multidisciplinary approach to the management of pregnant patients with end-stage renal disease. *J Perinat Neonatal Nurs* 8(1):12-19. doi: 10.1097/00005237-199406000-0003.

Peyvandi, S., Nguyen, T. A. T. T., Almeda-Jones, M., Boe, N., Rhee, L., Anton, T., Sklansky, M., Tarsa, M., Satou, G., Moon-Grady, A. J., and University of California Fetal Consortium (UCfC). (2017) Timing and Mode of Delivery in Prenatally Diagnosed Congenital Heart Disease-An Analysis of Practices within the University of California Fetal Consortium. *Pediatr. Cardiol.* 38(3):588-595. doi: 10.1007/s00246-016-1552-y.

Sebire, N.J. and Jauniaux, E. (2009) Fetal and placental malignancies: prenatal diagnosis and management. *Ultrasound Obstet Gynecol* 33(2): 235-244. doi: 10.1002/uog.6246.

Starfield, B. and Shi, L. (2004) The medical home, access to care, and insurance: a review of the evidence. *Pediatrics* 113(5 Suppl):1493-1498.

Stauffer, U.G. (1986) Management of prenatally diagnosed congenital malformations--actual problems and the importance of an interdisciplinary team approach. *Prog Pediatr Surg* 19:127-142. doi: 10.1007/978-3-642-70777-3_14.

Strickland, B., McPherson, M., Weissman G, van Dyck, P., Huang, Z. J., and Newacheck, P. (2004) Access to the medical home: results of the national survey of children with special health care needs. *Pediatrics* 113(5 Suppl):1485-1492.

About the Editors

Dr Amit Agrawal (MCh)

Department of Neurosurgery, All India Institute of Medical Sciences, Saket Nagar, Bhopal 462020, Madhya Pradesh, India

Dr Pradeep Chouksey (MCh)

Department of Neurosurgery, All India Institute of Medical Sciences, Saket Nagar, Bhopal 462020, Madhya Pradesh, India

Dr Adesh Shrivastava (MCh)

Department of Neurosurgery, All India Institute of Medical Sciences, Saket Nagar, Bhopal 462020, Madhya Pradesh, India

Dr Sumit Raj (MCh)

Department of Neurosurgery, All India Institute of Medical Sciences, Saket Nagar, Bhopal 462020, Madhya Pradesh, India

Dr Rakesh Mishra (MCh)

Assistant Professor, Department of Neurosurgery, Institute of Medical Sciences, Banaras Hindu University, Varanasi, Uttar Pradesh-221005, India

List of Contributors

Orlin Pavlov
Kalina Koleva
Kuntal Kanti Das
Kamlesh Rangari
Ashish Sharma
Priyadarshi Dikshit
Rashim Kataria
Mudit Mehrotra
Krishan K. Yadav
MS Sridhar
Pragya Gupta
Rudrashish Haldar
Ved Prakash Maurya
Arun Kumar Srivastava
Rajkumar
S. Shashivadhanan
M. Manoranjitha Kumari
R. Gopikrishnan
A. S. Ramesh
Aishik Mukherjee
Rupant Kumar Das
Dibyendu Kumar Ray
Kaushik Sil
Siddharth Mistri
Sandip Chatterjee
Gustavo Adolfo Gaitán-Herrera
Laura Marcela Acevedo-Aguilar
Iván David Lozada-Martínez
Mariana Hurtado-Pinillos

Yelson Alejandro Picón-Jaimes
Anant Mehrotra
Awadhesh Jaiswal
M. S. Sridhar
S. Shashivadanan
Bhawan Nangarwal
Vikas Dwivedi
Brig (Dr) S. Shashivadhanan
Shivangi Shashivadhanan
Balachandar D
Abhishek Kumar
Mohan Raj Sharma
Sagar Koirala
Hector E. James
Alexandra D. Beier

Index

B

C

D

F

G

J

K

L

N

O

P

Q

Y

Z